Monoclonal Antibodies in Cancer

Contemporary Biomedicine

MONOCLONAL ANTIBODIES IN CANCER

Edited by

STEWART SELL

*University of Texas Health Science Center,
Houston, Texas*

and

RALPH A. REISFELD

*Scripps Clinic and Research Foundation,
La Jolla, California*

Humana Press • **Clifton, New Jersey**

Library of Congress Cataloging in Publication Data

Main entry under title:

Monoclonal antibodies in cancer.

  (Contemporary biomedicine)
  Includes bibliographies and index.
  1. Tumor antigens—Analysis. 2. Antibodies,
Monoclonal. 3. Cancer—Diagnosis. I. Sell, Stewart,
1935-   . II. Reisfeld, Ralph A. III. Series.
[DNLM: 1. Antibodies, Monoclonal—immunology.
2. Antigens, Neoplasm—immunology. 3. Neoplasms—
immunology. QW 575 M75105]
RC268.3.M67 1985   616.99'4079   85-4735
ISBN 0-89603-068-7

© 1985 The Humana Press Inc.
Crescent Manor
PO Box 2148
Clifton, NJ 07015

Printed in the United States of America

CONTENTS

CHAPTER 1
Monoclonal Antibody Defined Antigens on Animal Tumors
Michael R. Price and Robert W. Baldwin

CHAPTER 4
Human Chorionic Gonadotropin Detection with
  Monoclonal Antibodies
**Paul H. Ehrlich, Zeinab A. Moustafa,
Alexander Krichevsky, and Ricardo Mesa-Tejada**

CHAPTER 5
Products of the Major Histocompatibility Complex on
  Tumor Cells
Gerald N. Callahan

CHAPTER 6

Monoclonal Antibodies: Probes for the Study of
   Malignant T Cells
**Elizabeth A. Harden, Thomas J. Palker, and
Barton F. Haynes**

CHAPTER 7

Antigenic Markers on Normal and Malignant B Cells
Stephen Baird

CHAPTER 8

Nonlymphoblastic Leukemia-Associated Antigens Identified
   by Monoclonal Antibodies
Robert G. Andrews and Irwin D. Bernstein

CHAPTER 9

Monoclonal Antibodies as Probes for the Molecular
  Structure and Biological Function of
  Melanoma-Associated Antigens
Ralph A. Reisfeld

CHAPTER 10

Lung Cancer Markers as Detected by
  Monoclonal Antibodies
James L. Mulshine, Frank Cuttitta, and John D. Minna

CHAPTER 11
Human Breast Cancer Markers Defined by
  Monoclonal Antibodies

**J. Schlom, J. Greiner, P. Horan Hand, D. Colcher,
  G. Inghirami, M. Weeks, S. Pestka, P. B. Fisher,
  P. Noguchi, and D. Kufe**

CHAPTER 15

Immunochemistry of Human Teratocarcinoma Stem Cells
Peter W. Andrews and Ivan Damjanov

CHAPTER 16

Use of Monoclonal Antibodies in
  Neurobiology and Neurooncology
Carol J. Wikstrand and Darell D. Bigner

CHAPTER 17
Human Monoclonal Antibodies: Humoral Immune
  Response in Patients with Cancer
Alan N. Houghton and Richard J. Cote

CONTRIBUTORS

PETER W. ANDREWS · *Wistar Institute of Anatomy and Biology, Philadelphia, Pennsylvania*

ROBERT G. ANDREWS · *Fred Hutchinson Cancer Research Center, Seattle, Washington*

STEPHEN BAIRD · *University of California, San Diego, California*

ROBERT W. BALDWIN · *University of Nottingham, Nottingham, Great Britain*

NEIL H. BANDER · *New York Hospital-Cornell Medical Center, New York, New York*

IRWIN D. BERNSTEIN · *University of Washington School of Medicine, Seattle, Washington*

DARELL D. BIGNER · *Duke University Medical Center, Durham, North Carolina*

GERALD N. CALLAHAN · *Colorado State University, Fort Collins, Colorado*

T. MING CHU · *Roswell Park Memorial Institute, Buffalo, New York*

D. COLCHER · *National Institutes of Health, Bethesda, Maryland*

CARLOS CORDON-CARDO · *Memorial Sloan-Kettering Cancer Center, New York, New York*

RICHARD J. COTE · *Memorial Sloan-Kettering Cancer Center, New York, New York*

FRANK CUTTITTA · *National Institutes of Health, Bethesda, Maryland*

IVAN DAMJANOV · *Hahnemann University School of Medicine, Philadelphia, Pennsylvania*

PAUL H. EHRLICH · *Columbia University, New York, New York*

P. B. FISHER · *Columbia University, New York, New York*

J. GREINER · *National Institutes of Health, Bethesda, Maryland*

ELIZABETH A. HARDEN · *Duke University, Durham, North Carolina*

BARTON F. HAYNES · *Duke University, Durham, North Carolina*

A. HOLLINGSWORTH · *Duke University, Durham, North Carolina*

P. HORAN HAND · *National Institutes of Health, Bethesda, Maryland*

ALAN N. HOUGHTON · *Memorial Sloan-Kettering Cancer Center, New York, New York*

G. INGHIRAMI · *National Institutes of Health, Bethesda, Maryland*

MARGARET KEANE · *Yale University, New Haven, Connecticut*

ALEXANDER KRICHEVSKY · *Columbia University, New York, New York*

D. KUFE · *Dana Farber Institute, Boston, Massachusetts*

RICHARD MESA-TEJADA · *Columbia University, New York, New York*

RICHARD S. METZGAR · *Duke University, Durham, North Carolina*

JOHN D. MINNA · *National Institutes of Health, Bethesda, Maryland*

ZEINAB A. MOUSTAFA · *Columbia University, New York, New York*

JAMES L. MULSHINE · *National Institutes of Health, Bethesda, Maryland*

P. NOGUCHI · *National Center for Drugs and Biologics, Food and Drug Administration, Bethesda, Maryland*

THOMAS J. PALKER · *Duke University, Durham, North Carolina*

S. PESTKA · *La Roche Institute of Molecular Biology, Nutley, New Jersey*

MICHAEL R. PRICE · *University of Nottingham, Nottingham, Great Britain*

RALPH A. REISFELD · *Scripps Clinic and Research Foundation, La Jolla, California*

GUSTAVO REYNOSO · *Norwalk Hospital, Norwalk, Connecticut*

MARY ANN REYNOSO · *Norwalk Hospital, Norwalk, Connecticut*

J. SCHLOM · *National Institutes of Health, Bethesda, Maryland*

STEWART SELL · *University of Texas Health Science Center, Houston, Texas*

M. WEEKS · *National Institutes of Health, Bethesda, Maryland*

CAROL J. WIKSTRAND · *Duke University, Durham, North Carolina*

Preface

This represents the third volume in a series on cancer markers published by the Humana Press. The first volume, published in 1980, stressed the relationship of development and cancer as reflected in the production of markers by cancer that are also produced by normal cells during fetal development. The concept that cancer represents a problem of differentiation was introduced by Barry Pierce in describing differentiation of teratocarcinomas. Highlighted were lymphocyte markers, alphafetoprotein, carcinoembryonic antigen, ectopic hormones, enzymes and isozymes, pregnancy proteins, and fibronectin.

The second volume, published in 1982 and coedited with Britta Wahren, focused on the diagnostic use of oncological markers in human cancers, which were systematically treated on an organ by organ basis. At that time, the application of monoclonal antibodies to the identification of cancer markers was still in a very preliminary stage. A general introduction to monoclonal antibodies to human tumor antigens was given there by William Raschke, and other authors included coverage of those markers then detectable by monoclonal antibodies in their chapters.

Since the appearance of the second volume there has been an exponential increase in the number of papers published in which monoclonal antibodies have been used to identify cancer markers. This justifies, in part, the award of the 1984 Nobel Prize in which Köhler and Milstein shared. In less than 10 years, the technique of cell hybridization described by Kohler and Milstein [*Nature* **256,** 495 (1975)] has been modified, adapted, transformed, and applied not only to the identification of cancer markers, but also to the identification of microbial and normal tissue molecules, as well as to the provision of highly specific tools for the unraveling of many biological and pathological processes. In view of the decisive impact made by monoclonal antibodies on biological research, it came as no surprise that Köhler and Milstein shared the 1984 Nobel Prize in medicine.

In this third volume, the editors have attempted to update the vast amount of new information that is rapidly accumulating because of the widespread application of monoclonal antibodies in the study, diagnosis, treatment, and prevention of cancer. The book begins with a brief review of the use of monoclonal antibodies in animals, and continues with the human system on which monoclonal antibodies have possibly made their greatest impact to date, that is, melanoma antigen. In this chapter the molecular characterization of melanoma markers made possible by monoclonal antibodies is presented by coeditor, Ralph Reisfeld, and the theme recurs with variations in subsequent chapters. In addition, the application of monoclonal antibodies to diagnosis is emphasized and the present status of the use of monoclonal antibodies in cancer therapy, now carried out in many laboratories, is presented.

A short history of cancer markers is given in the accompanying table. We feel that the main impact of monoclonal antibodies on cancer and cancer markers is still emerging, and many cancer markers of the future remain still to be discovered. In addition, monoclonal antibodies may also be used to understand the basic biology of cancer and carcinogenesis. As an example, our definition of cancer markers must now also include chromosomal changes that are currently being identified at new levels by ever more sophisticated methods. In the future, by probing for "oncogenes" or oncogene products, even more precise cancer markers should be found. In fact, monoclonal antibodies may prove to be an effective tool to identify oncogene products not yet identifiable.

Stewart Sell
Houston, Texas

Ralph Reisfeld
La Jolla, California

A Short History of Cancer Markers

Year	Author	Markers
1846	H. Bence-Jones	Bence-Jones protein
1928	W. H. Brown	Ectopic hormone syndrome
1930	B. Zondek	HCG
1932	H. Cushing	ACTH
1933	Gutmann and Gutmann	Prostatic acid phosphatase
1949	K. Oh-Uti	Deletion of blood group antigens
1959	C. Markert	Isozymes
1960	P. Newell	Philadelphia chromosome
1963	G. I. Abelev	Alphafetoprotein
1965	Gold and Freeman	Carcinoembryonic antigen
1969	Heubner and Todaro	Oncogenes
1975	Kohler and Milstein	Monoclonal antibodies
1980	Cooper, Weinberg, Bishop, etc.	Oncogene probes and transfection
1981	J. Yunis	Fragile sites

Chapter 1

Monoclonal Antibody Defined Antigens on Animal Tumors

MICHAEL R. PRICE AND ROBERT W. BALDWIN

Cancer Research Campaign Laboratories, University of Nottingham, University Park, Nottingham, UK

1. Introduction

Monoclonal antibodies to both experimental animal tumors and human tumors have been developed concurrently. Clearly most attention has focused upon human tumors, since antibodies specifically, or more commonly preferentially, reactive with these have diagnostic and therapeutic applications. However, because the basic immunology of experimental animal tumors, including the expression and occurrence of tumor-associated antigens, is considerably more defined, it is pertinent to assess the performance of monoclonal antibodies to these tumors.

Monoclonal antibodies represent powerful probes to dissect numerous problems in tumor immunology and the cellular and molecular biology of cancer, previously unapproachable using conventional methodology. However, since they are only tools for the researcher, they do not elaborate the concepts, but can only be employed for their resolution. The aim of this review therefore is to examine the application of monoclonal antibody technology in the study of antigens associated with experimental tumors and to identify those areas of research in which these reagents have proven or potential usage.

1

2. Antigen Expression on Chemically Induced Tumors

2.1. Murine Tumors

The expression of individually distinct, tumor specific antigens (TSA) on tumors induced by carcinogens remains somewhat of a paradox. Nevertheless, these antigens that invoke the rejection of viable tumor cells derived only from the immunizing tumor, have been demonstrated with tumors induced in the rat, mouse, and guinea pig by a variety of agents. These include sarcomas and carcinomas induced by polycyclic hydrocarbons, aminoazo dyes, aromatic amines, alkyl nitrosamines, hydrazines, and a number of physical agents (reviewed by Baldwin and Price, 1982).

It is unknown whether these antigens are products of genes that exist in the genome of all normal cells, being repressed under normal circumstances. Their derepression as a consequence of malignant transformation by chemical carcinogens may then lead to the expression of products at the cell surface that are recognized as tumor antigens. Alternatively, these genes may be normally expressed in a minority of cell lineages in the organism, perhaps at specific stages of differentiation, and become stabilized by malignant transformation (Greaves, 1979). These postulates infer that tumor antigens are normal cell products being expressed inappropriately in time or tissue. The converse of this concept is that tumor specific antigens are new cell products coded for by carcinogen-modified genes or by modified epigenetic control mechanisms governing gene expression.

Yet a further possibility stems from the work of Lennox et al. (1981), who attempted to produce monoclonal antibodies specific for 3-methylcholanthrene (MCA)-induced sarcomas in B10 mice. Initially, it appeared that five antibodies were specific for one particular tumor (MC6A), and one of these (4B1) was selected for further study. However, when tests for its detection were made more sensitive by increasing the number of target cells and the amount of radiolabeled antiglobulin added, the 4B1 antibody bound to several other B10 tumors. The same antibody also reacted with other B10 tumors grown from cells transformed in vitro with chemicals and viruses, and it was shown that antigens detected by the 4B1 anti-MC6A monoclonal antibody corresponded to those recognized by an anti-gp70 monoclonal antibody (Stone and Nowinski, 1980). In addition, 4B1 was shown to bind to a protein of about 70,000 daltons. Taken together, these observations suggest that the 4B1-defined antigen on MC6A sarcoma cells is related to murine leukemia virus gp70 molecules and since the original specificity of the 4B1 antibody indicated that it defined the MC6A TSA, it was postulated that this class of antigen, i.e., TSA, is represented by recombinant envelope glycoproteins of rodent leukemia viruses.

The actual difficulty in identifying differences between individual MCA-induced sarcomas in mice using biochemical rather than immunological techniques is illustrated by the two-dimensional gel electrophoretic studies of Koch and Smith (1983) who compared the Concanavalin A acceptor glycoproteins of the MC6A sarcoma (i.e., the tumor described by Lennox et al., 1981) with those of another B10 sarcoma, MC6B, and found that their glycoproteins were very similar if not identical. No differences were noted for glycoproteins in the region of 70,000 daltons that could represent TSA although in this case, there is evidence that these TSA are not Concanavalin A-binding glycoproteins (Sikora et al., 1979).

There has been a reluctance to accept that TSA of chemically induced tumors are recombinant envelope glycoproteins of rodent leukemia viruses since passenger viruses carried by long transplanted tumors have frequently confused the serological identification of TSA. Thus, Brown et al. (1978) examined a series of MCA-induced murine sarcomas for their capacity to induce tumor transplantation rejection and humoral antibody following immunization of syngeneic mice with irradiated tumor cells. In each case, rejection responses that were individually specific for the immunizing tumor were demonstrated, although only a proportion produced antibody. The antibody response was cross-reactive, and tumors which induced antibody or reacted with antibody were all MuLV-positive. It was clear that although mice were able to mount a rejection response against individual TSA, they predominantly produced antibodies to viral antigens. Simrell and Klein (1979) were among the first to attempt to clarify this situation by means of monoclonal antibodies. Many fusions were performed using the spleens of C57BL/6 mice bearing or immunized against syngeneic chemically induced tumors. Antibodies were produced that were reactive with the immunizing tumor and several virus preparations, but one antibody that reacted strongly with the immunizing tumor did not do so with the MuLV preparations tested. However, this antibody did react with other sarcomas so that tumor specificity was not established.

These studies illustrate the difficulties in the serology of chemically induced tumors in mice, although in other tests, individually distinct TSA have been demonstrated using conventional serological techniques. DeLeo et al. (1977, 1978) clearly identified cytotoxic tumor-specific antibodies in the sera from mice after prolonged immunization against the BALB/c sarcoma, Meth A. An advantage of this particular system is that the Meth A sarcoma is apparently negative for the expression of C-type viruses and viral antigens (DeLeo et al., 1978). The Meth A TSA was highly restricted to one of 20 sarcomas of BALB/c origin and was distinguishable from MuLV gp70 by its molecular weight and isoelectric point (Dubois et al., 1982; Law and Hopkins, 1982). Even so, in later studies, this antigen was also detected upon a Moloney murine sarcoma virus (Mo-MuSV)-transformed BALB/c 3T3 cell line designated 11A(v) (DeLeo et al., 1982). Infection of SC-1 cells with retroviruses present in culture filtrates of 11A(v) cells resulted in Meth A antigen expression. Thus, it was concluded that there were three possible mechanisms by which antigen expression in this system might occur: (1) the retrovirus codes for the Meth A antigen by capture of a cellular gene; (2) the retrovirus integrates near or adjacent to the Meth A coding region—this could result in a promotor insertion (Neel et al., 1981); or (3) the retrovirus codes for induction of the Meth A antigen (DeLeo et al., 1982). Despite the progress made with the Meth A sarcoma it is clear that the availability of monoclonal antibodies defining this determinant would more rapidly advance understanding of this system. This is particularly important since in transfection studies, using DNA from the Meth A sarcoma, there was a high frequency of transfer of the malignant phenotype and of the TSA as assayed in tumor rejection assays or serologically (Law and Hopkins, 1982).

Hellström et al. (1982) adopted a different approach for the preparation of monoclonal antibodies against mouse bladder carcinoma antigens. Rather than using lymphoid cells from mice bearing, or immunized against, syngeneic tumors, a rat was immunized against an MCA-induced mouse bladder carcinoma and later boosted with a pool of BALB/c bladder carcinomas as well as tissues from normal BALB/c urinary bladder. Thus, the sensitized spleen cells represented the products of a xenogeneic immunization and as such, the majority of the antibodies produced would not be expected to define antigens that were immunogenic in the syngeneic host. Two hybridomas were cloned that secreted antibodies to antigens more strongly expressed in mouse transitional-cell bladder carcinomas than in other mouse tumors or normal tissues. One antibody precipitated a protein of 140,000 dalton mol wt that was detected in cell membrane lysates from transitional-cell carcinoma and was more weakly expressed in normal bladder. The molecular nature of the antigen defined by the other antibody was not determined. This study with experimental tumors illustrates the feasibility of producing antibodies of restricted, and in this case, "tissue type" specificity, and the approach is analogous to that taken for the preparation of monoclonal antibodies against human tumors as described elsewhere in this volume.

2.2. Rat Tumors

With chemically induced tumors in the rat, as compared with those in mice, there is less evidence for the involvement of viruses contributing to TSA expression. Immunization of rats with syngeneic tumors has been shown to elicit tumor specific antibodies (Baldwin and Price, 1982) and, as in the studies on mouse sarcomas, it would be highly desirable to amplify the production of these antibodies using hybridoma technology. This may be achieved using the P3NS1 mouse myeloma to prepare rat–mouse hybrids with sensitized rat lymphoid cells or, more usefully, employing the Y3 Ag 1.2.3. rat myeloma to construct hybridomas producing rat antibodies. It should be recognized, however, that immunization of rats with syngeneic tumors, although inducing antibodies of the required tumor specificity, does not produce reagents of high titer. For this reason North et al. (1982) addressed themselves to the problem of defining the best method for producing monoclonal antibodies with tumor specificity. Spleen and lymph node cells from rats bearing tumors or from rats immunized against tumors served as the sources of antibody-producing cells. These were fused with the Y3 Ag 1.2.3. rat myeloma using polyethylene glycol. With lymph nodes cells the number of hybridomas obtained was lower than that given by equivalent fusions using spleen cells and very few hybridomas secreted antibodies that bound to cells derived from the immunizing tumor. Conversely, fusions performed using spleen cells from rats bearing, or hyperimmunized against, syngeneic sarcomas were more productive and, in the initial screen, there were generally at least one and up to four hybridoma colonies in each well. From 13 fusions, 88 hybridomas secreted antibodies binding to sarcoma target cells although only seven were of the IgG class, the remainder being IgM antibodies. Hyperimmune spleen cells yielded a greater number of antibody-secreting colonies compared with spleen cells from tumor bearers. After cloning selected hybridomas, two IgG_2 antibodies were obtained with tumor specificity and which were considered suitable for adjuvant therapy. Notably these were the products of tumor bearer spleens rather than from hyperimmune spleen cells, and North et al. (1982) recommended that the tumor bearer should be used as a source of lymphoid cells for fusion.

In order to obtain a better source of sensitized lymphoid cells, Dean et al. (1982) developed a procedure for preparing monoclonal allo-antibodies by antigen challenge in the Peyer's patches and collecting cells from the mesenteric nodes. Following on from these studies, syngeneic tumors were established in Peyer's patches in rats, and cells from the mesenteric nodes were fused with the rat myeloma Y3 Ag 1.2.3. This facilitated the preparation of a number of hybridomas secreting IgG_1 and IgG_2 antibodies with individual tumor specificity. Furthermore, by removing the mesenteric nodes 4–6 wk before tumor challenge, lymphoid cells leaving the Peyer's patches were obtained by cannulation of the thoracic duct, and these were found to be a useful source of IgA antibodies (Dean et al., unpublished findings).

Tumor-specific monoclonal antibodies have however been produced using spleen cells from rats immunized against a syngeneic tumor (Gunn et al., 1980), although , in this case, the tumor was a transplanted mammary carcinoma of unknown aetiology, termed Sp4. This tumor had previously been shown to express a TSA demonstrable in tumor transplant rejection tests (Baldwin and Embleton, 1969) or by membrane immunofluorescence techniques (Baldwin and Embleton, 1970). Spleen cells from a rat immunized against γ-irradiated Sp4 cells were fused with the mouse myeloma, P3NS1, to produce an interspecies rat–mouse hybridoma that yielded antibody (IgG_{2b}) specifically reactive with Sp4 tumor cells (Gunn et al., 1980). Analysis of the characteristics of the target antigen by sodium dodecyl sulfate polyacrylamide gel electrophoretic (SDS PAGE) separation of immune precipitates from ^{125}I-labeled tumor cells, monoclonal antibody, and an antiglobulin precipitating agent, failed to reveal a component identifiable as the TSA, although immunoadsorbent purification of papain digests of tumor cells yielded a peptide of 20,000 daltons. This may be taken to infer that the antigen was a cell surface protein or glycoprotein (Price et al., 1981).

2.3. Guinea Pig Tumors

The diethylnitrosamine (DENA)-induced, transplantable Line 10 hepatocarcinoma of strain 2 guinea pigs (Rapp et al., 1968) has proved to be a valuable model for tumor immunotherapy. In order to develop the model further for serotherapy, monoclonal antibodies were raised by immunizing BALB/c mice with viable Line 10 tumor cells and fusing splenic lymphocytes with the P3NS1 mouse myeloma (Key et al., 1983). After cloning, the products secreted by one hybridoma, D3, were selected for further study. Although radioimmunoassays on live cells revealed no cross-reactivity with normal tissues or with the control Line 1 hepatocarcinoma, immunoperoxidase staining of cryostat sections showed that the D3-defined antigen was expressed weakly upon some normal tissues (Bernhard et al., 1983a). The D3 monoclonal antibody reacted primarily with the Line 10 tumor, but some cross-reactivity with smooth muscle, placenta, fetal skeletal muscle, and fetal liver was evident. Radioimmunoprecipitation of detergent extracts of iodinated Line 10 cells showed that the antigen was present on the cell surface as a dimer of 290,000 daltons mol wt (unit size, 148,000 dalton mol wt). These basic characteristics of the D3 antibody and its associated antigen indicated that this system provided an appropriate model for evaluating monoclonal antibody serotherapy of solid tumors. This was proposed to be analogous to the treatment of human tumors with murine monoclonal antibodies, particularly since the immune responsiveness of guinea pigs closely approximates to that of humans (Bernhard et al., 1983a).

3. Use of Monoclonal Antibodies in Tumor Localization and Therapy

With human tumors, there is ample evidence that murine antitumor monoclonal antibodies localize to tumors when injected in patients (Farrands et al., 1982; Mach et al., 1981) or in immunocompromised mice (nude or immunodeprived mice) bearing human tumor xenografts (Pimm et al., 1982a; Ballou et al., 1979). This has most widely been developed using murine antibodies to CEA (e.g., Berche et al., 1982). In addition, there are a few reports evaluating therapeutic benefits derived from the administration of heterologous monoclonal antibodies to tumor patients (Miller et al., 1981; Ritz et al., 1981). There is further intense interest in preparing conjugates of antibody linked to cytotoxic agents (e.g., drugs or bacterial or plant toxins) and these have been shown to be selectively cytotoxic for human tumors in tissue culture or developing as human tumor xenografts (Thorpe and Ross, 1982; Garnett et al., 1983; Embleton et al., 1984). However, the use of monoclonal antibodies to experimental tumors has been explored to a lesser extent, even though such systems permit analyses of therapy in immunocompetent hosts.

3.1. In Vivo Localization of Monoclonal Antibodies in Experimental Tumors

In developing a pragmatic approach for the treatment of tumors with monoclonal antibodies or their therapeutic derivatives (drug–antibody conjugates, toxin–antibody conjugates), a number of studies have addressed the problem as to whether these antibodies localize to tumors in experimental animals. This has proven particularly successful with a monoclonal antibody prepared against the Rauscher virus envelope glycoprotein gp70 that was assayed for its localization to erythroleukemic cells in BALB/c mice (Scheinberg and Strand, 1982). In this study, papain digestion of the murine monoclonal antibody 103A generated $F(ab')_2$ fragments rather than Fab fragments (which was considered to be a peculiarity of this mouse IgG_1 immunoglobulin). These fragments were radioiodinated and injected into the peritoneal cavity of erythroleukemic mice. The spleens were removed later and cells were isolated, counted, and assayed for bound radioactivity. Up to 5% of the injected radioactivity was recovered in leukemic spleens, and mean uptake ratios of binding to leukemic over normal spleen cells ranged from greater than 70 at 7 h after injection to less than 10 at 40 h later.

With other solid tumors, notably with various experimental carcinomas, the localization of radiolabeled antibody within tumors has been assessed by determining the uptake of radioactivity in whole tissues and organs without dissociation into single cell suspensions. The validity of this approach was confirmed using a monoclonal antibody (Sp4/A4) against the rat mammary carcinoma Sp4 that was prepared by immunization of a rat with syngeneic tumor and fusion of spleen cells with the mouse myeloma P3NS1 (Gunn et al., 1980). The antibody selected for study exhibited tumor specificity in its reaction with Sp4 cells, and after immunoadsorbent purification, it was radiolabeled with [125]I. Intravenous injection of labeled antibody into rats bearing subcutaneous tumor produced preferential uptake of the radiolabel into the tumor compared with normal tissues (Pimm et al., 1982b). As shown in Fig. 1, the specificity of this effect was demonstrated by showing that there was no localization of labeled antibody to an unrelated tumor (mammary carcinoma, Sp15, or the azo dye-induced hepatoma, D192A) which had been established at a site contralateral to the Sp4 graft. The preferential localization of anti-Sp4 monoclonal antibody in subcutaneous deposits of the mammary carcinoma Sp4 has also been demonstrated by γ-camera scintigraphy of rats following injection of ^{131}I-labeled antibody (Baldwin, 1982). In this study, after acquisition of the ^{131}I image, rats were injected with indium-113M chloride to label the blood pool, and a computerized sub-

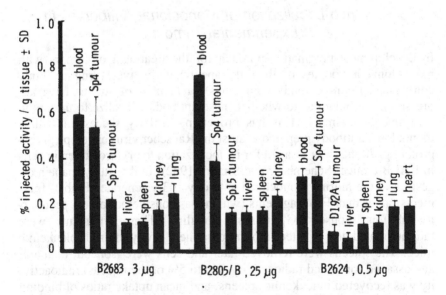

Fig. 1. In vivo distribution of ^{125}I-labeled Sp4/A4 monoclonal antibody preparations (batch numbers: B2683, B2805/B, and B2624) 2 to 3 d after injection into rats with growth of Sp4 and a second tumor (Sp15 or D192A) at a contralateral subcutaneous site. Rats were in groups of three or four. $P < 0.02$ for percentage injected activity/g Sp4 tumor compared with contralateral tumor in all three tests.

traction technique was used to accumulate a second image with which it was possible to visualize the tumor localization of ^{131}I-labeled antibody.

Comparable results have been obtained with the murine monoclonal antibody against the Line 10 hepatocarcinoma in guinea pigs. In animals bearing dermal Line 10 tumors in the thigh and Line 1 hepatocarcinoma in the contralateral thigh, the Line 10 tumors were visualized by immunoscintigraphy following intravenous injection of radiolabeled antibody, and tissue uptake of radiolabel was demonstrated to reside predominantly in the Line 10 tumor (Bernhard et al., 1983a).

3.2. Serotherapy Using Antitumor Monoclonal Antibodies

It is clear that radiolabeled monoclonal antibodies or their fragments may localize within tumor deposits following systemic administration. This being so, it is reasonable to propose that they have potential to exert direct therapeutic effects upon developing tumors or that antitumor conjugates constructed from antibodies and therapeutic agents may also limit tumor development and growth. Considering first the administration of antibody alone, suppression of tumor growth has been most evident using leukemia model systems rather than solid tumors. Thus, Bernstein et al. (1980 a, b) showed that a monoclonal antibody against the Thy-1 differentiation antigen on mature T cells can efficiently suppress the growth of thymic leukemia in mice without causing severe side-effects. Similarly, in humans the systemic administration of monoclonal antibodies against T-cell and common acute lymphocytic leukemia caused transient decreases in the number of tumor cells bearing these antigens (Miller et al., 1981; Miller and Levy, 1981; Ritz et al., 1981).

A particularly valuable model for the serotherapy of human leukemia was developed by Johnson and Shin (1983) who produced a monoclonal antibody against a normal differentiation antigen on human acute nonlymphocytic leukemia (ANLL) which cross-reacted with a rat ANLL. The antibody reacted with all ANLL tested as well as normal undifferentiated myelomonocytic cells. When employed therapeutically, it mediated complete tumor suppression in rats engrafted with 10^2–10^3 rat leukemic cells in vivo. Although this represents a particularly small burden of tumor, it was considered that this type of monoclonal antibody might be useful in the treatment of human ANLL after conventional therapy, which often eliminates most leukemic cells, leaving a small number of residual cells (Johnson and Shin, 1983).

Therapy with monoclonal antibodies against rodent leukemias is not always successful (e.g., Testorelli et al., 1983), and obviously the nature and stability of expression of the target tumor-associated antigen may be of significance and limit the efficacy of any particular treatment regimen. Antigenic modulation following interaction with antibody, or shedding of antigen, to neutralize antibody in the circulation may of course influence the potential of serotherapy (Price and Baldwin, 1977; Price and Robins, 1978). Young et al. (1983) addressed this problem by analyzing lymphomas developing in a few mice that had escaped protection following antibody administration. In this case, the antibody defined the glycolipid asialo GM2 antigen that is present on the lymphoma cell surface (Young and Hakomori, 1981). It was determined that asialo GM2-deficient variants arose in some of the mice that had been challenged with 1A1 lymphoma cells and treated unsuccessfully with monoclonal IgG$_3$ anti-asialo GM2 (Young and Hakomori, 1981). When these cells were used to challenge mice, anti-asialo GM2 had no effect on mouse survival. In nontreated tumor bearing mice, the lymphoma cells were found to consist of a mixture of asialo GM2-positive and -negative cells indicating the presence of selective pressures in these mice as well. Thus, since serotherapy was generally effective against this lymphoma, it was concluded that this form of treatment may complement a host antitumor response from which the asialo GM2-deficient cells can escape, although this was not considered to reflect resistance to natural killer cell lysis (Young et al., 1983).

Monoclonal antibody therapy of solid tumors has been less successful than with the rodent leukemias. However, North and Dean (1983) have examined monoclonal antibodies to a rat MCA-induced sarcoma to determine their value in influencing disseminated disease. The antibody employed was specific for the rat fibrosarcoma MC24 and it inhibited lung colonization when tumor cells were injected intravenously. In addition, when passively transferred into athymic MC24 tumor bearers, it prevented or considerably reduced the incidence of spontaneous lung metastases in more than half the treated animals (North and Dean, 1983).

3.3. Therapy Using Antitumor Monoclonal Antibodies Conjugated to Cytotoxic Agents

In order to enhance the therapeutic potential of monoclonal antibodies, a variety of cytotoxic agents have been linked covalently to antibodies reactive specifically or preferentially with tumor cells. There has been considerable interest in employing toxins as the cytotoxic component of conjugates, which has been provoked by their supreme potency. One molecule of the plant toxins, abrin or ricin, or of the bacterial exotoxin, diphtheria toxin, may be sufficient to kill a cell that it penetrates (Yamaizumi et al., 1978; Eiklid et al., 1980). This may however impose limitations for therapy since most monoclonal antibodies react to a greater or lesser extent with normal cells and tissues in addition to malignant cells. The preparation of these so-called "immunotoxins" and their applications in selectively killing tumor cells have been reviewed extensively elsewhere (Jansen et al., 1982; Thorpe and Ross, 1982; Bernhard et al., 1983b), and the modes of cytotoxic action of diphtheria toxin, abrin, and ricin have also been described in detail (Collier, 1976; Olsnes and Pihl, 1976; Pappenheimer, 1977; Gill, 1978). It is pertinent to consider the alternative approach using antitumor monoclonal antibodies, namely to assess their therapeutic effectiveness when coupled to broad spectrum cytotoxic drugs. The concept of employing drug–antibody conjugates for tumor therapy is a simple one, although only the availability of monoclonal antibodies permits its proper evaluation. As shown in Fig. 2, however, the development of appropriate conjugates for testing in vivo against developing tumors is more complex requiring interaction between several disciplines including chemistry, biochemistry, immunology, cell biology, and pharmacology. Nevertheless, progress has been evident using monoclonal antibodies against experimental tumors. This is exemplified in studies upon the rat mammary carcinoma, Sp4, and the Sp4/A4 monoclonal antibody that reacts specifically with this tumor (Gunn et al., 1980). As already described, in vivo organ distribution studies have indicated that the Sp4/A4 antibody localizes preferentially in tumor compared to normal organs in tumor bearing rats (Fig. 1). Also, this tumor is sensitive to adriamycin when tested by the suppression of subcutaneous tumor growth (Pimm et al., 1982b) or by inhibition of cellular DNA synthesis in cultured tumor cells. Conjugation of adriamycin (Doxorubicin) to Sp4/A4 antibody or normal rat IgG was effected through a dextran bridge using essentially the procedure developed by Hurwitz et al. (1975). Briefly, adriamycin is incubated with partially (25%) oxidized dextran and the resulting product is added to antibody at an equimolar ratio. After further incubation, the Schiff bases thus formed are reduced with sodium borohydride and the conjugates are separated from free adriamycin by gel filtration. This procedure yielded products with adriamycin:antibody molar ratios of up to 28:1 (Pimm et al., 1982b).

Retention of the composite biological activities of these conjugates was demonstrated: in indirect membrane immunofluorescence assays evaluated by flow cytofluorimetry, Sp4/A4–adriamycin conjugates bound to Sp4 cells, but not Sp15 tumor cells, while comparable conjugates of adriamycin and normal rat IgG bound to neither cell line (Fig. 3). In order to establish that adriamycin–Sp4/A4 conjugates retained antitumor activity, they were incubated in vitro (30 min at 37°C) with Sp4 tumor cells, and then after extensive washing, the cells were injected into normal rats. Treatment with adriamycin–Sp4/A4 antibody conjugate significantly suppressed tumor growth in comparison to that obtained with untreated cells or cells treated with adriamycin alone or adriamycin–normal IgG conjugates. Systemic treatment of Sp4 tumor-bearing rats with adriamycin–Sp4/A4 antibody conjugates also produced a therapeutic response and in five separate tests, conjugates significantly retarded

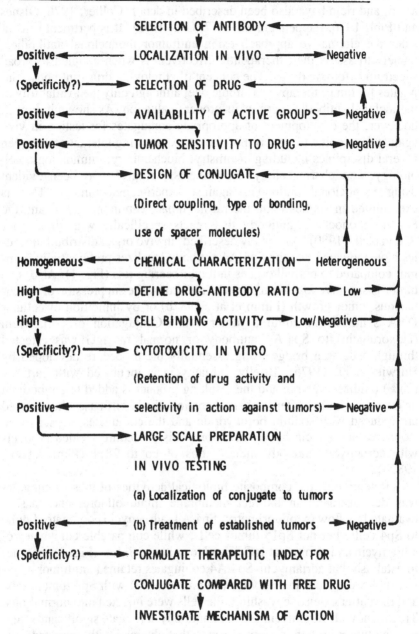

Fig. 2. Strategy for the production and evaluation of conjugates of cytotoxic drugs and antitumor monoclonal antibodies.

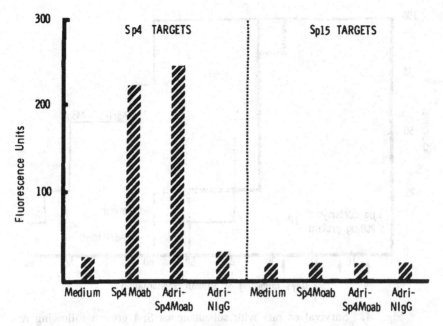

Fig. 3. Binding of Sp4/A4 monoclonal antibody and adri-amycin–antibody conjugates to Sp4 and Sp15 rat mammary carcinoma target cells as assessed by flow cytofluorimetry. Bound IgG was detected by indirect immunofluorescence using FITC-conjugated goat-anti-rat IgG. Moab = monoclonal antibody.

growth, with growth inhibition of between 37 and 56%. This therapeutic response was substantially greater than that achieved with free adriamycin or adriamycin–normal IgG, or free Sp4/A4 antibody alone. Comparably, a mixture of adriamycin and Sp4/A4 monoclonal antibody failed to modify tumor development in tumor-bearing rats (Pimm et al., 1982b). The therapeutic response of subcutaneous grafts of Sp4 to adriamycin and adriamycin conjugates is illustrated in Fig. 4. In this test, adriamycin and an adriamycin–normal rat IgG conjugate did not prolong survival, whereas a therapeutic response was obtained with the adriamycin–Sp4/A4 antibody conjugate.

4. Conclusion

The availability of monoclonal antibodies to antigens exclusively or preferentially restricted to tumors permits new approaches to be developed both for the analysis of these markers that may characterize malignant cells and for tumor diagnosis and therapy. Monoclonal antibodies also represent unique tools for the reevaluation of concepts concerning antigen expression and since this has been a contentious area, it is appropriate that efforts be directed towards further clarification.

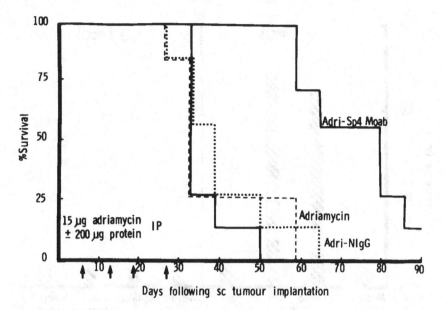

Fig. 4. Survival of rats with subcutaneous Sp4 growth following repeated treatment with adriamycin or adriamycin–immunoglobulin conjugates.
Each injection contained 15 μg adriamycin either free or conjugated to normal
rat IgG (Adr–NIgG) or Sp4/A4 monoclonal antibody (Adri–Sp4 Moab). Rats
were killed when tumors reached 3 cm mean diameter. Seven rats per group.

With regard to therapy, experimental animal tumors provide realistic
models for the development of new strategies. Their advantage, compared with human tumor xenograft systems, is that manipulations may be
attempted in immunocompetent hosts. This is particularly important since
therapy in cancer patients with xenogeneic antitumor monoclonal antibodies is becoming a practical possibility so that it will be essential to
define the limitations imposed by the administration of foreign
immunoglobulins and their therapeutic derivatives.

Acknowledgment

This work was supported by a grant from the Cancer Research Campaign,
London, UK.

References

Baldwin, R. W. (1982), *Proc. Roy. Soc. Edinburgh* **81**B, 261.
Baldwin, R. W., and M. J. Embleton (1969), *Int. J. Cancer* **4,** 430.
Baldwin, R. W., and M. J. Embleton (1970), *Int. J. Cancer* **6,** 373.

Baldwin, R. W., and M. R. Price (1982), in *Cancer: A Comprehensive Treatise*, Vol. 1, 2nd Edn. (F. F. Becker, ed.), Plenum Press, New York, p. 507.

Baldwin, R. W., M. J. Embleton, and M. R. Price (1981), in *Molecular Aspects of Medicine*, Vol. 4 (H. Baum, J. Gergely, and B. L. Fanburg, eds.), Pergamon Press, Oxford, p. 329.

Ballou, B., G. Levina, T. Hakala, and D. Solter (1979), *Science* **206**, 844.

Berche, C., J. P. Mach, J. D. Lumbroso, C. Langlais, F. Aubry, F. Buchegger, S. Carrel, P. Rougier, C. Parmentier, and M. Tubiana (1982), *Brit. Med. J.* **285**, 1447.

Bernhard, M. I., K. A. Foon, T. N. Oeltmann, M. E. Key, K. M. Hwang, G. C. Clarke, W. L. Christensen, L. C. Hoyer, M. G. Hanna, and R. K. Oldham (1983a), *Cancer Res.* **43**, 4420.

Bernhard, M. I., K. M. Hwang, K. A. Foon, A. M. Keenan, R. M. Kessler, J. M. Frincke, D. J. Tallam, M. G. Hanna, L. Peters, and R. K. Oldham (1983b), *Cancer Res.* **43**, 4429.

Bernstein, I. D., R. C. Nowinski, M. R. Tam, B. McMaster, L. L. Houston, and E. A. Clark (1980a), in *Monoclonal Antibodies, Hybridomas: A New Dimension in Biological Analyses* (R. H. Kennett, T. J. McKearn, and K. B. Bechtol, eds.), Plenum Press, New York, p. 275.

Bernstein, I. D., M. R. Tam, and R. C. Nowinski (1980b), *Science* **207**, 68.

Brown, J. P., J. M. Klitzman, I. Hellström, R. C. Nowinski, and K. E. Hellström (1978), *Proc. Nat. Acad. Sci. USA* **75**, 955.

Collier, R. J. (1976), in *Receptors and Recognition. Series B: The Specificity and Action of Animal, Bacterial and Plant Toxins* (P. Cuatrecasas, ed.), Chapman and Hall, London, p. 67.

Dean, C. J., L. A. Gyure, J. M. Styles, S. M. Hobbs, S. M. North, and J. G. Hall (1982), *J. Immun. Meth.* **53** 307.

DeLeo, A. B., S. S. Chang, N. A. Wivel, E. Appella, L. J. Old, and L. W. Law (1982), *Int. J. Cancer* **29**, 687.

DeLeo, A. B., H. Shiku, T. Takahashi, M. John, and L. J. Old (1977), *J. Exp. Med.* **146**, 720.

DeLeo, A. B., H. Shiku, T. Takahashi, and L. J. Old (1978), in *Biological Markers of Neoplasia: Basic and Applied Aspects* (R. W. Ruddon, ed.), Elsevier, New York, p. 25.

Dubois, G. C., L. W. Law, and E. Appella (1982), *Proc. Nat. Acad. Sci. USA* **80**, 1683.

Eiklid, K., S. Olsnes, and A. Pihl (1980), *Exp. Cell. Res.* **126**, 321.

Embleton, M. J., M. V. Pimm, M. C. Garnett, G. F. Rowland, R. G. Simmonds, and R. W. Baldwin (1984), *Behring Inst. Mitt.* **74**, 108.

Farrands, P. A., A. C. Perkins, M. V. Pimm, J. G. Hardy, R. W. Baldwin, and J. D. Hardcastle (1982), *Lancet* **i**, 397.

Garnett, M. C., M. J. Embleton, E. Jacobs, and R. W. Baldwin (1983), *Int. J. Cancer* **31**, 661.

Gill, D. M. (1978), in *Bacterial Toxins and Cell Membranes* (J. Jeljaszewicz and T. Wadstrom, eds.), Academic Press, London and New York, p. 291.

Greaves, M. F. (1979), in *Tumour Markers: Impact and Prospects* (E. Boelsma and Ph. Rümke, eds.), Elsevier, Amsterdam, p. 201.

Gunn, B., M. J. Embleton, J. Middle, and R. W. Baldwin (1980), *Int. J. Cancer* **26**, 325.

Hellström, I., N. Rollins, S. Settle, P. Chapman, W. Chapman, and K. E. Hellström (1982), *Int. J. Cancer* **29**, 175.

Hurwitz, E., R. Levy, R. Marom, M. Wilchek, R. Arnon, and M. Sela (1975), *Cancer Res.* **35**, 1175.

Jansen, F. K., H. E. Blythman, D. Carriere, P. Casellas, O. Gros, P. Gros, J. Laurent, F. Paolucci, B. Pau, P. Poncelet, G. Richer, H. Vidal, and G. A. Voisin (1982), *Immunological Rev.* **62**, 185.

Johnson, R. J., and H. S. Shin (1983), *J. Immunol.* **130**, 2930.

Key, M. E., M. I. Bernhard, L. C. Hoyer, K. A. Foon, R. K. Oldham, and M. G. Hanna (1983), *J. Immunol.* **130**, 1451.

Koch, G. L. E., and M. J. Smith (1983), *Brit. J. Cancer* **47**, 527.

Law, L. W., and N. Hopkins (1982), in *Tumour Progression and Markers* (K. Lapis, A. Jeney, and M. R. Price, eds.), Kugler Publications, Amsterdam, p. 351.

Lennox, E. S., A. O. Lowe, J. Cohn, and G. Evan (1981), *Transplant. Proc.* **13**, 1759.

Mach, J. P., F. Buchegger, M. Forni, J. Ritschard, C. Berche, J. D. Lumbroso, M. Schreyer, C. Girardet, R. S. Accolla, and S. Carrel (1981), *Immunology Today* **2**, 239.

Miller, R. A., and R. Levy (1981), *Lancet* **ii**, 226.

Miller, R. A., D. G. Maloney, J. McKillop, and R. Levy (1981), *Blood* **58**, 78.

Neel, B. G., W. S. Haywood, H. L. Robinson, J. Fang, and S. M. Astrin (1981), *Cell* **23**, 323.

North, S. M., and C. J. Dean (1983), *Immunology* **49**, 667.

North, S. M., J. M. Styles, S. M. Hobbs, and C. J. Dean (1982), *Immunology* **47**, 397.

Olsnes, S., and A. Pihl (1976), in *Receptors and Recognition, Series B: The Specificity and Action of Animal, Bacterial and Plant Toxins* (P. Cuatrecasas, ed.), Chapman and Hall, London, p. 129.

Pappenheimer, A. M. (1977), *Ann. Rev. Biochem.* **46**, 69.

Pimm, M. V., M. J. Embleton, A. C. Perkins, M. R. Price, R. A. Robins, G. R. Robinson, and R. W. Baldwin (1982a), *Int. J. Cancer* **30**, 75.

Pimm, M. V., J. A. Jones, M. R. Price, J. G. Middle, M. J. Embleton, and R. W. Baldwin (1982b), *Cancer Immunol. Immunother.* **12**, 125.

Price, M. R., and R. W. Baldwin (1977), in *Dynamic Aspects of Cell Surface Organization* (G. Poste and G. L. Nicolson, eds.), North Holland, Amsterdam p. 423.

Price, M. R., and R. A. Robins (1978), in *Immunological Aspects of Cancer* (J. E. Castro, ed.), M.T.P. Press, Lancaster, p. 155.

Price, M. R., R. G. Dennick, C. Y. Fang, D. Hannant, M. J. Embleton, B. Gunn, and R. W. Baldwin (1981), *Arch. Geschwulstforsch.* **51**, 302.

Rapp, H. J., W. H. Churchill, B. S. Kronman, R. T. Rolley, W. Hammond, and T. Borsos (1968), *J. Nat. Cancer Inst.* **41**, 1.

Ritz, J., J. M. Pesando, S. E. Sallan, L. A. Clavell, J. Notis-McCanarty, P. Rosenthal, and S. F. Schlossman (1981), *Blood* **58**, 141.

Scheinberg, D. A., and M. Strand (1982), *Cancer Res.* **42**, 44.

Sikora, K., G. Koch, S. Brenner, and E. Lennox (1979), *Brit. J. Cancer* **40**, 831.

Simrell, C. R., and P. A. Klein (1979), *J. Immunol.* **123,** 2386.
Stone, M. R., and R. C. Nowinski (1980), *Virology* **100,** 370.
Testorelli, C., G. Canti, P. Franco, A. Goldin, and A. Nicolin (1983), *Brit. J. Cancer* **47,** 353.
Thorpe, P. E., and W. C. Ross (1982), *Immunological Rev.* **62,** 119.
Yamaizumi, M., E. Makada, T. Uchida, and Y. Okada (1978), *Cell* **15,** 245.
Young, W. W., and S. Hakomori (1981), *Science (Wash. DC)* **211,** 487.
Young, W. W., Y. Tamura, H. S. Johnson, and D. A. Miller (1983), *J. Exp. Med.* **157,** 24.

Chapter 2

Monoclonal Carcinoembryonic Antigen Antibodies

GUSTAVO REYNOSO, MARGARET KEANE, AND
MARY ANN REYNOSO

*Department of Pathology, Norwalk Hospital, Norwalk, Connecticut,
and Yale University School of Medicine, New Haven, Connecticut*

1. Introduction

Carcinoembryonic antigen (CEA) is a useful test in clinical oncology. It is of proven value as a tumor marker, as a predictor of metastatic disease, and as a prognostic indicator of clinical remission or relapse. Serial CEA determinations are particularly useful in colorectal cancer, but good correlation with clinical stage and with survival has been observed also in breast carcinoma, gynecological, and other cancers. Potential usefulness is now well demonstrated in the histopathological evaluation of tumors capable of synthesizing CEA. The subject has been extensively reviewed (Westwood 1977; Freedman, 1977; Reynoso and Keane, 1979; Reynoso, 1981). A panel of experts assembled in August of 1977 (Norgaard-Pederson and Axelson, 1978) summarized the then current biochemical, immunological, methodological, and clinical aspects of the field and identified a series of questions to which no answers were then available. Paramount among the unanswered questions was the possible existence of epitopes in CEA molecules specific for cancer. It is the purpose of this chapter to review the contributions of hybridoma methodology to our understanding of the immunobiology of CEA and to analyze the progress so far made with monoclonal antibodies in the continuing goal of developing a cancer-specific CEA assay.

The reader is referred to the above reviews for details, but an article on the potential contribution of monoclonal antibodies to the CEA field cannot be written without at least a brief discussion of the problems of antigen and antibody heterogeneity, assay specificity, and clinical usefulness of CEA testing with conventional polyclonal antibodies.

CEA belongs to a family of closely related glycoprotein antigens present in many organs and tissues and detectable in significant amounts in malignant tumors originating therefrom. A summary of the antigen molecules cross-reacting with CEA, as determined by polyclonal antibodies, is presented in Table 1. There is extensive physicochemical, immunological, and other experimental data about many of the members of this family. It is probable that cross-reactive antigens one through six are all the same substance described under different names by different investigators and that the observed differences in physicochemical or immunological characteristics are due to methodological limitations and/or to post-translational heterogeneity. A review of the references in the original table suggests that cross-reacting antigens seven through twelve may indeed be immunologically different from each other, from the antigens in group one, and from tumor CEA. It is known that all of these antigens in the table share areas of physicochemical homology, but this does not exclude the possibility that they contain specific epitopes, or epitope groups, that are tumor specific. These potential cancer-specific epitopes, however, may be undetectable by polyclonal antibodies of the type obtained by immunizing animals with heterogeneous tissue extracts.

Most polyclonal antisera used in radioimmunoassay, histopathology, radioimaging, and other CEA detecting systems do contain

Table 1

Summary of Antigen Molecules Cross-Reacting with CEA as Determined by Polyclonal Antibodies[a]

No.		Name	Abbreviation
I	1	Normal glycoprotein	NGP
	2	Nonspecific cross-reacting antigen	NCA
	3	CEA-associated protein	CEX
	4	Colonic carcinoembryonic antigen-2	CCEA-2
	5	Colon carcinoma antigen III	CCA III
	6	Beta external protein	BE
II	7	Fetal sulfoglycoprotein antigen	FSA
III	8	Breast cancer glycoprotein	BCGP
IV	9	Second nonspecific cross-reacting antigen	NCA-2
V	10	Biliary glycoprotein	BGP-1
VI	11	Gastric CEA-like antigen	CELIA
VII	12	Pancreatic tumor ascites fluid glycoprotein	PAFG

[a]Source: Norgaard-Pedersen and Axelsen (1978), reproduced with permission.

antibodies reactive against epitopes shared by the various molecules. Absorption of antisera decreases, but does not eliminate shared cross-reactivity. The problem is complicated further by the fact that different degrees of cross-reactivity may be detected depending on the method of testing. For example, even though experimentally NCA shows 40–60% cross-reactivity with CEA, NCA is not an interfering antigen in the usual RIA systems in clinical practice.

The use of perchloric acid-extracted plasma for analysis minimizes nonspecific cross-reactivity, but does not eliminate the interference by cross-reacting molecules with shared determinants. Attempts to improve specificity by the use of particular species of CEA isolated by isoelectric focusing have not resulted in improved specificity (Edgington et al., 1975).

The use of serial CEA determinations in the monitoring of therapy in patients with CEA-producing tumors is widely accepted in clinical practice and in the postsurgical follow-up of patients with colorectal, breast, and other carcinomas (Reynoso and Keane, 1979). Rising CEA titers are indicative of recurrence and can be used to determine the need for second-look operations and further therapy, but the ultimate benefit of this approach, if any, has not been conclusively demonstrated (Balz et al., 1977).

Serial determinations of CEA do correlate with disease activity, but the correlation is not perfect and changes in serial CEA values, when interpreted by themselves, can be misleading in individual patients. In some series as many as 10% of the rising titers have been associated with a stable clinical condition and even with obvious clinical remission (Holyoke et al., 1975). Conversely, in other series, 10% of the patients in clinical relapse had normal or decreasing CEA levels (Reynoso and Keane, 1979).

Because polyclonal assays detect CEA in normal adult tissues and in the plasma of normal persons (Burtin et al., 1973; Chu and Reynoso, 1972a), CEA cannot be used as a screening test for cancer. Similarly, the variability of results and the high frequency of antigenemia in patients with inflammatory and degenerative diseases makes polyclonal CEA assays of little value in cancer diagnosis.

In histopathology the use of polyclonal antibodies often produces confusing results since it is here, even more than in serum assays, that NCA and the other antigens can interfere the most. In radioimaging, while much experimental data and many clinical trials are available, clinical progress has been slow. Nonspecific uptake by inflammatory masses, by benign tumors, and even by normal tissues makes interpretations of the images frought with difficulty.

Further progress requires a better understanding of the physicochemical nature of CEA, a more complete elucidation of the epitope distribution in cancer-associated and noncancer-associated cross-reactive anti-gens, and the eventual development of immunological reagents of defined epitope specificity suitable for clinical use. The progress that monoclonal methodology has made to the realization of these goals is discussed below.

2. The Development of Monoclonal CEA Immunoassays

2.1. General Concepts of Monoclonal Antibody Methodology

The development of hybridization methodology for the fusing of mye-loma cells with antibody-secreting cells by Kohler and Milstein (1975) offered the renewed hope of obtaining antibodies monospecific for antigen-determinant sites present exclusively on CEA molecules and not present in the cross-reacting molecules discussed above. Because the hybridoma method does not require extensive purification of antigen for immunization, and because most of the tedious and time-consuming steps associated with the absorption of conventional antisera can be eliminated, one can produce monospecific antibodies with documentable affinity for precisely defined antigens.

The basic principles of producing monoclonal antibodies by cell hy-bridization techniques are now well known. First a myeloma cell line, usually from mice, but rat and other sources including humans have also been used, is selected (Galfre et al., 1979; Olsson and Kaplan, 1980).

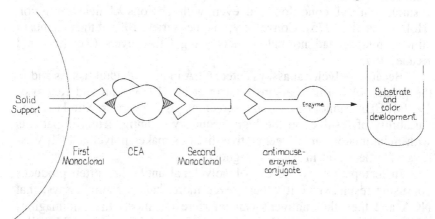

Fig. 1.   Diagrammatic representation of a double monoclonal immuno-assay for CEA. The first antibody on the surface of the solid support is used for isolation of antigen from the sample. Specificity is provided by the second monoclonal. Other assays use a polyclonal antibody as the primary antibody. Two or more monoclonals can be coated on the solid support for added sensitiv-ity (for references, see text).

The first step in selection consists in the isolation and propagation by tissue culture of cell lines with metabolic enzyme defects. The usual line is deficient in the enzyme hypoxanthine–guanine–phosphoribosyl transferase (HGPRT) or in thymidine kinase. In the absence of these enzymes, cells cannot synthesize nucleotides by the "salvage" pathway and must depend on the *de novo* synthesis of purines and pyrimidines, a folate-dependent pathway. When such enzyme-deficient cells are placed in a medium containing the folic acid antagonist aminopterin, they do not survive since their "salvage" pathway is lacking and their *de novo* pathway is blocked by aminopterin. The second cell line is obtained from animals that have been immunized with the antigen under study. Immunization techniques are relatively conventional and generally consist of a first immunizing dose that, as a rule, includes an adjuvant followed by a booster dose 5–7 d or as long as 2 mo later. Specifically stimulated B lymphocytes are harvested from the spleen (or from lymph nodes) 3–5 d after the booster immunization.

The two cell populations: one, the myeloma cell line and two, the specifically stimulated B cells are now ready for hybridization. The in vitro fusion of the cells is facilitated by the use of fusion-promoting agents of which several have been used. Certain viruses when added to the culture can promote fusion. In other instances, the antigen itself can act as a fusion promoting agent. Many laboratories have adopted the use of polyethylene glycol since the disruption of cell membranes by PEG is a reliable method producing high rates of hybridization in a variety of cell lines.

Several hybrid lines are generated under the usual experimental conditions, but the system is designed for the survival of the desired clones only. Original myeloma cells and myeloma–myeloma hybrids do not survive because of their deficient metabolic pathways. B cells and other nontumor cells from the immunized animal are not by their nature capable of survival in long term cultures and neither are the B–B hybrids that are formed. In theory then (and in practice since the system works), only hybrid cells that have acquired immortality from the myeloma cells and the specific enzymes for nucleotide synthesis from the normal, immunized B cells are capable of proliferation and survival in culture medium that contains hypoxanthine, aminopterin, and thymidine (HAT).

The next step consists of testing the surviving clones for antibody production followed by subcloning of the cells producing antibody in detectable amounts. Such subclones can be isolated and reinjected into the peritoneal cavity of mice where a permanent colony is established. The tumor colony is expected to produce ascites from which antibody can be obtained. Since the new cultures are monoclonal, they will continue to produce antibody of a single homogeneous class, usually IgG or IgM, but IgA hybridomas have been described (van Heyningen et al., 1982), and such monospecific antibodies, which are chemically and immuno-logically homogeneous, will continue to be produced in practically un-limited quantities provided the new cell line continues to be propagated and maintained.

Further details about hybridoma principles and methodology can be found in comprehensive reviews of the subject (Foster, 1982; Damjanov and Knowles, 1983). Suffice it to say here that the technology is now well established and that many investigators are now actively producing monoclonal anti-CEA antibodies. The hope remains that monoclonal anti-CEA antibodies will be produced that specifically react with the pos-tulated epitope or epitopes that confer to CEA molecules orginating in tumor tissue their tumor specificity, if indeed such an epitope exists. The final goal of producing monoclonal antibodies that are cancer and organ specific and that can be used in clinical practice remains.

2.2. Experimental and Clinical Experience with Monoclonal CEA Antibodies

Accolla and his group (Accolla et al., 1979) first reported the production of somatic cell hybrids capable of secreting monoclonal anti-CEA anti-bodies. They injected BALB/c mice with purified CEA obtained from hu-man colonic carcinoma. The spleen cells were fused with the myeloma cells P3-NSI/IAG4. Of the many hybrid lines studied, two were eventu-ally shown to produce monoclonal antibodies with high anti-CEA affinity when tested by a variety of techniques including radioimmunoassay and immunohistochemistry. Their two monoclonal antibodies showed only trace cross-reactivity with normal colon antigen (NGP). Extracts of nor-mal colon and lung reacted with the antibodies only at very high concen-trations, an observation consistent with the well-known existence of small amounts of CEA in these organs. This and similar work in other centers stimulated the efforts to produce other monoclonal antibodies potentially capable of selective reactivity with cancer specific epitopes and therefore of potential clinical usefulness.

Monoclonal antibodies that react with highly purified CEA but not with crude perchloric acid extracts of colonic carcinoma tissue have been described. Grunert and his group (1982) studied twenty antibody-producing clones by ELISA and by immunoprecipitation of radio-iodinated antigen. The object was to characterize the precipitated material by fingerprint analysis of the peptides obtained by digesting the immunoprecipitates. Two clones produced antibody that reacted with purified CEA only (180,000-dalton CEA) and three clones reacted only with determinant sites not present in the purified, 180,000-dalton CEA but the majority of the clones reacted with both. In their laboratory most of monoclonal antibodies, in a manner similar to conventional polyclonal antibodies, did not distinguish antigen determinant sites preferentially expressed in CEA from antigenic sites in other cross-reacting molecules.

Eight monoclonal antibodies produced by Hedin and his group have been extensively studied. All eight antibodies were IgG kappa and all had isoelectric points of between 6.5 and 7.5. By studying the pattern of reactivity of the eight antibodies, singly and in different combinations, against purified CEA in double diffusion plates, it can be deduced that there are at least six different epitopes present in the peptide moiety of CEA. Two of the antibodies cross-reacted with normal colon antigen (NCA) and none of the eight cross-reacted with biliary glycoprotein. A summary of the data is presented in Table 2 (Hedin et al., 1982a). Although Hedin and his group did not develop a radioimmunoassay for circulating antigen, their work provides a strong physicochemical and immunological framework for further development. The affinity constants they have described for their antibodies, as shown in Table 2, are well within the range needed for a sensitive radioimmunoassay.

Monoclonal antibodies of lesser binding activities exist. A mouse monoclonal serum described by Rogers (Rogers et al., 1981a) bound only 11% of a preparation of 125 I CEA. A conventional antibody bound 70% of the same CEA preparation. Interestingly, even though the antibody had relatively low binding affinity for CEA, it did show some selective affinities. For example, higher bindings were obtained when the antibody was incubated with antigen extracted from the serum of cancer patients than when incubated with perchloric acid extracts of tumors. Also, tissue extracts rich in normal colon antigen (NCA), such as normal lung and spleen, did not inhibit the binding of monoclonal antibody to tumor CEA any more strongly than extracts of normal colon. It is therefore possible that these types of monoclonal antibodies, even though of low binding capacity, may nevertheless have selective affinities for organs or tissues.

Monoclonals with affinity for CEA can be prepared by immunization with tumor tissue preparations other than colorectal tumors (Colcher et al., 1983). Mammary cell carcinoma metastatic to the liver was used to produce two monoclonals reactive with purified CEA. The two antibodies showed different reactivities against membrane-bound antigens in vitro. One reacted equally with melanoma, colonic, and human breast lines whereas the second not only did not react with melanoma, but showed different quantitative binding between breast and colon, strengthening the widely held belief that CEA preparations from different tissues contain specific epitopes for that organ or tissue. The importance of this finding for the eventual utilization of monoclonal CEA antibodies in cancer prognosis, tumor localization studies, and immunotherapy cannot be overlooked. If one analyzes monoclonals for reactivity against CEA and compares such reactivity with the simultaneously obtained results in reactions with two of the most frequently observed cross-reactive antigens: meco-

Table 2

Specificity and Binding Properties of Monoclonal Antibodies Against CEA[a]

Monoclonal antibody	Subclass	CEA	Reactivity against CEA (low)	NCA	CEA-epitope	No. of epitopes	K, M^{-1}
9	IgG$_{1k}$	+++++ (I)[b]	+++++ (I)	−	A	1	7.4×10^8
14	IgG$_{1k}$	+++++ (I)	+++++ (III)	+++	B	ND[c]	ND
27	IgG$_{1k}$	+++++ (I)	+++++ (I)	+−	C	≥2	3.3×10^8
47	IgG$_{1k}$	+++++ (I)	+++++ (III)	+++	E	ND	ND
48	IgG$_{1k}$	+++++ (I)	++++ (I)	+−	A	ND	ND
32S2	IgG$_{1k}$	+++ (II)	+++ (II)	−	Fφ	ND	ND
38S1	IgG$_{1k}$	++++ (III)	++++ (III)	−	D	2	1.2×10^8
46	IgG$_{1k}$	++++ (III)	++++ (III)	−	D	ND	ND

[a]Source: from Hedin et al., 1982, reproduced with permission.
[b]Denotes pattern of reactivity in ELISA.
[c]Not determined.

nium antigen (MA) and NCA, a pattern emerges that is consistent from laboratory to laboratory (Grunert et al., 1982; Hedin et al., 1982a; Kupchik et al., 1981). By a combination of classical competitive protein binding methodology and cross blocking experiments three classes of monoclonals can be postulated: class one shows identical or nearly identical affinities for CEA, NCA, and MA. Class II antibodies do not react with NCA, but do with MA and CEA. Class III antibodies react with CEA alone. The distribution of epitopes that would explain the differences in reactivity among these classes in the experiments performed by Primus et al. (1983b) are not inconsistent with the pattern of epitopes suggested by Hedin.

Even though CEA is a potent immunogen in rabbits, goats, and mice (Gold and Freedman, 1965; Chu and Reynoso, 1972b; Rogers, 1981a), many fusions must be performed and several hundred clones and subclones must be analyzed for antibody production before a few clones capable of long term survival as ascitic tumors and capable of synthesizing antibody continuously can be obtained (Accolla et al., 1979; Kupchik et al., 1981). Often, upon subcloning the products of a single hybridization experiment, several antibodies of different specificities and different binding capacities will be obtained indicating that, in fact, each monoclonal is specific for a single epitope. Accolla and his group (1979), using two internally labeled monoclonals, were able to show by cross-inhibition experiments that the binding of purified CEA by their antibody VII-37-a that had been internally labeled with H-3-leucine was not inhibited by coincubation with an excess of nonlabeled VII-23-e, an antibody produced by a subclone of the same original fusion. Further, the titer of the two antibodies when tested for their capacity to bind CEA was different: antibody 23 bound up to 80% of the purified CEA in the system versus a maximum of only 65% for monoclonal 37. Both antibodies showed only minimal cross-reactivity with NGP or with perchloric acid extracts of normal colon or lung.

Kupchik and his group, on the other hand, have produced from a single hybridization experiment a family of monoclonals that upon cross-incubation experiments show no additive effects when the various antibodies are mixed indicating that at least one of their clones, the one designated by them as 5-E-9, was capable of reacting with a spectrum of antigenic sites. None of their clones produced antibody with binding capacity greater than 30–40% of the binding obtained with a goat polyclonal antibody. Such monoclonal antibodies, even though they may show specificity for certain forms of CEA and little or no cross-reactivity with non-CEA antigens are, because of their low affinity, unlikely to be useful in conventional immunoassays for the detection and quantitation of CEA in serum or other biological fluids (Kupchik et al., 1981). A summary of the affinities observed by different investigators is shown in Table 3.

Table 3
The Binding Affinity of Several Anti-CEA Monoclonal Antibodies

Antibody	Affinity	Reference
Mab 9	$7.4 \times 10^8 \, M^{-1}$	Hedin, 1982a
Mab 27	$3.3 \times 10^8 \, M^{-1}$	Hedin, 1982a
Mab 38 SI	$1.2 \times 10^8 \, M^{-1}$	Hedin, 1982a
Clone 23	$1.4 \times 10^8 \, M^{-1}$	Accolla, 1979
Clone 37	$1.1 \times 10^7 \, M^{-1}$	Accolla, 1979
Mab IE9	$1.0 \times 10^8 \, M^{-1}$	Kupchik, 1981
Polyclonal Ab (goat)	$1.9 \times 10^9 \, M^{-1}$	Kupchik, 1981

A number of workers have developed monoclonal-based immuno-assays suitable for early clinical trials. Buchegger, working in Dr. Jean Pierre Mach's laboratory, designed a double solid phase assay using polyclonal goat anti-CEA in a solid support to isolate CEA from heat-extracted serum. The CEA bound to the support by the polyclonal is then detected by incubation with a mouse monoclonal followed by a final en-zyme immunoassay step. In 134 normal individuals and 380 serum samples from patients with cancer and other diseases (colorectal cancer, 208; gastric adenocarcinoma, 10; breast cancer, 17; and liver cirrhosis, 15) correlation coefficients between the new monoclonal enzyme immunoassay and a conventional polyclonal radioimmunoassay were be-tween 0.85 and 0.92. The sensitivity of the monoclonal assay is of the order of 0.6 ng/mL of serum. No differences were found in the correla-tion when normal samples and samples from colorectal cancer or other cancers were analyzed separately. The investigators concluded that even though their new assay is convenient, fast, and reproducible, it does not offer any additional sensitivity or specificity over conventional radioimmunoassays (Buchegger et al., 1982b). An additional refinement by the same group in which two monoclonal antibodies were attached to the solid phase for the isolation step and a third mouse monoclonal was used for the detection step, did not contribute materially to the specificity or sensitivity of the assay or to the ability, in preliminary clinical trials, to differentiate the CEA in samples from patients with malignancy from the antigen present in samples from normal individuals or patients with inflammatory or degenerative diseases (Buchegger et al., 1982a).

A high affinity mouse monoclonal antibody capable of reacting with CEA in unextracted serum has been described by Lindgren (Lindgren et al., 1982a). The antibody does not react with NCA and has a binding affinity comparable to that of a polyclonal rabbit anti-CEA antiserum. There is no published clinical experience using this assay.

Another double monoclonal enzyme immunoassay has recently been described. The two antibodies had previously been shown not to cross-react with NCA or BGP. Further analysis showed no significant cross-reactivity with NCA II either. One of the two monoclonals (38-S-1) was coupled to the solid phase and the other, Mab 27, was used to prepare an enzyme conjugate for detection of the CEA bound to the solid phase by the primary antibody. The limit of sensitivity in serum is 0.5 $\mu g/L$. A summary of the clinical results in 180 samples from patients with and without malignant disease is shown in Table 4. The results are most encouraging provided the additional specificity for cancer samples shown by this assay can be confirmed in a larger series of patients (Hedin et al., 1983).

It must be recognized that even if monoclonal assays of sufficient sensitivity can be developed, and even though the results of such assays correlate with results obtained by polyclonal assays (Buchegger et al., 1982a), or even if they improve upon their specificity and sensitivity (Hedin et al., 1983), nevertheless, the two types of assays recognize different sets of epitopes. Furthermore, epitope heterogeneity may be observed within the same patient as the disease progresses clinically or the treatment affects the physicochemical or immunological characteristics of circulating CEA (Rogers et al., 1981b). This additional complication, if confirmed, may require a complete reevaluation of the design of monoclonal assays to be used in clinical practice.

3. Monoclonal Antibodies in the Immunohistological Evaluation of CEA

There is considerable interest in and accumulated experience with the tissue localization and distribution of CEA by immunohistological methods. The extensive literature on the results of such studies with the use of polyclonal antibodies will not be reviewed here. Comprehensive reviews

Table 4
Clinical Results from Patients with and Without Malignant Disease[a]

	Total samples	RIA		MEIA	
		Normal[b]	Increased	Normal	Increased
Healthy individuals	40	35	5	40	0
Nonmalignant liver disease	45	19	26	43	2
Ulcerative colitis	25	20	5	25	0
Carcinoma (colon, pancreas, lung, breast)	60	5	55	6	54
Other malignancies	10	4	6	8	2

[a]Prepared from data in (Hedin, 1983).
[b]Up to 5 ng/mL in both assays.

with experimental data, methodological details, and clinical results have been published (Primus et al., 1981; Lindgren et al., 1982b; Bordes et al., 1973). Immunoperoxidase assays using the PAP technique can be quite sensitive for CEA. The limits of detection are 3 μg CEA/g of tissue for ethanol-fixed material and 3–5 μg/g for formalin-fixed tissue (Goldenberg et al., 1976).

Using fresh frozen tissue or formalin-fixed and either fluorescence or any of the variations of the peroxidase technique, CEA and other cross-reacting substances have been detected in many organs and tissues. In most series, colonic adenocarcinoma is positive 80–100% of the time. Somewhat lower percentages are seen in other cancers of the gastrointestinal tract. In the female reproductive system, positive staining has been shown in mucinous ovarian carcinomas, cervical cancer (both squamous and adenocarcinoma), and endometrial adenocarcinoma. In breast cancer as many as 66% of the tumors are positive and similarly high positivity rates have been seen in lung cancer and in medullary thyroid carcinoma (van Nagell et al., 1982; Primus et al., 1981). All of the reports are based on studies using polyclonal antibodies and because of that, and in spite of careful absorption of the antisera to eliminate cross-reactivity with CEA-like molecules, there is no assurance that the substance stained in the tissues is indeed CEA. Even the most highly purified polyclonal antibodies have been shown in careful studies to cross-react with NCA II and other mucin-related antigens from normal and pathological tissues.

It is reasonable to expect that further refinements in the determination of circulating CEA for monitoring and diagnosis will be based on and correlated with the tissue distribution of the antigen, but up to now the correlation has been poor as reported in the published literature. Although a number of reasons can be adduced for such poor correlation, the multiplicity of epitopes in CEA and the corresponding heterogeneity of the polyclonal antisera are the major obstacles for better correlation. Here as elsewhere it is hoped that monoclonal antibodies of defined epitope specificity will provide the tools needed.

There are few reported series on immunohistochemical localization of CEA with monoclonal antibodies. An antibody described by Gatter (Gatter et al., 1982) reacts with normal colon and stomach epithelium and with adenocarcinoma of colon, breast, and stomach but not with other glandular epithelia. This type of monoclonal can be useful to pathologists and clinicians in evaluating tumors when histopathology alone is not sufficient. Often a metastatic adenocarcinoma will offer no clue by routine histology as to the site of the primary tumor, but positive staining with a high-affinity anti-CEA antibody may help in eliminating some organs or tissues from consideration. In other situations, a normal serum CEA that does not correlate with a positive-staining tumor may be explained on the basis of nonspecificity of tissue staining by a polyclonal antibody.

Many monoclonal antibodies show high titers when tested for their ability to stain tissue sections, but the pattern of results has not been different from the patterns obtained with polyclonal antisera regardless of whether one considers the tissue distribution or the cellular localization of the antigen (Lindgren et al., 1982b).

Four monoclonals that may define four different epitopes by immunocytochemical studies have been described. One reacts with CEA, NCA, and NGP. Two other monoclonals cross-react with NGP only and the fourth recognizes a subpopulation of CEA molecules only. Whereas antibodies 1, 2, and 3 stain most colonic adenocarcinomas and their metastases, only 30% of primary tumors reacted with monoclonal 4 (Primus et al., 1983a). These results are promising. If more such selective monoclonals can be found their patterns of tissue reactivity, singly or in combination, may help elucidate the relationship of tissue antigen with serology, tumor behavior, and clinical outcome. Two classes of tumor antigens identified by monoclonals are produced by tissue cultures. One class is abundantly released into the culture fluid and the other can be detected in cells, but not in the supernatant fluid (Steplewski et al., 1981). From such studies an understanding may come about the correlation between tissue antigens, circulating tumor markers, and tumor behavior. By combining several monoclonals, patterns of reactivity characteristic for certain organs or tissue may be observed, or, within the same tumor, particular subpopulations of cells with different reactivities to monoclonals may be associated with differences in response to therapy and clinical outcome. Work in these areas is already in progress in many laboratories (van Nagell et al., 1982).

4. Monoclonal Anti-CEA Antibodies in Tumor Imaging

The use of radiolabeled tumor antibodies for the radiological detection of human cancer was first proposed over twenty years ago by Pressman and others (1957). However, this early work was limited by the use of antibodies directed against poorly defined tumor antigens. Carcinoembryonic antigen, a well-defined tumor marker purified from colorectal carcinoma, was proposed as a target for tumor localization studies soon after its identification in 1965 (Gold and Freedman, 1965). Success rates using radiolabeled polyclonal goat antibodies directed against CEA in radioimmunodetection techniques have varied widely, ranging from up to 50% success by one set of investigators (Mach et al., 1978; Mach et al., 1980b) to 90% in other centers (Goldenberg et al., 1978; Goldenberg et al., 1980).

The major reason for the wide range in success rates using polyclonal CEA antibodies must be attributed to the well known variability of specificity and to the heterogeneity of binding affinities of the antibody preparations used for injection. Conventional polyclonal antibodies, as previously discussed, are directed against a variety of determinants in the CEA molecule, only some of which may be truly CEA-specific (Hedin et al., 1982a). However, discrepancies may also be due to differences in photoscanning techniques and/or to differences in the subjective interpretation of results (Mach et al., 1980b).

Some of the problems of sensitivity and specificity may be eliminated by the recent advances in hybridoma technology, but problems inherent in imaging technology remain and the use of monoclonals may itself produce a new set of problems.

The monoclonal antibodies are homogeneous and directed against individual epitopes of the CEA molecule and are also easier to purify than the polyclonals that require extensive absorptions in order to remove nonspecific and cross-reacting immunoglobulins. Even though some purification of ascitic fluid antibodies is required, absorption steps are unnecessary in hybridoma-produced antibodies. Finally, unlike the polyclonal antibodies, the individual monoclonal CEA antibodies are available in unlimited amounts.

Monoclonal CEA antibodies are not entirely advantageous for use in radioimmunodetection techniques. If a CEA-producing tumor contains low levels of the particular epitope the radiolabled monoclonal antibody is directed against, the tumor may go undetected. Rather than using individual preparations, it may therefore be preferable to use antibody mixtures that are directed against different epitopes of the same antigen (Primus et al., 1983b) or against different antigens of the same tumor cells (Gaffar et al., 1981). Recent findings have also shown that the bivalent F(ab')$_2$ antibody fragment of a monoclonal against CEA may be better than either the intact antibody or the monovalent Fab fragment for I-131 tumor imaging (Wahl et al., 1983). This method also appears to facilitate the clearance of antibody from the circulation and from nontarget tissue without interfering with antibody uptake or the amount of antibody accretion by the tumor, thereby resulting in improved tumor imaging.

In one tumor immunolocalization study, three different monoclonal antibodies (Mabs) against separate protein determinants in CEA were evaluated for their ability to detect CEA-producing human tumors grown in nude mice (Hedin et al., 1982b). The monoclonals were isolated from the ascitic fluids of hybridoma-bearing BALB/c mice and designated as Mab 38S1, Mab 9, and Mab 48. After extensive dialysis, each antibody was labeled with 1–2 mCi NaI-131 per 200 μg of purified antibody (Hedin et al., 1982a).

Nude mice (BALB/c nu/nu) were injected with tissue-culture-grown living tumor cells from the following human tumor cell lines: colon adenocarcinoma LS 174T (Kahan et al., 1976), colon adenocarcinoma HT-29 (Fogh, 1975), pharynx carcinoma Detroit 562 (Peterson et al., 1971) and non-CEA-producing rhabdomyosarcoma RD (McAllister et al., 1969). Tumor were detectable 10–14 d after the injection of tumor cells. The mice were then injected with 10–20 μCi of ^{131}I-labeled monoclonal antibody in a single dose. Control mice were given the same dose of ^{131}I-labeled normal mouse IgG or NaI-131. In the first series of experiments, mice carrying tumor LS 174T were given 1–2 μg of ^{131}I-labeled mab 38S1 and then killed on d 1–6 after injection. Concentration ratios (concentration of radioactivity in specific tissue/mean concentration of radioactivity in the mouse) for the tumor and other tissues were determined. Tumor ratios increased up to days four and five whereas ratios for the other tissues decreased with time. Thereafter, all mice were killed 4 d after injection and subjected to either scintigraphy or complete dissection.

The best results were seen in mice carrying LS 174T tumors and injected with ^{131}I-labeled Mab 38S1. In the most favorable experiment, the whole mouse contained 7.6% of the injected dose of radioactive antibody with 5.6% of the injected dose (equal to 74% of the total radioactivity at d 4) being found in the tumor. In the ten mice bearing LS 174T and injected with I-131-Mab 38S1, the mean concentration ratio of labeled antibody was at least seven times higher in the tumor than in any other tissue, including blood. In mice bearing one of the other three tumors and injected with labeled Mab 38S1, the concentration ratios of labeled antibody were highest in the tumor and blood. Only in the LS 174T tumor, however, was the ratio higher in the tumor than in the blood. Since LS 174T tumors had the highest concentration of CEA as compared to the other tumors, as determined by a double antibody radioimmunoassay (Zimmerman, 1979), the investigators concluded that the concentration of CEA in the tumor ''at least partly determines the extent of tumor localization obtained with anti-CEA antibodies.'' As a control, nude mice carrying a non-CEA producing human sarcoma were also injected with the radiolabeled antibody. No selective uptake of antibody in the tumor tissue was seen.

Mab 48 and Mab 9 were also chosen for study because they were CEA-specific, were strongly reactive with CEA, and were directed against different epitopes in the CEA molecule from the one recognized by Mab 38S1. Results indicated that Mab 48 showed relatively good localization whereas Mab 9 reacted poorly to the tumor. The reason for the differences in reactivity of the antibodies was not understood since all three were fully immunoreactive after purification and all were of the same IgG subclass (i.e., IgG_1).

In another study giving the first clinical results using radiolabled monoclonal antibodies against CEA, tomoscintigraphy was employed to detect gastrointestinal and medullary thyroid cancers (Berche et al., 1982). The monoclonal anti-CEA antibodies were produced by two mouse hybridoma lines in ascitic form and labeled with ^{131}I. Nineteen patients with a history of primary cancer were included in the study (six with medullary thyroid carcinomas and 13 with a variety of gastrointestinal carcinomas). Two of the patients (one from each group) were in complete remission when the study was performed. Rectiliner scintigraphy was performed on 18 patients and tomoscintigraphy on all 19 after injection with the radiolabeled antibodies.

Ninety-four percent of the tumor sites studied were detected by tomoscintigraphy whereas only 44% were detected by rectilinear scintigraphy. The only tumor site not detected by tomoscintigraphy was large (110 cm^3). This negative result and a low serum CEA level in the patient indicated that the tumor was not producing CEA. The poor sensitivity rate of rectilinear scintigraphy may occur because this technique mainly detects tumors larger than 50 cm whereas tomoscintigraphy detects tumors as small as a few cubic centimeters. In addition, the specificity rate (true positive versus false positive) was better for tomoscintigraphy (84%) than for rectilinear scintigraphy (78%).

The investigators concluded that immunotomoscintigraphy allows the detection of smaller tumors whereas the clinical use of rectilinear scintigraphy for immunoscintigraphy appears limited to the detection of large tumors. Therefore, the first method "may represent an efficient diagnostic technique for detecting occult CEA-producing tumors preoperatively, and, in particular, for localizing recurrences or metastases of medullary thyroid carcinomas."

It seems evident that the discovery of the highly sensitive and specific monoclonal antibodies has led to a renewed interest in the development of radioimmunodetection as a standard detection technique. However, single antibody preparations are not as effective as antibody mixtures, as discussed above. With CEA, the answer may be to use mixtures of monoclonals that are directed against different determinants of the CEA molecule in order to produce a more effective cancer detection agent. Goldenberg refers to these mixtures as "engineered polyclonal antibodies" (Goldenberg, 1983). The corresponding advancements in imaging instrumentation (i.e., computerized tomoscintigraphy) also contribute to the use of radioimmunodetection in both the detection and staging of cancer. In turn, the ability to use these antibodies for detection may lead to using the same antibodies for therapy.

5. Immunotherapy with Monoclonal CEA Antibodies

A therapeutic approach that is receiving considerable attention experimentally is the use of antitumor agents which can be selectively delivered to target tissue by coupling the agent to an antitumor antibody. Such agents may be chemotherapeutic drugs, radioisotopes, toxins, and so on (Hellstrom et al., 1982). The conjugates have been prepared with whole antibody molecules or with Fab and F(ab')$_2$ fragments.

Polyclonal anti CEA antibodies conjugated with ^{131}I have been used in the experimental treatment of a Hamster model bearing a CEA-producing tumor. At a dose of 1 mCi, growth inhibition and increased survival were achieved (Goldenberg et al., 1981). Studies using monoclonal antibodies against other colon antigens have been reported. The antibody was conjugated to the A chain of ricin, a plant toxin consisting of an alpha chain and a beta chain (Gilliland et al., 1980). The approach may not be completely successful because single toxin chains do not deliver full cytotoxicity to the target cells and because of nonspecific binding of toxins to noncancer cells. A novel solution to this problem is discussed below.

There are other complications with the use of injected antibodies. The foreign immunoglobulin may be toxic to the host, or the host may develop antibodies to the injected mouse immunoglobulin. However, the experience with the administration of antibodies in vivo for radioimmunodetection suggests that such complications may be less frequent than suspected (Goldenberg et al., 1981). The problems of specificity may be solved when more epitope specific monoclonals are used to prepare the conjugates, but this may result in decreased sensitivity, as discussed in the section of immunodetection.

Recent advances in our understanding of how proteins and other high-molecular weight substances enter cells may contribute to further advances in this field. Monoclonal antibodies against membrane receptors have been prepared and used to deliver antibody–toxin conjugates (immunotoxins) selectively to target cells. A toxin such as ricin can be separated into its composing A and B chains. Each chain can be conjugated separately to an antireceptor monoclonal antibody. The antibodies deliver the individual chains to the target cell for intracellular recombination and full cytotoxic activity. The monoclonal antibodies perform two functions: one, they deliver toxin to the target cells and two, they prevent free chains from binding to nontarget cells (Vitetta et al., 1983).

6. Summary

Monoclonal antibody technology has already contributed much to our understanding of the pathobiology of carcinoembrionic antigen. Such important data as the localization of key epitopes to the polypeptide moeity of the molecules; the corroboration of the fact that some epitopes are conformation dependent; the confirmation that monoclonal antibodies with potential tumor specificity react preferentially with high mol wt (186,000 daltons) CEA and not as well with the low mol wt CEAs are all advances in our understanding of CEA immunochemistry that, although already known or postulated by studies with polyclonals, are now more firmly established on the basis of data obtained with monoclonal antibodies.

Further advances will come when the pattern of epitopes giving the molecules their tumor specificity is fully elucidated, but some progress has already been made by using the monoclonals as proving tools. With polyclonal antibodies as many as 10–20 epitopes had been postulated on CEA (Hammarstrom et al., 1976). In fact, the real number may be smaller, closer to four or six than to 20. Furthermore, it may be possible to allocate the epitope distribution to no more than three families of glycoprotein antigens (Primus et al., 1983a).

Most of the data so far obtained has been obtained from hybridization experiments in which the primary immunogen is colorectal carcinoma metastatic to the liver, but the fact that at least one set of monoclonals has been prepared with metastatic breast cancer as the immunogen is an important additional insight. Indeed such CEA-reacting monoclonals subcloned from a mouse immunized with a breast tumor extract are strong encouragement to continue to pursue CEA as a discrete molecule with tumor-specific epitopes. Several tissues may synthesize a molecule in which the specificity is to the malignant cell and not necessarily to the site of origin. The possibility of such molecule or molecules existing has been contemplated for many years.

In practice, the specificity has been less than expected and much work remains to be done in this area. Further, the affinities of the monoclonals for CEA, although of very high order when expressed as constants derived from Scatchard or reciprocal plot data (Table 3), are lower when their binding capacity is compared to that of polyclonals in immunoassay systems, monoclonals often showing as little as 20–30% of the binding capacity of conventional polyclonals. This low sensitivity is of course a definite limitation for the development of useful immunoassays. In radioimmunological detection techniques the problem is twofold: the low binding affinity is complicated by the increased specificity of the monoclonals since a monoclonal antibody against a single epitope may miss a tumor that might have been detected, however nonspecifically, by the polyclonal.

Few monoclonal systems have reached the stage of clinical trials. The available early data is confirmatory of the traditional work done with polyclonals, but only limited success has been reported in the overriding goal of improving cancer and/or tissue specificity.

In several series the correlation of results of polyclonals versus monoclonals has been excellent, and parallel results have been obtained when the same patients have been followed by simultaneous serial determinations (Buchegger et al., 1982b; Rogers et al., 1981b; Kupchik et al., 1981). In one laboratory a sandwich immunoassay using two monoclonal antibodies bound to a solid phase for antigen isolation, and a third monoclonal for detection, did show lesser reactivity with the serum of healthy individuals and patients with nonmalignant disease than conventional radioimmunoassay while preserving comparable sensitivity for detecting hyperantigenemia in cancer patients (Table 4). It is reasonable to hope for further developments along this encouraging line. The monoclonal immunoassays do not lack for analytical sensitivity since their detection limits of about 0.5 ng/mL are equal to those of polyclonal radioimmunoassays. Analytical specificity has been shown experimentally to be better in monoclonal than in polyclonal assays but the clinical specificity has not improved significantly.

The immunohistochemical characterization of CEA-producing tumors is slowly becoming a routine component of histopathology and clinical oncology. The contributions of monoclonal technology to this field are also already evident. There is a better understanding of the cellular localization of the antigens; of the influence of tissue processing techniques on the variability of the results and of the relative distribution, tissular and cellular, of CEA and the cross-reacting antigens. Perhaps here, in immunocytochemistry, monoclonals have the most to offer to our understanding of fundamental tumor biology and to the eventual development of histochemical assays that will provide clinical information about malignant potential, staging, and therapy. Similar statements can be made about radioimaging techniques with CEA monoclonals. The literature is extensive and experimental data are encouraging, but few studies using monoclonal radioimaging have appeared, and the promise of more specific radioimages remains a promise.

The hope of developing a cancer-specific CEA assay remains viable, not in small part because of the contributions of monoclonal methodology.

Acknowledgment

We thank Ms. Dawn M. Devaney for her skillful editorial assistance.

References

Accolla, R. S., S. Carrel, and J. P. Mach (1980), *Proc. Natl. Acad. Sci. USA* **77,** 563.

Accolla, R. S., S. Carrel, M. Phan, D. Heumann, and J. P. Mach (1979), *Protides Biol. Fluids Proc. Colloq.* **27,** 31.

Balz, J. B., E. W. Martin, and J. P. Minton (1977), *Rev. Surg.* **34,** 1.

Berche, C., J. P. Mach, J. D. Lumbroso, C. Langlais, F. Aubry, F. Buchegger, S. Carrel, P. Rougier, C. Parmentier, and M. Tubiana (1982), *B. Med. J.* **285,** 1447.

Bordes, M., R. Michiels, and F. Martin (1973), *Digestion* **9,** 106.

Buchegger, F., C. Mettraux, R. S. Accolla, S. Carrel, and J. P. Mach (1982a), *Immunol. Lett.* **5,** 85.

Buchegger, F., M. Phan, D. Rivier, S. Carrel, R. S. Accolla, and J. P. Mach (1982b), *J. Immunol. Meth.* **49,** 129.

Burtin, P., S. von Kleist, M. C. Sabine, and M. King (1973), *Cancer Res.* **33,** 3299.

Chu, T. M., and G. Reynoso (1972a), *Nature* **238,** 152.

Chu, T. M, and G. Reynoso (1972b), *Clin. Chem.* **18,** 918.

Colcher, D., P. H. Hand, M. Nuti, and J. Schlom (1983), *Cancer Invest.* **1,** 127.

Damjanov, I., and B. B. Knowles (1983), *Lab. Invest.* **48,** 510.

Edgington, T. S., R. W. Astarta, and E. F. Plow (1975), *N. Eng. Jour. Med.* **293,** 103.

Fogh, J. (1975), *Human Tumor Cells in Vitro,* Plenum Press, New York, N.Y.

Foster, C. S. (1982), *Cancer Treat. Rev.* **9,** 59.

Freedman, S. O. (1977), *Tumor Markers,* University Park Press, Baltimore, MD.

Gaffar, S. A., K. D. Pant, D. Shochat, S. J. Bennett, and D. M. Goldenberg (1981), *Int. J. Cancer* **27,** 101.

Galfre, G., C. Milstein, and B. Wright (1979), *Nature* **277,** 131.

Gatter, K. C., Z. Abdulaziz, P. Beverley, J. R. F. Corvalan, C. Ford, E. B. Lane, M. Mota, J. R. G. Nash, K. Pulford, H. Stein, J. Taylor-Papadimitriou, C. Woodhouse, and D. Y. Mason (1982), *J. Clin. Pathol.* **35,** 1253.

Gilliland, D. G., Z. Steplewski, R. J. Collier, K. F. Mitchell, T. H. Chang, and H. Koprowski (1980), *Proc. Natl. Acad. Sci. USA* **77,** 4539.

Gold, P., and S. O. Freeman (1965), *J. Exp. Med.* **122,** 467.

Goldenberg, D. M. (1983), *J. Nucl. Med.* **24,** 360.

Goldenberg, D. M., F. Deland, E. Kim, S. Bennett, F. J. Primus, J. R. van Nagell, N. Estes, P. DeSimone, and P. Rayburn (1978), *N. Eng. J. Med.* **298,** 1384.

Goldenberg, D. M., S. A. Gaffar, S. J. Bennett, and J. L. Beach (1981), *Cancer Res.* **41,** 4354.

Goldenberg, D. M., E. E. Kim, F. H. Deland, S. Bennett, and F. J. Primus (1980), *Cancer Res.* **40,** 2984.

Goldenberg, D. M., R. M. Sharkey, and F. J. Primus (1976), *J. Natl. Cancer Inst.* **57,** 11.

Grunert, F., K. Wank, G. A. Luckenback, and S. von Kleist (1982), *Oncodevel. Biol. Med.* **3,** 191.

Hammarstrom, S., T. Svenberg, and G. Sundblad (1976), *Oncofetal Development Gene Expression,* Academic Press, New York, 559 pp.

Hedin, A., L. Carlsson, A. Berglund, and S. Hammarstrom (1983), *Proc. Natl. Acad. Sci. USA* **80,** 3470.

Hedin, A., S. Hammarstrom, and A. Larsson (1982a), *Mole. Immunol.* **19 (12),** 1641.

Hedin, A., B. Wahren, and S. Hammarstrom (1982b), *Int. J. Cancer* **30,** 547.

Hellstrom, K. E., I. Hellstrom, and J. P. Brown (1982), *Springer Semin. Immunopath.* **5,** 127.

Holyoke, E. D., T. M. Chu, and G. P. Murphy (1975), *Cancer* **25,** 830.

Kahan, B., L. Rutzky, B. Bulin, J. Tomita, F. Wiseman, S. LeGrue, H. Noll, and B. Tom (1976), *Cancer Res.* **36,** 3526.

Kohler, G., and C. Milstein (1975), *Nature* **256,** 495.

Kupchik, H. Z., V. R. Zurawski, J. G. Hurrell, N. Zamchek, and P. Black (1981), *Cancer Res.* **41,** 3306.

Lindgren, J., B. Bang, M. Hurme, and O. Makela (1982a), *Acta Path. Microbiol. Immunol. Scand. Sect.* C **90,** 159.

Lindgren, J., T. Wahlstrom, B. Bang, M. Hurme, and O. Makela (1982b), *Histochemistry* **74,** 223.

Mach, J. P., S. Carrel, M. Forni, J. Ritschard, A. Donath, and P. Alberto (1980a), *N. Engl. J. Med.* **303,** 5.

Mach, J. P., S. Carrel, C. Merenda, D. Heumann, and U. Roenspies (1978), *Eur. J. Cancer* (Suppl. 1), **44,** 113.

Mach, J. P., M. Forni, J. Ritschard, F. Buchegger, S. Carrel, S. Widgren, A. Donath, and P. Alberto (1980b), *Oncodevel. Biol. Med.* **1,** 49.

McAllister, R. M., J. Melnyk, J. Z. Sinkelstein, E. C. Adams, Jr., and M. B. Gardner (1969), *Cancer* **24,** 520.

Norgaard-Pedersen, B., and N. H. Axelson (1978), *Scand. J. Immunol.* Supp. No. 8, **8,** 27.

Olsson, L., and H. S. Kaplan (1980), *Proc. Natl. Acad. Sci. USA* **77,** 5429.

Peterson, W., C. Stulberg, and W. Simpson (1971), *Proc. Soc. Exp. Biol. (N.Y.)* **136,** 1187.

Pressman, D., E. D. Day, and M. Blau (1957), *Cancer Res.* **17,** 845.

Primus, F. J., C. A. Clark, and D. M. Goldenberg (1981), *Diagnostic Immunohistochemistry,* Masson, New York, p. 263.

Primus, F. J., W. J. Kuhns, and D. M. Goldenberg (1983a), *Cancer Res.* **43,** 693.

Primus, F. J., K. D. Newell, A. Blue, and D. M. Goldenberg (1983b), *Cancer Research* **43,** 686.

Reynoso, G. (1981), *Diag. Med.* **4,** 41.

Reynoso, G., and M. Keane (1979), *Immunodiagnosis of Cancer,* Part I, Marcel Dekker, New York, p. 239.

Rogers, G. T., G. A. Rawlins, and K. D. Bagshawe (1981a), *Br. J. Cancer* **43,** 1.

Rogers, G. T., G. A. Rawlins, P. A. Keep, E. H. Cooper, and K. D. Bagshawe (1981b), *Br. J. Cancer* **44,** 371.

Steplewski, Z., T. H. Chang, M. Herlyn, and H. Koprowski (1981), *Cancer Res.* **41,** 2723.

van Heyninger, V., L. Barron, D. J. H. Brock, D. Crichton, and S. Laurie (1982), *J. Immunol. Meth.* **50**, 123.
van Nagell, J. R., S. Hudson, E. C. Gay, E. S. Donaldson, M. Hanson, D. F. Powell, and D. M. Goldenberg (1982), *Cancer* **49**, 379.
Vitetta, E. S., K. A. Krolick, M. Miyama-Inaba, W. Cushley, and J. W. Uhr (1983), *Science* **219**, 644.
Wahl, R. L., C. W. Parker, G. W. Philpott (1983), *N. Nucl. Med.* **24**, 317.
Westwood, J. H. (1977), *Tumor Markers,* University Park Press, Baltimore, p. 15.
Zimmerman, B. (1979), *J. Immunol. Meth.* **25**, 311.

Chapter 3

Monoclonal Antibodies to Alphafetoprotein and Regulation of AFP Gene Expression

STEWART SELL

Department of Pathology and Laboratory Medicine, University of Texas Health Science Center in Houston, Medical School, Houston, Texas

1. Introduction

The modern era of tumor markers began with the discovery of alphafetoprotein (AFP) by Garri I. Abelev of the Soviet Union in 1963 (Abelev et al., 1963; Abelev, 1971). He found, by immunodiffusion, that a protein was present in fetal mouse sera and in sera from adult mice with hepatocellular carcinomas that was not detectable in normal adult mouse sera. This discovery rekindled an interest in products produced by tumors that could be useful for diagnosis. AFP has served as the prototype for a growing number of tumor markers, and has been studied extensively in animal models and in human disease. The results of previous studies have been reviewed in previous editions of this series (Sell, 1980, 1982). Important findings regarding the normal physiology and the pathologic associations for AFP are listed in Table 1, and will not be reviewed in detail here (see earlier reviews: Abelev, 1971; Ruoslahti et al., 1974; Abelev, 1975; Adinolfi et al., 1975; also Sell and Becker 1978; Sell, 1981; Sell et al., 1983).

41

Table 1

Major Observations on the Physiology and Pathologic Associations of AFP

AFP is synthesized in yolk sac and fetal liver, and to a much lesser extent in the GI tract.

AFP crosses the placenta to produce elevation in maternal serum AFP levels during pregnancy.

Abnormally high maternal or amniotic fluid levels are predictive of open spinal cord defects.

A specific physiologic function has not been identified; claims for immuno-suppressive activity controversial.

Rodent, but not AFP of other species, binds estrogen at high affinity.

Sustained elevations in adult are associated with hepatocellular and germinal cell (yolk sac) tumors, elevations less frequent with GI, lung, and breast carcinomas.

Temporary elevations occur following liver injury; AFP is synthesized by dividing hepatocytes during restitutive proliferation.

Transient elevations occur early during exposure of rats to chemical hepato-carcinogens, before hepatocellular carcinoma develops; AFP found in new cell populations at this time (oval cells, atypical hepatocytes), but not in "neoplastic nodules."

---

2. Monoclonal Antibodies to AFP

A listing of monoclonal antibodies to AFP is given in Table 2. With the development of the hybridoma technology required to produce mono-clonal antibodies (Kohler and Milstein, 1975), it was not surprising that one of the first set of monoclonal antibodies made would be to AFP since it was better characterized than other tumor markers and relatively easy to isolate and assay (Ruoslahti et al., 1974). Up to four epitopes have been identified on AFP using monoclonal antibodies (Micheel et al., 1983). Most of the monoclonal antibodies produced did not provide the level of sensitivity in ELISA or RIA as did conventional antisera. However, se-lection of monoclonal antibodies with high affinities for AFP resulted in assays that were essentially as sensitive as those using conventional antisera. The major advantage of monoclonal antibodies was the ability of two monoclonal antibodies that recognized different epitopes to be used in a one-step sandwich ELISA.

2.1. ELISA Using Monoclonal Antibodies

The one step ELISA is performed by coating assay plates with one monoclonal antibody, then inculating the sample containing AFP and the second monoclonal antibody labeled with enzyme at the same time (Uotila et al., 1981; Ruoslahti and Engvall, 1982). Since the monoclonal

Table 2
Monoclonal Antibodies to AFP

Observation	Reference
Three Mabs to human AFP characterized and used for RIA with essentially same sensitivity as conventional antisera; Mabs did not distinguish among Con A variants.	Uotila et al., *Molec. Immunol.* 17:791, 1980
Two Mabs to different AFP determinants used for one-step sandwich ELISA.	Uotila et al., *J. Immunol. Methods* 42:11, 1981, Ruoslahti and Engvall, *Clin. Immunol. Newsletter* 3:139, 1982
Three Mabs to human AFP pooled and used in RIA not as sensitive as conventional antisera, low affinity Abs used for purification. Polyethylene glycol needed for RIA with Mab.	Heyningen et al., *J. Immunol. Methods* 50:123, 1982
Labeled Mab used for immunoradiometric assay. RIA sensitivity using conventional Ab similar but requires shorter incubation period.	Hunter et al., *J. Immunol. Methods* 50:133, 1982
Immobilized Mab in conjunction with peroxidase conjugated conventional or Mab used for sandwich assay in one-step assay.	Brock et al., *Clinica Chemica Acta* 122:353, 1982
Two-site one-step sandwich RIA sensitivity decreased at high AFP concentrations because of binding of labeled antibody to AFP not bound to immunobilized antibody.	Nomura et al., *J. Immunol. Methods* 56:13, 1983
Three antigenic determinants on human AFP detected by Mabs. Combination of one and two labeled Mabs used for three-site sandwich RIA; higher sensitivity than two-site.	Nomura et al., *J. Immunol. Methods* 58:293, 1983
Four epitopes on human AFP detected by Mabs.	Micheel et al., *Eur. J. Can. Clin. Oncol.* 19:1239, 1983
Sixteen Mabs with different affinities to human AFP produced. RIA using Mab with highest affinity more sensitive (1 ng/mL) than conventional antisera.	Yamazaki et al., *Hokkaido U. Med. Library Series* 15:163, 1983

antibody bound to the assay plate and the enzyme-linked monoclonal antibody react with different epitopes on the sample, they do not compete with each other. The amount of enzyme-linked antibody bound to the plate after washing is directly related to the amount of sample (AFP) added if the amount of sample does not exceed the binding capacity of the antibody bound to the assay plate. The amount of enzyme labeled antibody bound is then determined by addition of a colorless substrate for the enzyme linked to the second antibody. The amount of substrate converted by the enzyme during a selected period of time is quantitated colorimetrically and converted to the amount of AFP in the sample by comparison to a standard curve.

At high concentrations of AFP in an unknown sample the amount of AFP measured may be erroneously low because the labeled antibody binds to excess AFP that is not bound to the immobilized antibody. The labeled antibody is removed by the washing step as it is not held by the immobilized antibody (Nomura et al., 1983a). The sensitivity may be further increased by the use of two labeled monoclonal antibodies that each react with a different epitope that is in turn different from the epitope with which the immobilized antibody reacts (Nomura et al., 1983b). Yamazaki et al. (1983) were able to develop a radioimmunoassay using one of their monoclonal antibodies that is more sensitive than one using a conventional horse antiserum. In any case, when all is said and done, it appears that ELISAs using monoclonal antibodies to AFP do not offer great advantages over assays that employ conventional antibodies.

2.2. Immune Localization Using Anti-AFP

Other than their use in immunoassays for AFP, this author is not aware of other applications for monoclonal antibodies to AFP. However, the use of conventional antibodies to AFP in tumor localization and tumor therapy deserves further comment. Parks et al. in 1974 demonstrated localization of radiolabeled rabbit anti-mouse-AFP to transplanted AFP-producing hepatocellular carcinoma BW7757 in vivo, and many authors have reported the cellular localization of AFP in tissue sections of AFP-producing tumors. Thus it was of interest to attempt to localize tumors in vivo using immunescintigraphy.

2.3. Radioimmunescintigraphy

Studies using radiolabeled antibody to AFP to localize tumors in vivo are listed in Table 3. There has been much less work with localization with radiolabeled antibody to AFP than with labeled antibody to CEA (Kim et al., 1980a). Koji et al. (1980) demonstrated localization of sites of tumor growth in a mouse model employing a transplantable hepatocellular carcinoma and isolated radiolabeled horse Fab fragments of antibody to mouse AFP. The labeled Fab selectively localized in tumor lesions even though

Table 3

In Vivo Localization of AFP Producing Tumors by Radioimmunescintigraphy

System	Observation	Reference
Rats; [125]I Fab horse anti-AFP Ab; Yoshida ascites transplantable hepatoma	Localization of radioactivity in tumors relatively selective for antibody, normal IgG also localized to a lesser extent.	Koji et al., *Cancer Res.* 40:3013, 1980
Human (16 pts), ^{131}I goat IgG anti-AFP, computer assisted processing, various tumors	12/12 sites in AFP-positive patients localized, 6/16 sites in AFP-negative patients localized.	Kim et al., *Cancer Res.* 40:3008, 1980
Human (5 Pts), ^{131}I goat anti-AFP, testicular tumors	Immune scintigraphy with anti-AFP not better than conventional radiologic detection.	Javadpour, et al. *J. Amer. Med. Assn.* 246: 45, 1981
Human (15 pts), ^{131}I horse anti-AFP, [131]I Mab	Localization in 6/12 pts with horse Ab; 1/3 pts with Mab.	Nishi et al., in *Nuclear Medicine and Biology Advances* (C. Raynaud, ed.) Pergamon Press 1983, p. 2304

AFP was present in the circulation of the animals. Apparently the formation of immune complexes in the blood does not block localization of the antibody to the tumor. This also appears to be true for localization of CEA-producing tumors in patients with circulating CEA (Primus et al., 1980). Kim et al. (1980b) were able to demonstrate localization of radiolabeled anti-AFP in twelve metastatic sites in five patients with AFP-producing hepatocellular carcinomas or teratocarcinomas. It is of interest that localization of radiolabeled anti-AFP also was seen in six of sixteen lesions in patients that had tumors that did not produce detectable AFP. Javadpour et al. (1981), using antibody to human chorionic gonadotropin or to AFP, were able to localize germinal cell tumor lesions. These lesions were also detectable using conventional radiologic techniques. Nishi et al. (1983) observed localization in 1/3 patients with an Mab compared to 6/12 with horse antibody. They suggest that an appropriate Mab could be more effective than conventional antibody, but this has not yet been demonstrated. Further studies are now underway at a number of medical centers using different antibodies to tumor markers. The use of ^{111}In-labeled monoclonal antibodies is proposed to give better localization the iodine-labeled antibodies (Halpern et al., 1983). In general, radioimmunescintigraphy has shown promise, but requires a high degree of sophistocated technology, is not cost effective, and may not be superior to more advanced computerized tomography or nuclear magnetic resonance procedures now available. Radiolocalization does suggest that labeled antibodies to antigens on tumors can be effective in selectively delivering the antibody to the tumor in vivo and supports the possible application of labeled antibodies to deliver radioactivity or drugs to tumor sites for therapy.

2.4. Immunotherapy

Active immunization with AFP and passive immunization with anti-AFP has been attempted as immunotherapy for AFP-producing tumors (Table 4). The results in experimental systems reveal differences using different systems. In the mouse, anti-AFP has been shown to kill some AFP-producing tumor cell lines in the presence of complement in vitro; other tumor lines are not killed, but in some growth is inhibited. In the rat, little or no effect of anti-AFP was noted on transplantable Morris Hepatoma 7777 in vitro. The injection of anti-AFP into rats or mice bearing transplantable AFP-producing tumors has an inconsistent effect. Mizejewski and Allen (1974) noted a reduction in the size of transplanted BW7756 hepatoma in mice, but no cures. We found reversal of tumor growth in 3/14 rats when anti-AFP was administered at the time of transplantation of hepatoma 7777 (Sell et al., 1976b). Wepsic et al. (1980) reported inhibition of growth in rats bearing AH66 hepatoma and treated with horse anti-AFP. Rats (Gousev and Yaskova, 1974; Sell et al., 1976b) and mice (Engvall et al., 1977) actively immunized with AFP also show inconsistent effects. Gousev and Yazkova (1974) noted regression of tumors in 4/10 actively immunized rats bearing the Zajdela hepatoma. Sell et al. (1976b) found regression in only 1/9 rats inoculated with hepatoma 7777. Engvall et al. (1977) found no effect of active immunization in mice injected with hepatoma BW7756. When the cytotoxic drug daunomycin was conjugated to horse anti-AFP and injected into Donryu rats bearing the AH66 hepatoma, partial inhibition of growth was observed and in vitro cytotoxicity was enhanced (Tsukada et al., 1982a). Horse anti-human-AFP partially suppressed the growth of a human hepatoma transplanted into nude mice (Kuwahara et al., 1978), and a preliminary trial in ten patients with advanced liver cancer revealed that anti-AFP depressed the elevated serum AFP seen in these patients, but no conclusive effects on tumor growth were found (Hirai et al., 1981).

The use of a Mab-daunomycin conjugate proved to be essentially of the same effectiveness in killing tumor cells in vitro and in prolonging survival of rats injected with AHGG hepatoma cells as horse anti-AFP in the same system (Tsukada et al., 1982b). To the best of the author's

Table 4
Effects of Anti-AFP on AFP-Producing Tumors

System	Observation	Reference
Rat hepatoma AH66, horse anti-AFP, immunofluorescence	Inhibits growth of tumor cells in vitro; there is selection for low AFP-producing cells that grow slowly when transplanted; AFP is on cell membrane.	Tsukada et al., *Int. J. Cancer* 13:187, 1974
Rabbit anti-mouse and human AFP, BW7756 hepatoma	Anti-AFP cytotoxicity not C mediated; no suppression of tumor growth in vivo; labeled Ab localized to tumor.	Parks et al., *Ann. Surg.* 180:599, 1974
Rats immunized to mouse AFP produce antibodies to rat AFP; Zajdela hepatoma	Involution of transplantable hepatomas in 4/10 actively immunized rats.	Gousev and Yazkova, in *Coll. Inserm,* Paris, 1974, p 255
C57BL mice, BW7756 hepatoma, rabbit antisera	32% Reduction in size of transplanted hepatoma; in vitro cytotoxicity not C dependent; lymphoid cell infiltrate seen.	Mizejewski and Allen, *Nature* 250:52, 1974
BW7756 in vitro	In vitro growth inhibited by anti-AFP.	Mizejewski et al., *J. Natl. Cancer Inst.* 36:476, 1975
Rat hepatoma 7777, goat anti-AFP (passive), also active immunization to rat AFP	Reversal of tumor growth in 3/14 rats passively immunized; 1/9 actively immunized; no effect of anti-AFP in vitro.	Sell et al., *Cancer Res.* 36:476, 1976
BW7756 in vitro, rabbit anti-ALB, rabbit-anti-AFP	Anti-AFP C-dependent cytotoxicity, as well as non-C-dependent growth inhibition in vitro.	Allen and Ledford, *Cancer Res.* 37:696, 1977
BW7756, rabbit anti-AFP	As above, postexcision sera block cytotoxicity; AFP in cytoplasm and membrane by IF.	Mizejewski and Allen, *Cell Immunol. and Immunopath.* 11:307, 1978

(continued)

Table 4 (*continued*)

System	Observation	Reference
BW7756, rabbit anti-AFP	Partial suppression of hepatoma growth by passive anti-AFP.	Mizejewski and Dillon, *Arch. Immunol. et Therap. Exp.* 27:655, 1979
Mice BW 7756, active immunization	Anti-AFP toxic in vitro, active immunization fails to affect tumor growth.	Engvall et al., *J. Natl. Cancer Inst.* 59:277, 1977
AH66, horse anti-AFP, DEN carcinogenesis	Cytotoxic in vitro; inhibits growth in vivo (prolonged survival); inhibits development of tumors in carcinogen-treated rats.	Hirai, in *Carcino-Embryonic Protein*, Elsevier, 1979, p. 527
Human testicular tumors in nude mouse	Suppressed growth.	Ibid.
Donryu rats, AH66 tumor, horse anti-AFP	Inhibition of growth in 7/24 rats; subcutaneous tumor; 15/35 IP; regressors resist rechallenge.	Wepsic et al., *Int. J. Cancer* 26:655, 1980
10 Patients with hepatoma, affinity purified horse-anti-AFP	Depression of serum AFP levels; effects on tumor not conclusive; serum sickness noted in 2 patients.	Hirai et al., Report of Found. Basic Res. in Oncology, Tokyo, Japan, June 1981
Daunomycin conjugated to horse Ab to rat AFP, AH 66 tumor in Donryu rats	Partial inhibition of growth in vivo and cytotoxicity in vitro enhanced.	Tsukada et al., *Proc. Natl. Acad. Sci.* 79:621, 1982
Daunomycin conjugated to Mab to rat AFP, AH 66 tumor in Donryu rats	Both Mab and horse anti-AFP equally cytotoxic in vitro and equally effective in prolonging survival of rats injected with tumor.	Tsukada et al., *Proc. Natl. Acad. Sci.* 79:7896, 1982

knowledge, therapeutic studies using monoclonal antibodies to human AFP have not been reported although trials are underway in Japan. The above experience using conventionally derived antibodies to a well defined tumor marker indicate that it may be difficult to obtain consistent therapeutic effects with monoclonal antibodies.

3. Control of AFP Gene Expression

3.1. AFP and Albumin Gene Expression During Development

There have been a number of studies on the molecular mechanisms of control of the AFP gene. Because of the basic importance of this subject, it will be reviewed briefly herein. A listing of these studies is given in Table 5. A brief summary of the salient findings is as follows: AFP was first synthesized in a cell-free system using polysomes from rat ascites hepatoma AH66 by Kanai et al. (1974). Synthesis of a complementary DNA probe using reverse transcriptase was reported by Innes and Miller (1977), by Tse et al. (1978) and by Sala-Trepat et al. (1979a). In a number of systems it was found that the rate of synthesis of AFP by normal liver cells, normal yolk sac cells, and tumor cells correlated closely with the amount of messenger RNA for AFP present in the cells either by rates of translation in vitro or by R_0t analysis using cDNA probes (*See* Table 5). Tilghman and Belayew (1982) report parallel increases in AFP and albumin mRNA in the liver of fetal mice during development and that the decrease in AFP after birth was due to a decrease in rate of AFP transcription. In rats it was found that mRNA for AFP increases earlier than mRNA for albumin and that there is a correlation between the postnatal decrease in AFP synthesis and mRNA levels for AFP (Sell et al., 1979; Sala-Trepat et al., 1979a; Sell et al., 1980; Sellem et al., 1984). Other than a species difference, the reason for this apparent difference in concordance of mRNA AFP and mRNA ALB production during embryonic development remains unexplained. Peters et al. found that in vitro synthesized AFP contains a twenty-amino-acid leader sequence not found in serum AFP (Peters et al., 1979).

Using a highly sensitive plasmid-derived cDNA probe, Boulter et al., (1982) found that fetal tissues not usually thought of as producing AFP, such as kidney, intestine, lung, and heart, actually contained a few hundred copies of mRNA for AFP per cell. Fetal brain or adult tissues contain less than 10 molecules/cell of mRNA for AFP. Undifferentiated embryonal carcinoma cells contain no mRNA for AFP, but mRNA for AFP appears when these cells are induced to differentiate (Buc-Caron et al., 1983). In earlier in vitro studies (Sell et al., 1975), it was clearly demonstrated that AFP synthesis occurs in dividing fetal hepatocytes, and that AFP production could be demonstrated in adult hepatocytes that are stimulated to proliferate in vivo (Sell et al., 1976a) or in vitro (Leffert et al., 1978). Whatever precursor to mRNA that is made in the nucleus for AFP and albumin appears to be rapidly processed since essentially all of the mRNA in cellular fractions is found in the polysomal RNA fraction (Nahon et al., 1982). Probing of the DNA from producing and nonproducing cells and restriction endonuclease analysis revealed no evidence

Table 5
Summary of Studies on AFP Gene Expression

System	Observation	Reference
Mouse liver RNA	Cell free synthesis of albumin by RNA extracted from polysomes.	Faber et al., *Can. J. Biochem.* 52:429, 1973
Ascites rat hepatoma AH66	Polysomes synthesize AFP in cell free system; activity in membrane-bound polysomes.	Kanai et al., *Cancer Res.* 34:1813, 1974
Fetal mouse liver	Rate of synthesis related to translation activity of polysomal RNA during development.	Koga et al., *Nature* 252:495, 1977
Rat hepatoma 7777 cDNA AFP	Preparation of cDNA AFP using anti-AFP precipitation of polysomal RNA and reverse transcription; hybridization with hepatoma and liver RNA.	Innis and Miller, *J. Biol. Chem.* 252:8469, 1977
Rat 7777 normal liver cDNA ALB	Translational assays and cDNA hybridization show mRNA AFP to be 10% of total liver RNA; mRNA ALB fourfold less in hepatoma 7777; no change in ALB gene frequency.	Tse et al., *Biochemistry* 18:3121, 1978
Rat cDNA AFP, cDNA, ALB, synthesis in vitro	Isolation of mRNA AFP; synthesis of cDNA; AFP serum levels in developing rats correlate with synthesis rates and mRNA levels in liver.	Sell et al., in *Carcino-Embryonic Proteins*, Vol. I, Elsevier, p. 121, 1979
Four transplantable hepatomas, cDNA, translation	Levels of mRNA AFP and mRNA ALB correlate with protein synthesis rates in	Sell et al., *Biochim. Biophys. Acta* 564:173, 1979

(*continued*)

Table 5 (*continued*)

System	Observation	Reference
	vitro, serum levels in vivo and intensity of immunofluorescence of cytoplasm.	
Rat hepatoma 7777 cDNA AFP and cDNA ALB	1–2 ALB genes and 2–3 AFP genes/haploid genome in 7777 and normal liver; restriction endonuclease maps of 7777 and liver identical; cDNA AFP and cDNA ALB do not cross hybridize with respective mRNAs.	Sala-Trepat et al., *Proc. Natl. Acad. Sci.* 76:695, 1979
In vitro cell free translation, mouse	In vitro synthesized AFP contains a 20 AA N-terminal peptide not seen in serum AFP = PRE − AFP "leader sequence."	Peters et al., *Cancer Res.* 39:3702, 1979
Plasmid pBR322 rat cDNA AFP	Amplification of fragment of cDNA AFP by bacterial cloning.	Innis et al., *Arch. Biochem. Biophys.* 195:128, 1979
Mouse yolk sac	Isolation of mRNA AFP from yolk sac polysomal RNA by immunoprecipitation. Synthesis of cDNA; analysis of mRNA AFP in fetal and adult liver.	Miura et al., *JBC* 254:5515, 1979
Rat hepatoma 7777 cDNA AFP, cDNA ALB	Isolation of mRNA and synthesis of cDNA ALB and cDNA AFP, mRNA ALB 2265 nucleotides; mRNA AFP 2235; mRNA ALB has 330 noncoding bases, mRNA AFP, 385; mRNA AFP in devel-	Sala-Trepat et al., *Biochemistry* 18:2167, 1979

(*continued*)

Table 5 (*continued*)

System	Observation	Reference
	oping liver falls after birth; mRNA ALB stays high; mRNA in 7777 10^3-fold higher than in normal liver.	
Rat hepatoma 7777	Isolation of mRNA AFP, synthesis of cDNA; AFP high in hepatoma 7777, 10 day liver.	Belanger et al., *Cancer Res.* 39:2141, 1979
Rat ALB genomic DNA, R loop analysis	Rat ALB gene isolated from recombinant library and cloned. Contains 14 exons and 13 introns in 14.5 kilobases of DNA.	Sargent et al., *Proc. Natl. Acad. Sci.* 76:3256, 1979
Mouse mRNA cDNA	Isolation of mRNA AFP from yolk sac; cDNA synthesized; construction of cloned plasmids; 3 Eco RI fragments of genomic DNA hybridize with cDNA on at least 2 introns.	Tilghman et al., *J. Biol. Chem.* 254:7393, 1979
Rat hepatoma 7777	In vitro synthesis of AFP by 7777 correlates with mRNA AFP levels; mRNA AFP more stable in rapidly dividing cells.	Innis and Miller, *J. Biol. Chem.* 254:9148, 1979
Rat ALB, AFP	Review of synthesis, mRNA, serum levels in developing and adult liver; transplantable hepatomas; calculation of gene frequencies, gene location, subcellular distribution of mRNA (essentially all in polysomes).	Sell et al., *Cell Biol. Int. Reports* 4:235, 1980

Table 5 (*continued*)

System	Observation	Reference
Mouse	Insertion of cDNA for yolk sac mRNA into plasmid pBR322; screened for cDNA to mRNA AFP and cDNA AFP isolated.	Law et al. *Gene* 10:53, 1980
Mouse	Isolation of genomic Eco RI fragments of DNA AFP cloned. Restriction endonuclease mapping and EM indicates 11 noncoding DNA sequences.	Gorin and Tilghman, *Proc. Natl. Acad. Sci.* 77:1351, 1980
Rat	DNA sequence of 3' terminal 540 bases reveals COOH-terminal homology to albumin (40%).	Innis and Miller, *J. Biol. Chem.* 255:8944, 1980
Rat	AFP and ALB mRNA levels in yolk sac and liver cell sap by cDNA and translation; mRNA AFP 25% of yolk sac poly A+RNA, 10-fold less in fetal liver; mRNA AFP remains high in fetal liver until 2 wk after birth then falls; mRNA ALB is rising during this time and is 85% of adult liver by 2 wk of age; mRNA ALB in yolk sac is 400-fold less than in fetal liver.	Liao et al., *J. Biol. Chem.* 255:10036, 1980
Mouse	Nucleotide sequence of mRNA AFP and 3 overlapping cDNA segments used to deduce AA sequence of protein. There is 32% conservation with al-	Gorin et al., *J. Biol. Chem.* 256:1954, 1981

(*continued*)

Table 5 (*continued*)

System	Observation	Reference
	bumin. AFP has 3 structural domains similar to albumin.	
Mouse genomic clones, RE mapping	Genomic DNA for AFP and ALB each contain 15 coding segments and 14 intervening segments. Number of nucleotides in coding segments and sizes and sequences of intervening sequences different. The coding sequences in each gene consist of three repeated domains, each containing 4 coding segments.	Kioussis et al., *J. Biol. Chem.* 256:1960, 1981
Rat	Sequences of cDNA for AFP and ALB determined in plasmid inserts, mRNA's have 50% homology in introns; deduced protein structure has 34% homology. Postulate duplication of a common ancestral gene.	Jagodzinski et al., *Proc. Natl. Acad. Sci* 78:3521, 1981
Mouse	AFP and ALB genes mapped to chromosomes 5. Using a DNA probe containing flanking sequences indicates AFP and ALB genes are in tandem with ALB gene on the 5′ side of the albumin gene. ALB gene is undermethylated in some cells that do not express the gene.	Ingram et al., *Proc. Natl. Acad. Sci.* 78:4694, 1981
Mouse	Somatic cell hybrids containing mouse and	D'Eustachio et al., *Somatic Cell Genetics*

Table 5 (*continued*)

System	Observation	Reference
	hamster chromosomes; hybrids containing mouse chromosome 5 had both AFP and ALB genes; hybrids not containing chromosome 5 had neither.	7:289, 1982
Rat, thioacetamide	mRNA not increased when ALB synthesis increased after thioacetamide. Conclude that translational activity increased.	Chakrabartty et al., *Cancer Res.* 42:421, 1982
Novikoff hepatoma	Lack of mRNA ALB by translation and cDNA hybridization. No deletions, insertions, or rearrangements of gene.	Capetanaki et al., *Molec. Cell. Biol.* 2:258, 1982
Human DNA clone to mRNA AFP	cDNA sequence reveals homology with albumin.	Beattie and Dugaiczyk, *Gene* 20:415, 1982
cDNA to mouse AFP and ALB	Parallel increase of mRNA AFP and mRNA ALB during late gestation, followed by decrease in mRNA AFP after birth. Ratios to total RNA used, not quantitative.	Tilghman and Belayew, *Proc. Natl. Acad. Sci.* 79:5254, 1982
EcoRI maps of ALB gene	Different banding in Sprague-Dawley vs Buffalo rats. F1 has both; hepatomas show same pattern as strain of origin.	Lucotte et al., *Biochem. Genet.* 20:1105, 1982
Rat, DAB carcinogenesis	Increased mRNA AFP in livers of rats exposed to 3' MDAB.	Schwartz et al., *Biochem. Biophys. Res. Cancer* 107:239, 1982

(*continued*)

Table 5 (*continued*)

System	Observation	Reference
ALB, rat hepatoma	5′ End of albumin gene undermethylated in hepatoma cells. This is necessary but not sufficient for expression. Undermethylation does not appear to determine expression during development.	Ott et al., *Cell* 30:825, 1982
Rat liver and tumors cDNA	Essentially all cellular mRNA ALB and mRNA AFP is in polysomal RNA. Essentially no detectable mRNA sequences in nuclei or post-polysomal structure.	Nahon et al., *Nucleic Acid Res.* 10:1895, 1982
Rat cDNA	Nick translated plasmid derived cDNA probe; mRNA AFP found in low levels in fetal kidney, intestine, lung, and heart (few hundred copies per cell), but not in fetal brain, not in adult tissues (<10 copies per cell).	Boulter et al., 13th Int. Cancer Cong., Seattle, Sept. 1982
Rat cDNA	Increased mRNA AFP occurs 24 h after peak of DNA synthesis in regenerating liver. Increased mRNA AFP in livers of rats exposed to ethionine.	Petropoulos et al., *J. Biol. Chem.* 258:4901, 1983
Mouse AFP "Minigene"	AFP-SV40-pBR322 recombinant DNA in Hela cells. TATA located 30 BP upstream from cap site needed for direction of AFP transcription. No upstream promotor	Scott and Tilghman, *Molec. Cell. Biol.* 3:1285, 1983

(*continued*)

Table 5 (*continued*)

System	Observation	Reference
	needed but may be needed in vivo.	
Rat fetal liver AFP, albumin	Methylation patterns of AFP and albumin genes in fetal and adult liver by Hpa II and Msp. I. Albumin gene transcribed whether methylated or not. AFP gene heavily methylated in fetal liver and develops unmethylated regions at 3' end of the gene in the adult.	Kunnath and Locker, *Embo J*. 2:317, 1983
Rat hepatomas, carcinogenesis, fetal	Arrangement and methylation patterns of AFP and ALB genes not different in producing and non-producing tissues. AFP and ALB genes in carcinogen-exposed livers are methylated normally.	Boulter et al., AACR Meeting, May, 1983 San Diego
Human cDNA, cloned	Nucleotide sequence of genomic DNA and cDNA determined, there is 66% homology with mouse AFP; 39% homology with human AFP.	Morinaga et al., *Proc. Natl. Acad. Sci.* 80:4604, 1983
Rat, high resolution blot hybridization, plasmid probes	Low amounts of mRNA AFP in adult rat liver are mature moleucles.	Gal et al., *Anal. Biochem*. 132:190, 1983
Rat teratocarcinoma, dot hybridization	No mRNA AFP in undifferentiated embryonal CA cells; mRNA AFP appears during differentiation. Some differentiated F9 cultures contain	Buc-Caron et al., *CSHC on Cell Proliferation* 10:411, 1983

(*continued*)

Table 5 (continued)

System	Observation	Reference
	mRNA, but do not produce measurable protein.	
Rat liver	Methylation patterns of AFP in fetal and adult hepatocytes analyzed by HpaII and MspI isoschizomers not associated with changes in gene activity.	Vedel et al., Nucl. Acids Res. 11:4335; 1983
Rat and mouse fetal liver and yolk sac, rat and mouse cDNA probes	High levels of albumin mRNA in mouse but not in rat yolk sac.	Sellem et al., Develop. Biol., in press, 1984
Inbred strains of rat, AFP cDNA probes	Different Eco RI and Hind III restriction pattern for the AFP gene in Sprague-Dawley and Buffalo rats. Existence of two structural variants of the AFP gene in different inbred strains of rat demonstrated.	Gal et al., Molec. General Genet. in press, 1984

for gene duplication or rearrangement in producing cells as compared to nonproducing cells (Sala-Trepat et al., 1979b).

3.2. AFP and Albumin Gene Structure

The albumin gene was found by Sargent et al. (1979, 1981) to contain 15 coding segments and 14 introns. In a series of publications from Tilghman's laboratory (Gorin and Tilghman, 1980; Gorin et al., 1981; Kioussis et al., 1981), it was found that the AFP and albumin genes each contained 15 coding segments and 14 introns. Both genes were mapped to chromosome 5 in the mouse, where the genes were discovered to be in tandem with the AFP gene on the 5' side of the albumin gene (Ingram et al., 1981; D'Eustachio et al., 1981). The restriction endonuclease banding of DNA from transplantable hepatocellular carcinoma revealed that albumin and AFP genes are the same as the normal liver of the strain of rat in which the tumor originated. All tumors from a given strain of rat reveal the same banding pattern (Sell et al., 1980; Lucotte et al., 1982; Gal et al., 1984), but there are two different banding patterns for the albumin gene and also for the AFP gene in different strains of rat (Lucotte et al., 1982; Gal et al., 1984). Although several groups have reported some nucleotide sequence homology between the AFP and albumin genes (Innis and Miller, 1980; Gorin et al., 1981; Beattie and Dugaiczyk, 1982), there is no cross hybridization between the cDNAs for AFP and albumin and their respective isolated mRNAs (Sala-Trepat et al., 1979a).

3.3. AFP and Albumin Gene Expression and Methylation

The possible relationship between degree of methylation of the AFP and albumin gene and expression of the gene is not clear. Ingram et al. (1981) reported that the ALB gene is undermethylated in some cells that do not express the gene. The 5′ end of the albumin gene was found to be undermethylated in some hepatoma cells, but this was not sufficient for expression of the gene (Ott et al., 1982). Undermethylation does not appear to control expression of the albumin gene during development (Ott et al., 1982). We have found that the arrangement and methylation patterns of the AFP and albumin genes are not different in producing and nonproducing tissues and that AFP and albumin genes are methylated normally in livers of carcinogen-exposed rats (Boulter et al., 1983). The mRNA for AFP is increased in the livers of rats exposed to chemical hepatocarcinogens (Schwartz et al., 1982; Petropoulos et al., 1983). Scott and Tilghman (1983) found that a TATA box located 30 base pairs upstream for the AFP gene cap site is required for direction of transcription in Hela cells. In contrast, most other genes tested in Hela cells need TATA and approximately 100 bps upstream for efficient transcription. The methylation patterns of the AFP gene in fetal and adult hepatocytes, analyzed by HpaII and MspI isoschizomers, are not changed with changes in gene activity (Vedel et al., 1983).

4. Summary

Monoclonal antibodies to human alphafetoprotein have led to identification of at least four epitopes on the AFP molecule and have been applied to developing rapid ELISA assays using a one-step sandwich technique. Conventional anti-AFP has been shown to be effective in localization of tumors in vivo using radioimmunescintigraphy, and it induces some regression of growth of AFP-producing tumors in experimental systems. Daunomycin-conjugated monoclonal antibodies to AFP are as effective as conventional antibody in a rat system, but the results of clinical trials using Mab for therapy in humans have not yet been published.

Control of AFP gene expression is at the level of transcription, but the mechanism of control of transcription remains undefined. The state of methylation of the AFP gene does not appear to correlate directly with expression of the gene. AFP and albumin genes are located in tandem on chromosome 5 of the mouse and are structurally similar. Coordinate expression of AFP and albumin may occur in the mouse, whereas levels of AFP mRNA rise earlier in the fetal rat liver than do the levels of albumin mRNA. Albumin mRNA remains high in adult liver (>40,000 copies/cell), whereas that of AFP falls to less than 10 copies/cell within a few weeks after birth.

Note Added in Proof

Bellet et al. (*Proc. Natl. Acad. Sci.* **81**, 3869, 1984) have described a one-hour "simultaneous sandwich" radioimmunoassay for human AFP using monoclonal antibodies that is similar to the assays described in this review. They claim that their assay is "more sensitive and more specific" than assays using conventional antisera. However, no direct comparison of standard curves of their assay and a conventional assay is shown and the direct comparison of both assays on 17 selected cancer patients reveals no significant difference.

References

Abelev, G. I. (1971), *Adv. Cancer Res.* **14**, 1295.

Abelev, G. I. (1975), *Trans. Rev.* **20**, 3.

Abelev, G. I., S. D. Perova, N. I. Khramokova, Z. A. Prostnikova, and I. S. Irin (1963), *Transplant* **1**, 1974.

Adinolfi, A., M. Adinolfi, and M. H. Lessof (1975), *J. Med. Genet.* **12**, 138.

Allen, R. P. and B. E. Ledford (1977), *Cancer Res.* **37**, 696.

Beattie, W. G. and A. Dugaiczyk (1982), *Gene* **20**, 415.

Belanger, L., P. Commer, and J.-F. Chiu (1979), *Cancer Res.* **39**, 2141.

Boulter, J. and S. Sell (1982), 13th Int. Cancer Cong., Seattle, Washington.

Boulter, J., K. Evans, M. A. Longley, and S. Sell, AACR annual meeting, San Diego, CA, (1983).

Brock, D. J. H., L. Barron, and V. Van Heyningen (1982), *Clin. Chim. Acta* in Elsevier Biomedical Press **122**, 353.

Buc-Caron, M. H., M. Darmon, M. Poiret, C. Sellem, J. M. Sala-Trepat, and T. Erdos (1983), in *Cold Spring Harbor Conferences on Cell Proliferation*, vol. 10, p. 411.

Capetanaki, Y. G., C. N. Flytzanis, and A. Alonso (1982), *Molec. Cell. Biol.* **2**, 258.

Cassio, D., M. C. Weiss, M.-O. Ott, J. M. Sala-Trepat, J. Fris, and T. Erdos (1981), *Cell* **27**, 351.

Chakrabartty, P. K., S. K. Chattopadhyay, and W. C. Schneider (1982), *Cancer Res.* **42**, 421.

D'Eustachio, P., R. S. Ingram, S. M. Tilghman, and F. H. Ruddle (1981), *Somatic Cell Genetics* **7**, 289.

Engvall, E., H. Pihko, H. Jalanko, and E. Ruoslahti (1977), *J. Natl Cancer Inst.* **59**, 277.

Faber, A. J., S. H. Miall, and T. Tamaoki (1973), *Can. J. Biochem.* **52**, 429.

Gal, A., J.-L. Nahon, and J. M. Sala-Trepat (1983), *Anal. Biochem.* **132**, 1.

Gal, A., J.-L. Nahon, G. Lucotte, and J. M. Sala-Trepat (1984), *Molec. General Genet.*, in press.

Gorin, M. B., D. L. Cooper, F. Eiferman, P. van de Rijn, and S. M. Tilghman (1981), *J. Biol. Chem.* **256**, 1954.

Gorin, M. B. and S. M. Tilghman (1980), *Proc. Natl. Acad. Sci.* **77**, 1351.

Gousev, A. and A. Yazova (1974), in *Colloques L'Inserm L'alpha-Fetoprotein* (R. Masseyeff, ed.), Paris, France, p. 255.

Halpern, S. E., P. L. Hagan, P. R. Garver, J. A. Koziol, A. W. N. Chen, J. M. Frincke, R. M. Bartholomew, G. S. David, and T. H. Adams (1983), *Cancer Res.* **43**, 5347.

Hirai, H. (1981), in *Report of the Research Group Working with Alpha-Fetoprotein Antiserum*, The Foundation for Basic Research in Oncology, Tokyo, Japan, p. 1.

Hunter, W. M., J. G. Bennie, D. J. H. Brock, and V. Van Heyningen (1982), *J. Immunol. Methods,* Elsevier Biomedical Press **50**, 133.

Ingram, R. S., R. W. Scott, and S. M. Tilghman (1981), *Proc. Natl. Acad. Sci.* **78**, 4694.

Innis, M. A., M. M. Harpold, and D. L. Miller (1979), *Arch. Biochem. Biophy.* **195**, 128.

Innis, M. A. and D. L. Miller (1977), *J. Biol. Chem.* **252**, 8469.

Innis, M. A. and D. L. Miller (1979), *J. Biol. Chem.* **254**, 9148.

Innis, M. A. and D. L. Miller (1980), *J. Biol. Chem.* **255**, 8994.

Jagodzinski, L. L., T. D. Sargent, M. Yang, C. Glackin, and J. Bonner, (1981), *Proc. Natl. Acad. Sci.* **78**, 3521.

Javadpour, N., E. E. Kim, F. H. DeLand, J. R. Salyer, U. Shah, and D. M. Goldenberg (1981), *J. Amer. Med. Assn.* **246**, 45.

Kanai, K., Y. Endo, T. Oda, and N. Tanaka (1974), *Cancer Res.* **34**, 1813.

Kim, E. E., S. DeLand, R. L. Casper, R. L. Corgan, F. J. Primus, and D. Goldenberg (1980a), *Cancer* **45**, 1243.

Kim, E. E., F. H. DeLand, M. O. Nelson, S. Bennett, G. Simmons, E. Alpert, and D. M. Goldenberg (1980b), *Cancer Res.* **40**, 3008.

Kioussis, D., F. Eiferman, P. van de Rijn, M. B. Gorin, R. S. Ingram, and S. M. Tilghman (1981), *J. Biol. Chem.* **256**, 1960.

Koga, K., D. W. O'Keefe, T. Iio, and T. Tamaoki (1974), *Nature* **252**, 459.

Kohler, G., and C. Milstein (1975), *Nature* **256**, 459.

Koji, T., N. Ishii, T. Munehisa, Y. Kusumoto, S. Nakamura, A. Tamenishi, A. Hara, K. Kobayashi, Y. Tsukada, S. Nishi, and H. Hirai (1980), *Cancer Res.* **40**, 3013.

Kunnath, L., and J. Locker (1983), *Embo J.* **2**, 317.

Kuwahara, T., J. Uchino, K. Manabe, Y. Une, Y. Hata, A. Kakita, Y. Kasal, Y. Tsukada, and H. Hirai (1978), *Igakunoayui* **107**, 96.

Law, S., T. Tamoaki, F. Kreuzaler, and A. Dugaiczyk (1980), *Gene,* Elsevier/North-Holland Biomedical Press **10**, 53.

Leffert, H., T. Moran, S. Sell, H. Skelly, K. Ibsen, M. Mueller, and I. Arias (1978), *Proc. Natl. Acad. Sci.* **75**, 1834.

Liao, W. S. L., A. R. Conn, and J. M. Taylor (1980), *J. Biol. Chem.* **255,** 10036.

Lucotte, G., A. Gal, J.-L. Nahon, and J. M. Sala-Trepat (1982), *Biochem. Genetics* **20,** 1105.

Micheel, B., H. Fiebach, U. Karsten, A. I. Goussev, A. K. Jazova, and J. Kopp (1983), *Eur. J. Cancer & Clin. Oncol.* **19,** 1239.

Miura, K., S. W. T. Law, S. Nishi, and T. Tamaoki (1979), *J. Biol. Chem.* **254,** 5515.

Mizejewski, G. J. and R. P. Allen (1974), *Nature* **250,** 50.

Mizejewski, G. J. and R. P. Allen (1978), *Clin. Immunology Immunopath.* **11,** 307.

Mizejewski, G. J. and W. R. Dillon (1979), *Arch. Immunol. Therap. Exp.* **27,** 655.

Mizejewski, G. J., S. R. Young, and R. P. Allen (1975), *J. Natl. Cancer Inst.* **54,** 1361.

Morinaga, T., M. Sakai, T. G. Wegmann, and T. Tamaoki (1982), *Oncodevel. Biology Med.* **3,** 301.

Nahon, J. L., A. Gal, M. Frain, S. Sell, and J. M. Sala-Trepat (1982), *Nucleic Acds. Res.* **10,** 1895.

Nishi, S., H. Yamazaki, H. Hirai, N. Ishii, T. Koji, and S. Nagatakl (1983), in *Nuclear Medicine and Biology Advances* (C. Raynaud, ed.), Pergamon Press, Oxford, p. 2304.

Nomura, M., M. Imai, K. Takahashi, T. Kumakura, K. Tachibana, S. Aoyagi, S. Usuda, T. Nakamura, Y. Miyakawa, and M. Mayumi (1983a), *J. Immunol. Methods* **58,** 293.

Nomura, M., M. Imai, S. Usuda, T. Nakamura, Y. Miyakawa, and M. Mayumi (1983b), *J. Immunol. Methods,* Elsevier Biomedical Press **56,** 13.

Ott, M.-O., L. Sperling, D. Cassio, J. Levilliers, J. Sala-Trepat, and M. C. Weiss (1982), *Cell,* **30,** 825.

Parks, L. C., A. N. Baer, M. Pollack, and G. M. Williams (1974), *Ann. Surg.* **180,** 599.

Peters, E. H., S. Nishi, K. Miura, F. L. Lorscheider, G. H. Dixon, and T. Tamaoki (1979), *Cancer Res.* **39,** 3702.

Petropoulos, C., G. Andrews, T. Tamaoki, and N. Fausto (1983), *J. Biol. Chem.* **258,** 4901.

Primus, F. J., S. J. Bennett, E. E. Kim, F. H. DeLand, M. C. Zahn, and D. Goldenberg (1980), *Cancer Res.* **40,** 497.

Ruoslahti, E., and E. Engvall (1982), *Clinical Immun. Newsletter* **3,** 139.

Ruoslahti, E., H. Pihko, and M. Seppala (1974), *Transplant Rev.* **20,** 38.

Sala-Trepat, J. M., J. Dever, T. D. Sargent, K. Thomas, S. Sell, and J. Bonner (1979a), *Biochem.* **18,** 2167.

Sala-Trepat, J. M., T. D. Sargent, S. Sell, and J. Bonner (1979b), *Proc. Natl. Acad. Sci.* **76,** 695.

Sargent, T. D., L. L. Jagodzinski, M. Yang, and J. Bonner (1981), *Mol. Cell. Biol.* **98,** 503.

Sargent, T. D., L. L. Jagodzinski, M. Yang, and J. Bonner (1978), *Proc. Natl. Acad. Sci. USA* **76,** 3256.

Schwartz, C. E., T. Gabryelak, C. J. Smith, J. M. Taylor, and J.-F. Chiu (1982), *Biochem. Biophy. Res. Commun.* **107**, 239.

Scott, R. W. and S. M. Tilghman (1983), *Molec. Cellular Biol.* **3**, 1295.

Sell, S. (1981), *Human Pathology* **12**, 959.

Sell, S. (1980), in *Cancer Markers: Developmental and Diagnostic Significance* (Sell, S., ed.), Humana Press, New Jersey, p. 249.

Sell, S. (1982), in *Human Cancer Markers* (Sell, S. and Wahren, B., eds.), Humana Press, New Jersey, p. 133.

Sell, S., F. Becker, H. Leffert, K. Osborn, J. Salman, B. Lombardi, H. Shinozuka, J. Reddy, E. Ruoslahti, and J. Sala-Trepat, (1983), in *Application of Biological Markers to Carcinogen Testing* (Millman, H. and Sell, S., eds.), Plenum Press, New York, p. 271.

Sell, S., and F. F. Becker (1978), *J. Natl Cancer Inst.* **60**, 19.

Sell, S., F. F. Becker, H. L. Leffert, and H. Watabe (1976a), *Cancer Res.* **36**, 4239.

Sell, S., J. M. Sala-Trepat, T. D. Sargent, K. Thomas, J.-L. Nahon, T. A. Goodman, and J. Bonner (1980), *Cell Biol. Inter. Rep.* **4**, 235.

Sell, S., H. W. Sheppard, Jr., R. Nickel, D. Stillman, and M. Michaelsen (1976b), *Cancer Res.* **36**, 476.

Sell, S., and H. Skelly (1975), *Annals NY Acad. of Sci.* **259**, 45.

Sell, S., K. Thomas, M. Michaelson, J. Scott, and J. Sala-Trepat (1979), *Carcino-Embryonic Proteins*, Elsevier/North-Holland Biomedical Press, **1**, 11.

Sellem, C., M. Frain, T. Erdos, and J. M. Sala-Trepat (1984), *Develop. Biol.*, in press.

Tilghman, S. M. and A. Belayew (1982), *Proc. Natl. Acad. Sci., Biochemistry* **79**, 5254.

Tilghman, S. M., D. Kioussis, M. B. Gorin, J. P. G. Ruiz, and R. S. Ingram (1979), *J. Biol. Chem.* **254**, 7393.

Tse, T. P. H., H. P. Morris, and J. M. Taylor (1978), *Biochemistry* **18**, 3121.

Tsukada, Y., W. K.-D. Bischof, N. Hibi, H. Hirai, E. Hurwitz, and M. Sela (1982a), *Proc. Natl. Acad. Sci.,* **79**, 621.

Tsukada, Y., E. Hurwitz, R. Kashi, M. Sela, N. Hibi, A. Hara, and H. Hirai (1982b), *Proc. Natl. Acad. Sci.* **79**, 7896.

Tsukada, Y., M. Mikuni, H. Watabe, S. Nishi, and H. Hirai (1974), *Int. J. Cancer* **13**, 187.

Uotila, M., E. Engvall, and E. Ruoslahti (1980a), *Molec. Immunol.* **17**, 791.

Uotila, M., E. Ruoslahti, and E. Engvall (1981), *J. Immunol. Methods,* Elsevier/North-Holland Biomedical Press **42**, 11.

Van Heyningen, V., L. Barron, D. J. H. Brock, D. Crichton, and S. Lawrie (1982), *J. Immunol. Methods,* Elsevier Biomedical Press **50**, 123.

Vedel, M., M. Gomez-Garcia, M. Sala, and J. M. Sala-Trepat (1983), *Nucleic Acids Res.* **11**, 4336.

Wepsic, H. T., Y. Tsukada, N. Takeichi, S. Nishi, and H. Hirai (1980), *Int. J. Cancer* **25**, 655.

Yamazaki, H., S. Nishi, and H. Hirai (1983), *Hokkaido Univ. Med. Library Series* **15**, 163.

Chapter 4

Human Chorionic Gonadotropin Detection with Monoclonal Antibodies

PAUL H. EHRLICH,[1] ZEINAB A. MOUSTAFA,[1]
ALEXANDER KRICHEVSKY,[1] AND RICARDO MESA-TEJADA[2]

*Departments of Medicine[1] and Pathology[2], and the Institute of
Cancer Research[2], College of Physicians and Surgeons of Columbia
University, New York, New York*

1. Introduction: hCG Chemistry and Immunochemistry with Antisera

Hormone production in cancer can result from the presence of transformed endocrine cells that continue to secrete or, as in the case of human chorionic gonadotropin, the hormone can also be considered an onco-developmental gene product and thus may be produced by many different types of tumors. The use of hormones as cancer markers has been previously reviewed (Sell and Wahren, 1982). This article will concentrate on hormone detection using monoclonal antibodies, particularly those aspects of monoclonal antibodies against human chorionic gonadotropin that differ from antisera.

Many of the potential advantages of monoclonal antibodies for clinical use are well known—availability of an unlimited supply of easily purified antibodies of uniform quality; the ability to utilize impure antigens (including cell surface proteins); and the potential for unusual specificity. In the cases of human chorionic gonadotropin and many other hormones, the molecules have been purified and antisera have been raised in large quantities. Therefore, since one of the major advantages of monoclonal antibodies (the use of impure antigen) is irrelevant, the use of monoclonal antibodies against these hormones will depend on learning if (1) monoclonal antibodies can adequately replace antisera so that the advantages of chemical standardization and supply dictate the use of the monoclonal antibodies; (2) the ability of monoclonal antibodies to probe individual antigenic sites results in unique specificities that are useful; and (3) the ability to mix monoclonal antibodies of predetermined characteristics and in optimized ratios, i.e., the production of artificial antisera, can result in superior characteristics to those of the antibody mixtures present in antisera. We will show that for several areas in the detection of hormone cancer markers, monoclonal antibodies are the reagents of choice.

Human chorionic gonadotropin is a glycoprotein hormone with a mol wt of 36,700 (Birken and Canfield, 1980). It is composed of two subunits: α with a mol wt of 14,500 and β with a mol wt of 22,200. Carbohydrate comprises 29–31% by weight of the hormone, 26–32% of the α subunit, and 28–36% of the β subunit (Birken and Canfield, 1980). The α subunit is identical with the subunit of the other glycoprotein hormones including luteinizing hormone, thyroid stimulating hormone, and follicle stimulating hormone. The β subunit confers biological specificity with respect to receptor binding. However, even this subunit retains substantial homology among the different hormones, with an 80% homology between the β subunits of hLH and hCG (the two hormones bind to the same receptor). The β subunit of hCG also has a unique 30-amino-acid addition to its COOH-terminus that is not found in any of the other hormones (Birken and Canfield, 1980). Sequencing of the hCGβ gene has led to the hypothesis that this addition is the result of a mutation of a stop codon in an ancestral gene that allowed transcription of additional DNA (Fiddes and Goodman, 1980).

Animals immunized with the complete hCG hormone produce antisera that are highly cross-reactive with hLH in part because of the anti-α subunit antibodies (Vaitukaitis et al., 1972). Even antisera raised against the β subunit are frequently cross-reactive, although occasionally there are somewhat specific antisera raised in this way (Vaitukaitis et al., 1972; Birken et al., 1982). The COOH-terminal peptide of the β subunit, when conjugated to a large protein, is an ideal immunogen for raising specific antisera since this amino acid sequence has no analogue on the other glycoprotein hormones. Indeed antisera raised against the peptide obtained by protease cleavage of the hormone (Chen et al., 1976) or synthetic peptide (Matsuura et al., 1979) have essentially no cross-reactivity with hLH. The affinity of most of these antisera is high (10^9–10^{11} L/M) with the anti-COOH-terminal β antisera usually being in the low end of this range.

2. Description of Monoclonal Antibodies to hCG

Several groups have reported extensively on the production of monoclonal antibodies to hCG (Moyle et al., 1982; Ehrlich et al., 1984; Stahli et al., 1983; Bosch et al., 1981; Kofler et al., 1982). In addition, there are many reports characterizing what are probably the authors' most interesting clones (Khazaeli et al., 1981). We will describe the numerous monoclonal antibodies produced with an emphasis on the stereochemical relationship of their epitopes and the determination of the similarity of the antibodies produced by different investigators.

2.1. Affinity, Isotype, Subclass, and Cross-Reactivity of Antibodies

We have produced many clones that secrete antibodies to hCG (Ehrlich et al., 1984) both with complete hormone and subunits as immunogen. Immunization with the complete hormone seems to result in many more antibody-producing colonies. A summary of some of the characteristics of the antibodies produced by the clones is shown in Table 1. There is a very wide range of affinity for hCG, from 10^7 to 10^{11} M^{-1}. This is probably biased since lower affinity antibodies (10^5 to 10^7 M^{-1}) would not be detected in the liquid phase double antibody radioimmunoassay employed in these studies. In fact, colonies that are positive in a solid phase immunoradiometric assay that is capable of detecting low affinity antibodies are often negative in the liquid phase assay. Thus, we and others (Ehrlich et al., 1984) have been able to detect very low affinity antibodies. The range of cross-reactivities is also great—from antibodies that react almost exclusively with the intact hCG, to antibodies that are completely cross-reactive with the respective hCG subunit and other glycoprotein hormones. All of the monoclonal antibodies against hCG that have been described are IgG. However, this may have arisen solely by the methods used to detect anti-hCG-producing colonies. Most of the antibodies are of the IgG_1 subclass but several IgG_{2b} antibodies have been isolated.

2.2. Topological Mapping of Monoclonal Antibodies: Relative Orientation of Epitopes

Figure 1 shows the relative orientation of the epitopes of the monoclonal antibodies described in Table 1. This is a modification of a figure shown in Moyle et al. (1982). There appear to be four major regions of binding of anti-hCGβ subunit antibodies and probably four major regions for anti-hCGα antibodies. Within these regions the antibodies can vary greatly in

Table 1
Characteristics of Several Monoclonal Anti-hCG Antibodies

Antibody	K_{hCG}, M^{-1}	Cross-reactivity in % relative to hCG[a], for			Antibody can bind simultaneously with antibodies
		hCG Subunit	hLH	hTSH	
B101	7×10^8	9	2	<0.1	B102, B103, B105, A109
B102	3×10^7	200	11	[c]	B101, B105, B106, B107, A102, A103, A109
B103	2×10^8	50	90	12	B101, B106, B107, A102, A103, A109
B105	1.5×10^{11}	100	100	7	B101, B102, B106, B107, A102, A103, A109
B106	2×10^{10}	0.1	1.6	<0.1	B102, B103, B105
B107	4×10^{10}	0.1	<0.5	<0.1	B102, B103, B105
A102	2×10^8	25	[c]	100[b]	B102, B103, B105, A103
A103	2×10^8	150	[c]	[c]	B102, B103, B105, A102, A109
A109	3×10^7	1200	[c]	[c]	B101, B102, B103, B105, A103

[a]The cross-reactivities were determined using the double antibody radioimmunoassays with ^{125}I-hCG by comparing the amount of hCG needed to inhibit 50% of the binding of the antibody to radiolabeled hCG with the amount of the other molecule needed to inhibit 50%. In the cases where cross-reactivity is less than 1%, the inhibition of antibody binding used for this determination was less than 50%.

[b]Cross-reactivities of anti-hCGα have not generally been tested since the α subunit is identical in hCG, hLH, and hTSH. In the one case in which these assays have been performed, A102, the cross-reactivity was indeed 100%. However, clones could theoretically exist that differentiate between the α subunit bound to different β subunits. Strickland and Puett (1980) have reported that the β subunit from hCG, oLH, and pLH induces different conformations when recombined with oLH α subunit.

[c]Not tested.

both affinity and cross-reactivity. We define a major region of the molecule by the epitopes of those monoclonal antibodies that cannot bind simultaneously to the hormone and have a generally similar spectrum of simultaneous binding with other monoclonal antibodies. The fact that the cross-reactivities of antibodies in the same region differ and the spectra of simultaneous binding with other antibodies are not identical indicates that each region is made up of subregions. The anti-α antibodies, each represented by a single antibody (most investigators have not characterized their anti-hCGα antibodies), are distinguished by their ability to bind simultaneously with other monoclonal antibodies (relative orientation of epitopes) and their cross-reactivity with intact hormone and α subunit. Thus, A102 binds α subunit less strongly than intact hormone and cannot bind simultaneously to hCG with many anti-hCGβ monoclonal antibodies (B101, B106, B107), whereas A109 binds α subunit much better than intact hormone and can bind simultaneously to hCG with many anti-hCGβ antibodies. A103 has intermediate properties. Another interesting hCGα epitope has been described by Kofler et al. (1982). They have detected several monoclonal antibodies against hCGα that appear to bind hFSH and hTSH better than hCG and hLH. Stuart et al. (1983) described

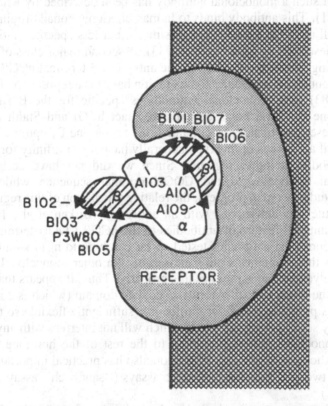

Fig. 1. Relative orientation of the epitopes of some monoclonal antibodies against human chorionic gonadotropin and the rat Leydig cell receptor. Triangles (which are symbols for the epitopes) that are close together, such as those for B102 and B103, indicate that the two antibodies cannot bind simultaneously to hCG. Triangles that are far apart, such as those for B101 and B102, indicate that the two antibodies can bind simultaneously to hCG. Antibodies that cannot bind simultaneously to hCG but have a different spectrum of simultaneous binding with other monoclonal antibodies, such as A102 and B101, are symbolized by an intermediate distance between the triangles representing their epitopes.

a monoclonal antibody that binds the α subunit of hCG but not the intact hormone. Miggiano et al. (1980) have reported on an anti-hCGα antibody that does not bind ^{125}I-hCG. These antibodies may represent a class for which we have no representative since we screen for antibody-producing colonies with radiolabeled hCG. However, it should be noted that A103 has low but significant reactivity with ^{125}I-hCG and therefore could be similar to the antibody described by Miggiano et al. (1980).

The epitopes of the anti-hCGβ antibodies can be compared with monoclonal antibodies from several different laboratories. One major class of antibodies that is not represented in Fig. 1 is antibodies that can bind only to the individual subunits but not to the intact hormone. One example of such a monoclonal antibody has been described by Khazaeli et al. (1981). This antibody binds to human chorionic gonadotropin only ¼₀₀ as well as the hCGβ subunit. A similar, but less specific, antibody has been described by Stuart et al. (1983). A second major class of antibody binding sites is represented by the anti-COOH-terminal hCGβ antibodies. Monoclonal antibodies to this region have been reported by Bellet et al. (1983) (one monoclonal antibody is specific for the β subunit whereas one can bind both subunit and intact hCG) and Stahli et al. (1983) (these investigators have named this region the $β_1$ epitope; their monoclonal antibodies of this type generally have lower affinity for hCG than antibodies to other regions). Since we did not have access to monoclonal antibodies to the COOH-terminal sequence while our mapping studies were in progress, the relative orientation of this region of the molecule was determined with an antiserum (Birken et al., 1982). One very unusual feature of antibodies to the hCGβ COOH-terminus is that all monoclonal antibodies tested so far can bind to hCG simultaneously with the antibodies in this antiserum. No other monoclonal antibody or polyclonal antiserum has this property. Thus, it appears that this region of the molecule either forms a separate domain (which is consistent with its probable genetic origin) or it is sufficiently flexible so that it can occupy several positions one of which will not interfere with any particular monoclonal antibody binding to the rest of the hormone. This characteristic of antibodies to this region also has practical importance in designing two-site immunoradiometric assays ("sandwich" assays) (see Section 3.).

A third major region includes the epitopes of antibodies B101, B106, and B107. These antibodies block the interaction of the hormone with its receptor and interfere with the binding of many anti-hCGα monoclonal antibodies to intact hormone. A distinctive characteristic of these antibodies is their low cross-reactivity with the hCGβ subunit—B101 binds this subunit only about 9% as well as hCG, whereas B106 and B107 have such low cross-reactivity that they may not bind the individual subunit at all. Useful properties of these antibodies are their

weak interaction with human luteinizing hormone (hLH) and their generally high affinity for hCG. The characteristics of these antibodies seem to
coincide with some monoclonal antibodies raised by other investigators.
Bosch et al. (1981) reported on monoclonal antibodies that had low cross-
reactivity with hLH and bound only the intact hormone; these antibodies
were named $\alpha\beta$. Similar antibodies were described by Kofler et al.
(1982). Stahli et al. (1983) also isolated antibodies that did not bind individual subunits (and named their epitope "h"). However, these antibodies also bound to hLH, although somewhat less well than hCG.

The fourth major region of monoclonal antibody binding to hCG
comprises the B102-B103-B105 epitopes. These antibodies are characterized by their binding both hCG and hCGβ subunit with approximately the
same affinity. However, they vary in their cross-reactivity with hLH,
from totally cross-reactive to about 11%. The P_3W_{80} hybridoma antibody
(courtesy of Wampole Laboratories; described in Gupta and Talwar,
1980, and Gupta et al., 1982) binds to this region also and has a cross-
reactivity for hLH of less than 1%. Miggiano et al. (1980) have reported
five different classes of monoclonal anti-hCG antibodies that bind to the
β subunit with varying cross-reactivities to hLH. Presumably, these antibodies bind in the same region as B102-B103-B105. However, one of
these classes of antibody will not bind to ^{125}I-hCG which may indicate
that its epitope is not in the same region. Bosch et al. (1981) have described two monoclonal antibodies against hCG that bind hCGβ and have
some specificity for hCG over hLH. These antibodies could also bind in
this fourth region of antibody binding. Kofler et al. (1982) and Miggiano
et al. (1980) have also described antibodies that can bind both hCG and
hCGβ. These have been named B-MCA and group numbers D, E, and F,
respectively.

2.3. Biological Effects of Monoclonal Antibodies Against hCG

Human chorionic gonadotropin binds to the same receptor as hLH and
will stimulate the production of steroids, and, at high concentrations,
cAMP. When hCG is bound to the rat Leydig cell receptor, it induces
testosterone synthesis. The ability of monoclonal antibodies to affect this
response was determined (Moyle et al., 1982). Seven monoclonal antibodies were tested (five reported in Moyle et al. (1982) and two subsequently in unpublished observations) with very different results. Three
antibodies (B101, B107, and A102) greatly inhibited the production of
testosterone stimulated by hCG incubation with the cells. It was concluded that the epitopes of these antibodies are at or near the receptor
binding site of the hormone. Since antibodies to both subunits can inhibit
binding it appears that both hCG subunits may participate in receptor

binding. It was also shown that an antibody (B101) that inhibited the formation of the hormone–receptor complex could not inhibit testosterone production or promote hCG–receptor dissociation once the complex was formed, indicating that it did not alter the stability of the hCG–receptor complex. Four anti-hCG monoclonal antibodies (B102, B103, B105, and A103) do not inhibit binding of hCG to receptor. Radiolabeled B102, B103, and B105 can bind to the receptor–hormone complex indicating that part of the β subunit remains exposed. However, radiolabeled A103 cannot bind to the hCG–receptor complex, which is unexpected considering its inability to inhibit testosterone production. It is possible that the region on hCG that is bound by antibody A103 undergoes a conformational change when the hormone is bound to receptor or the orientation of the hormone in the receptor complex changes.

Monoclonal antibody P_3W_{80} has also been tested for its effect on the biological activity of hCG (Gupta et al., 1982). The production of testosterone by mouse Leydig cells induced by hCG was greatly inhibited by P_3W_{80} ascites fluid (an 800,000 dilution neutralized one-half of the hCG activity). The antibody was also inhibitory in an in vivo assay. The increase in wet weight of the mouse uterus induced by hCG was completely inhibited by dilutions of the P_3W_{80} ascites fluid up to a dilution of 1:1000. As expected from the above experiments, preliminary studies indicate that P_3W_{80} antibody could induce spontaneous abortions in mice. Thus, this antibody has been shown to inhibit the biological activity of hCG by three methods.

The map shown in Fig. 1 can be used to predict which antibodies can bind to hCG in the hCG–receptor complex. However, this should be approached with caution since antibody P_3W_{80}, the epitope of which is very near that of B102, B103, and B105, inhibits the hCG-receptor interaction. In general, it appears that antibodies that can bind both the intact hormone and the β subunit are more likely to be able to bind to the hormone–receptor complex. It is not known if any anti-α subunit antibodies can bind to hCG simultaneously with the receptor since only two monoclonal antibodies have been tried.

There has been a large effort in the last decade to determine if immunization with hCG could be used as a fertility control method (Talwar et al., 1979; Stevens, 1976; Hearn, 1976). It has been generally concluded that passive and active immunization are successful in reducing fertility. However, the mechanism of action is unknown. Monoclonal antibodies such as B101 could probably block the physiological effects of the hormone thus interfering with the support of the corpus luteum that hCG normally provides. Alternatively, antibodies such as B103 could bind to receptor-bound hCG and activate the complement system so that any cells that bind hCG would be destroyed. In addition, either class of antibody might bind to hCG in the trophoblast and activate the complement system, thus killing the fetus directly. Further research must be performed to determine the actual mechanism. The use of monoclonal antibodies in immunodetection and therapy of hCG-secreting tumors could also benefit from a similar approach. The orientation (if there is a preferred orientation) of the hCG near or on the tumor cells that secrete the hormone could determine whether B101-like or B103-like antibodies are optimal (also see Section 4 below).

2.4. Special Properties of Monoclonal Antibodies to hCG: Synergistic Effects

Monoclonal antibodies against hCG have been shown to exhibit synergistic effects in that a monoclonal antibody will be more likely to bind hCG in the presence of certain other monoclonal antibodies (Ehrlich et al. 1982; Ehrlich and Moyle, 1983; Ehrlich et al., 1983a). This has also been found to be true for antibodies to several other molecules (Tosi et al., 1981; Holmes and Parham, 1983). The mechanism of enhancement is the formation of a circular complex consisting of two antigen and two antibody molecules, as shown in Fig. 2A (Moyle et al., 1983a, b). For an antigen that has several copies of a determinant, one monoclonal antibody to this epitope should also be capable of forming a circular complex.

We and others have studied extensively the properties of the mixtures of monoclonal antibodies. As described above, the apparent affinity of the antibodies for hCG rises. For example, under the normal conditions of a double antibody radioimmunoassay for hCG employing monoclonal antibodies B101 and B102, the inhibition curve with nonradiolabeled hCG is about eight times more sensitive than the curve for the higher affinity individual antibody (B101). When one of the antibodies is digested to the monovalent F(ab) fragment this cooperativity is removed. Thus, it is unlikely that conformational effects could cause the synergism since the F(ab) fragment should also be able to induce a similar conformational change. In addition, F(ab')$_2$ fragments are synergistic suggesting that the Fc region of the antibody is not involved in cooperativity. Not all pairs of antibodies that can bind hCG simultaneously can act synergistically in a liquid phase assay (B101 and B103 are not synergistic; however, the synergism is a common characteristic of antibody pairs that can bind simultaneously to hCG). In contrast, when one antibody is bound to a solid phase, all pairs of antibodies that can bind simultaneously to hCG that have been tested are synergistic (Ehrlich et al., 1983a). Mathematical modeling studies have suggested that the conditions under which the solid phase assays are performed enhance the detection of cooperative interactions. Two antibodies bound to a solid phase can also cooperate in binding hCG (Stahli et al., 1981; Ehrlich et al., 1982). The synergistic interaction is not a special property of a certain,

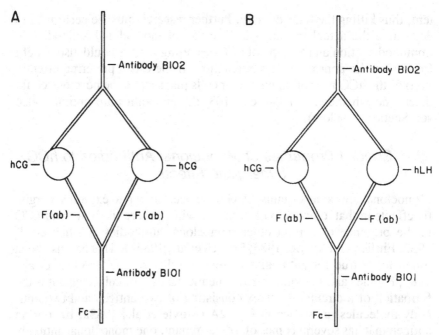

Fig. 2.   A, Circular complex consisting of two different monoclonal antibodies and two antigen (hCG), molecules; B, Circular complex consisting of two
different monoclonal antibodies, one antigen molecule (hCG), and one cross-
reacting molecule (hLH). Complexes such as this may contribute to higher cross-
reactivity of cooperative immunoassays since the low cross-reactivity of the individual antibodies may be overcome by the free energy of formation of the
complex. However, if a structure such as this is unlikely to form because of the
geometry of the cross-reactive molecule, then the specificity of a cooperative
immunoassay could be much improved over what is expected from the individual
antibodies.

subclass of IgG (Ehrlich et al., 1983a), but it is not known whether antibodies of other isotypes are capable of this effect.

There are several lines of evidence linking the synergistic binding of
antigen to a circular complex (Moyle et al., 1983a) besides the dependence on bivalent antibody. A high-molecular-weight complex can be isolated on polyacrylamide gels, gel filtration columns, and HPLC columns
that is only present when the antigen and correct pair of monoclonal antibodies are present. The high molecular weight complex, which has the
molecular weight expected for two antigen and two antibody molecules,
is removed by the presence of excess antigen. This is expected since the
formation of antigen-saturated antibodies will prevent formation of the
circular complex. The ratio of antibody molecules to antigen molecules in
the high molecular weight complex determined by radiolabeling these reagents is also what would be predicted by the model in Fig. 2. Finally,

the high-molecular-weight complex is the only component that is not absorbed on affinity columns containing B101 or B102 or hCG when hCG, monoclonal antibody B101, monoclonal antibody B102, or mixtures containing two or three of these reagents are chromatographed on these columns. This is consistent with none of the antibody binding sites or relevant epitopes on hCG being available for binding, as is the case with the circular complex.

When liquid-phase radioimmunoassays are performed under certain conditions with a synergistic pair of monoclonal antibodies, the addition of unlabeled antigen first causes a rise in antibody-bound radiolabeled antigen and then, only on addition of larger amounts of antigen is the typical inhibition curve detected (Ehrlich and Moyle, 1983). A similar phenomenon termed a "hook" effect, has been observed with antisera (Weintraub et al., 1973). This positive cooperativity occurs at low concentrations of antigen so that very low concentrations of radiolabeled antigen must be present in the assay. This is the reason why normal conditions in the hCG radioimmunoassay resulted in apparently typical inhibition curves. The increase in antibody-bound hCG with a mixture of B101 and B102 occurs at an hCG concentration 100–1000 times lower than the concentration detectable with antibody B101 alone. Thus, this part of the curve can be used as the basis for a very sensitive immunoassay named the cooperative immunoassay or CIA. Computer calculations (Ehrlich and Moyle, 1983) suggest that extremely sensitive immunoassays can be constructed by mixing the correct monoclonal antibodies and that the limiting factor in the sensitivity will not be the affinity of the antibodies but the specific activity and nonspecific background activity of the tracer. Although higher affinity antibodies contribute to a more sensitive CIA, an important parameter is also the ability of the mixture of two antibodies and antigen to form the circular complex (this binding constant has been termed K'). B101 and B102 have a high K' (i.e., formation of the circular complex is highly favored), whereas B101 and B103 have a low K'. In general, the larger the value of K', the greater the sensitivity of an assay. In fact, two monoclonal antibodies with low affinity for antigen but very high K' will result in the optimal CIA since the binding by the individual antibodies will be low. This third parameter in the CIA (the first two being the affinity constants of the individual antibodies) can vary so as to either improve or degrade the quality of an immunoassay in another important aspect—the specificity of the assay. If K' for a cross-reactive molecule (such as hLH or hTSH in an hCG immunoassay) were less for the cross-reactive molecule than for the molecule to be measured, then the specificity of the immunoassay would increase. As indicated in Fig. 3, this is apparently the case for one pair of anti-hCG antibodies we have studied (A102 and B103) in which the cross-reactivity of both antibodies for hTSH is very high but a cooperative assay results in very little binding

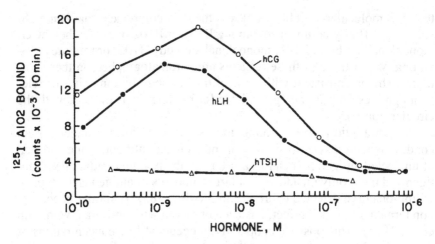

Fig. 3. Immunoassays for hCG, hLH, and hTSH utilizing monoclonal antibodies directed agsinst hCG. Antibody B103 was adsorbed to plastic microtiter wells. The antibody was removed and the wells incubated with 10% horse serum in phosphate-buffered saline for two hours at 20°C. The horse serum was removed and then the wells were incubated with 16,200 cpm ^{125}I-A102, 1% horse serum in phosphate-buffered saline, and the indicated amounts of hormone for 18 h at 20°C. The liquid was then removed, the wells rinsed three times with distilled water, and the wells were counted. An inhibition assay utilizing solid-phase B103 and ^{125}I-hCG indicated that this antibody could bind hCG about eight times better than hTSH. A102 bound hCG and hTSH with about the same affinity, as expected since the α subunit is identical on both hormones. However, as shown here, a cooperative immunoassay utilizing both of these highly cross-reactive monoclonal antibodies is very specific for hCG.

to hTSH (Ehrlich et al., 1983b). K' is probably close to zero in the hTSH, A102, B103 immunoassay. Conversely, it is also possible that K' could be higher for the cross-reactive molecule than for the molecule to be measured, and therefore, the immunoassay would be less specific. An even more important problem in degrading the specificity of the CIA is the formation of the hybrid circular complex shown in Fig. 2B. Even if the K' for hLH or hTSH were less than that for hCG, the K' for the hybrid circular complex may be significant. The resulting immunoassay may not only be less specific than expected, but concentrations of cross-reacting molecules in the presence of the antigen may give misleading values of antigen using standard curves derived with a pure antigen. Thus, whereas the CIA offers great possibilities in the increase of specificity and sensitivity in immnnoassays, special care must be taken in the choice of monoclonal antibodies. At present there is no known method for predicting the K' of any particular pair of monoclonal antibodies or for stimulating the production and isolation of monoclonal antibodies of high K'.

The cooperative immunoassay has another potential useful characteristic—the possibility of expanding or contracting the range of measurement. Figure 4A shows that varying the ratio of two monoclonal antibodies in a double antibody radioimmunoassay can greatly increase the usable range of antigen concentration. This probably occurs because the circular complex consists of one molecule of each antibody and any excess of either antibody will have the same effect on radioimmunoassay data as adding a lower affinity antibody. A unique feature of the cooperative immunoassay is shown in Fig. 4B. These data are replotted from previously published work (Ehrlich et al., 1983a) and shows that the dose–response curve can be increased in slope. Theoretical data (Ehrlich and Moyle, 1983) have shown that the increase is related to K'. This property may have use in qualitative immunoassays in which a yes-or-no answer is required. For example, in an ELISA assay, color could be generated by the presence of a predetermined amount of antigen but the assay solution remain completely colorless with just a slightly lower amount of antigen. The generation of color is a step-function of the amount of antigen.

Another interesting consequence of the formation of the circular complex is the kinetics of formation and dissociation of the antibody–antigen interaction. The practical consequences of these results are discussed in Section 4 in relation to the in vivo detection of hCG-producing tumors. The circular complex appears to be extremely stable. Holmes and Parham (1983) have shown that two monoclonal antibodies that can form a circular complex with radiolabeled HLA-A2 had no detectable loss of antigen in 100 min, whereas an HLA-A2 single antibody complex had a half-life of about 10 min.

3. Immunoassays with Monoclonal Antibodies to hCG

Although immnnoassays for hCG with antisera have reached levels of sensitivity (Vaitukaitis et al., 1972) and specificity (Chen et al., 1976) that are excellent compared to assays for many other biomolecules, there is still a need for improved assays due to the low levels of hCG in early pregnancy and some cancers and the occasionally high levels of hLH. Monoclonal antibodies can offer not only the possibility of high affinity and high specificity without the presence of antibodies of lower quality, but the larger amounts and ease of purity of monoclonal antibodies has enabled investigators to consider the possibility of alternative designs in

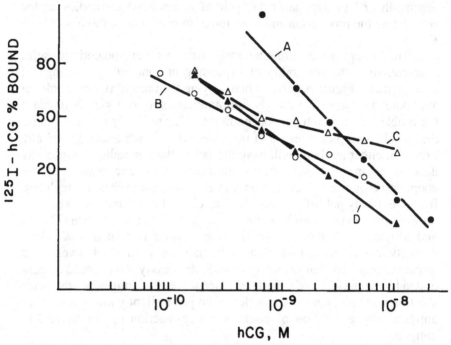

Fig. 4A. Double antibody radioimmunoassay with antibody B101 and varying ratios of antibody B101 and B102. Percent ^{125}I-hCG bound to antibody is plotted vs the amount of unlabeled hCG added to the assay. The slope of the dose-response curve varies greatly with the ratio of the two antibodies. A, antibody B101; B, equal volumes of stock solutions of antibodies B101 and B102; C, the same stock solutions of antibodies B101 and B102 mixed in the proportion 1:9; D, the same stock solutions of antibodies B101 and B102 mixed in the proportion 4:1.

immunoassays. A major trend has been the movement from traditional competitive radioimmunoassays to two-site immunoradiometric assays (IRMA). The latter assay consists of a solid-phase-bound antibody and a labeled (enzyme, radiolabeled, etc.) second liquid-phase antibody. The more antigen present in a sample, the higher the amount of labeled antibody will be bound to the solid through an antigen bridge and, therefore, a higher signal will be present. For molecules that can simultaneously bind two monoclonal antibodies, there are usually several advantages to the two-site immunoradiometric assay, both in theory (Miles and Hales, 1968) and in practical use (Hunter and Budd, 1981). Since the two-site IRMA is an excess reagent assay, i.e., there can be high concentrations of antibodies present in the assay, the affinity of the antibodies for the antigen is not as decisive in determining assay sensitivity as in radioimmunoassays. Several other potential advantages are: (1) pure antigen is

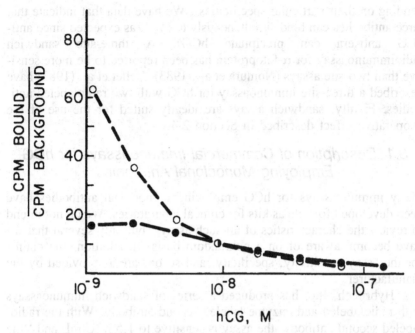

Fig. 4B. The effect of a second monoclonal antibody on the slope of the dose response curve. The slope is greatly increased. These results are from a solid phase assay with antibody B102 adsorbed to the plastic and ^{125}I-hCG and unlabeled hCG in the liquid phase. The amount of radioactivity bound to the plastic in experiments with liquid-phase B101 (1.4 µg/mL; open circles) or without liquid-phase antibody B101 (filled circles) divided by the amount of radioactivity bound in the presence of saturating concentrations of unlabeled hCG is plotted vs the amount of unlabeled hCG.

not necessary for labeling; (2) antibodies can generally be labeled without interfering with activity, whereas some antigens are easily denatured in the labeling process; (3) antibodies are more stable than many antigens; (4) assay range is often increased since this is related to the amount of antibody present and is not limited by the reliability of detecting a given amount of inhibition; (5) measurements are made by an increase in signal above a low background rather than a decrease from a high level; and (6) the specificity of the assay may be increased (Haber et al., 1981) since the specificities of both antibodies contribute to the assay specificity. From the data in Section 2.2, it can be seen that there are many possible combinations of two monoclonal antibodies that can bind simultaneously to hCG. This allows for some variation depending on the exact goal of the assay. For example, a two-site IRMA based on one monoclonal antibody to the α subunit and one to the β subunit would only measure intact hormone. This may not necessarily be true for two anti-hCGβ antibodies (depending on their particular specificities). We have data that indicate that three antibodies can bind simultaneously to hCG (as expected since anti-hCG antisera can precipitate hCG). A three-site sandwich radioimmunoassay for α-fetoprotein has been reported to be more sensitive than two-site assays (Nomura et al., 1983). Bellet et al. (1983) have described a three-site immunoassay for hCG with two radiolabeled antibodies. Finally, sandwich assays are ideally suited for the use of the cooperative effect described in Section 2.4.

3.1. Description of Commercial Immunoassays for hCG Employing Monoclonal Antibodies

Many immunoassays for hCG employing monoclonal antibodies have been developed for sale as kits for clinical laboratories. We do not intend to review the characteristics of all such assays, but only several that we have become aware of on a nonrandom basis. In addition, the claims for the assay sensitivity, specificity, and so on, are as provided by the manufacturer.

Hybritech, Inc. has produced a series of sandwich immunoassays with radiolabeled and enzyme-labeled second antibody. With the radiolabeled second antibody, the assay is sensitive to 1.5 mIU/mL and "the highest concentration of LH, FSH, and TSH routinely reported for abnormal patients should not interfere with results." The assay can be performed quantitatively with either 1- or 2-h incubations and the upper limit of detectable concentrations are then, respectively, up to 100 and 400 mIU/mL. With enzyme-labeled second antibody, the minimum detectable concentration is 2.5 mIU/mL and the cross-reactivity with hLH is reported to be 0.23%, and with hFSH and hTSH it is 0.00%. Both assays are available for qualitative tests and an enzyme-labeled test can be used for a visual assay. A group from Hybritech has also published an article describing a sandwich assay that utilizes one anti-hCGβ and one anti-hCGα antibody so that only the whole hormone is measured (Shimizu et al., 1982).

Wampole Laboratories has produced a radioimmunoassay named Genesis β-hCG employing a monoclonal antibody. This test is sensitive to 5 mIU/mL. One difference from the Hybritech assays is that free β subunit can be detected in addition to intact hormone.

Monoclonal Antibodies, Inc. has released the Model urine hCG assay, a sandwich immunoassay with a solid-bound anti-α antibody and an enzyme-labeled anti-hCGβ antibody. This test can be performed in 60 min, is sensitive to 50 mIU/mL, and is read by the amount of visual color development. As expected from the design of the assay, only intact hormone will be detected. A research group from this corporation has also published a description of a very sensitive enzyme immunoassay for hCG (Wada et al., 1982). Although sensitive to 0.2 ng/mL, the problem with this assay, which is a sandwich assay employing a solid phase monoclonal antibody to the α subunit incubated simultaneously with a liquid phase anti-hCGβ monoclonal antibody, is that there is 8% cross-reactivity with hLH. A loss of specificity may have been caused through cooperative effects as described in Section 2.4 since the anti-hCGβ monoclonal antibody is less than 1% cross-reactive in a competitive radioimmunoassay. However, other explanations are possible.

Leuvering et al. (1983) from the Organon Scientific Development Group have described a homogeneous sol particle immunoassay (SPIA) for hCG. The assay, which is not sensitive since it is intended for routine pregnancy testing, employs two monoclonal antibodies because agglutination with antibody-coated particles will not occur with just one monoclonal antibody and an antigen with nonrepeating epitopes. Both spectrophotometry and visual reading can be used for detection.

As can be seen by the limited sample described above, immunoassays for hCG have been produced with a whole range of characteristics similar to the products available with polyclonal antisera. The one exception may be the Hybritech immunoradiometric assay that appears to be more sensitive than the standard radioimmunoassay with antisera to hCGβ (Vaitukaitis et al., 1972). However, the ease of producing large quantities of monoclonal antibodies and their potential superior performance in sandwich assays are significant advantages in this field.

3.2. Research Immunoassays for hCG

Much effort has been devoted to the development of exceptionally sensitive, specific, and/or rapid assays for hCG. Most of these assays are only available in the laboratories that have reported them and have been designed to answer specific research questions or prove the utility of some new technologies.

An exceptionally sensitive and specific immunoassay has been developed with a monoclonal solid-phase antibody (B101) and radiolabeled affinity purified rabbit anti-hCGβ COOH-terminal peptide antibody (Canfield et al., 1983). The assay was reported to have a sensitivity of approximately 0.02 ng hCG/mL of urine, which is about the concentration of hormone excreted by some normal individuals. The cross-reactivity with hLH was negligible. One disadvantage of the assay is the long incubation times that are required—the assay takes several days. However, the sensitivity and specificity are such that several clinical research questions, such as the extent of hCG production by various tumors, can be answered definitively. Already, this assay has resulted in the finding of relatively higher concentrations of hCG in postmenopausal females than in other "normals."

A monoclonal antibody has also been used to develop an assay with the opposite goal—a relatively insensitive test that is very rapid (Stenman et al., 1981). This assay is an inhibition radioimmunoassay that can be performed in about 2 h and is sensitive to 5 IU/L. Although these investigators may not have screened many monoclonal antibodies to optimize the speed of the assay, this could be done in principle and indicates one of the advantages of monoclonal antibody technology—the antibody can be chosen on the basis of the exact use for which it is desired.

The same anti-hCGβ monoclonal antibody as used by Stenman et al. (1981) was also incorporated into a fluorescence sandwich immunoassay (Pettersson et al., 1983). This assay, which is very sensitive (0.7 IU/L) and rapid (as fast as 1 h), is based on a tracer of europium complexed to an EDTA-derivative that is then conjugated to one of the antibodies. The lanthanide chelate offers several advantages over conventional fluorescent probes (Pettersson et al., 1983; Soini and Kojola, 1983), among which are the long decay times of the lanthanide fluorescence (which allows one to distinguish tracer from background fluorescence in the biological samples) and high quantum yield.

4. In Vivo Immunodetection of Tumors

Tumors secreting human chorionic gonadotropin have been detected by photoscanning after injection of ^{131}I-labeled goat anti-hCG IgG (Goldenberg et al., 1980). It was not clear that similar results could be obtained with monoclonal antibodies since some doubts have been raised about their effectiveness in nuclear imaging of tumors (Fairweather et al., 1982; Sfakianakis and DeLand, 1982). One preliminary report describing the utilization of a monoclonal antibody directed against hCG for immunodetection of tumors has appeared (Bellet et al., 1982).

There have been several criticisms of the use of monoclonal antibodies in imaging. It has been claimed that the results with monoclonal antibodies are no better than polyclonal antisera in the case of antibodies to carcinoembryonic antigen (Fairweather et al., 1982), that "mouse antibodies may not distribute uniformly in normal tissues" (Fairweather et al., 1982), that the signal may be weaker with monoclonal antibodies (Sfakianakis and DeLand, 1982), and that the activity concentration ratio (T/NT, i.e., target-to-nontarget ratio: the ratio of counts in the tumor compared to an equivalent area of the body) for monoclonal antibodies may be greater only for the first 24–48 h after injection, but less at later times (Sfakianakis and DeLand, 1982) [the results of Levine et al. (1980) who obtained the best images with a monoclonal antibody 48 h postadministration, offer a counter argument]. It has been proposed by Sfakianakis and DeLand (1982) that a mixture of monoclonal antibodies may overcome some of these disadvantages. More radiolabeled antibody will be taken up by the tumor with a mixture because more epitopes will become available, i.e., there may be a limiting amount of one epitope on a tumor that a monoclonal antibody will react with, and this may not be enough for a strong, long-lasting signal. Though we believe this idea has merit, we would like to propose a modification. Results described in Section 2.4 indicate that the half-life of the antibody–antigen interaction is much longer if a circular complex is formed than if there is only a single antibody. This could explain the difference between polyclonal antisera and monoclonal antibodies in radioimaging experiments. It should be noted that bivalent binding of a monoclonal antibody to two antigen molecules on a cell surface will also result in a long-lived complex but this may not always be possible, may be inhibited by soluble antigen in the serum, and may still be shorter lived than a circular complex. Figure 5 shows two ways in which a circular complex could be formed after administration of two antibodies. In Fig. 5A, only surface bound antigen is required. Figure 5B shows how a circular complex could be formed that is composed of both cell surface and soluble antigen. This may explain why high serum concentrations of tumor antigens do not interfere with imaging experiments (as shown by Goldenberg et al., 1980)—the soluble antigen may actually aid in forming the image by helping to build an antibody–antigen aggregate. It is unlikely that preformation of a circular complex with two monoclonal antibodies, either in vitro or by simultaneous injection of both antibodies, would increase the T/NT ratio since the circular complex is so stable it is unlikely that it would reform near the tumor after forming in the serum.

We therefore propose that one monoclonal antibody be administered and then, following a rest period that must be experimentally determined, the second antibody be injected so that the circular complex can be formed. This procedure should theoretically overcome several of the objections to the use of monoclonal antibodies in radioimaging: (1) the long-lived circular complex should result in the antibodies remaining in the tumor long enough for the background radiation to decrease; (2) the T/NT ratio should also be increased by the presence of antibodies to more than one epitope; and (3) the specificity of the interaction can be increased by extrapolation of the results described for cooperative immunoassays in Section 2.4. Thus, our proposal includes injection of the "poly-monoclonal antibody preparations" described by Sfakianakis and DeLand, but the monoclonal antibodies must be of the proper type, i.e., complementary and preferably synergistic. Evidence for the usefulness of this proposal may have been provided by Hughes-Jones et al. (1983). They have reported that the synergistic lysis of cells by monoclonal antibodies is caused by both the presence of two antibodies binding to each antigen molecule and the formation of antibody–antigen aggregates.

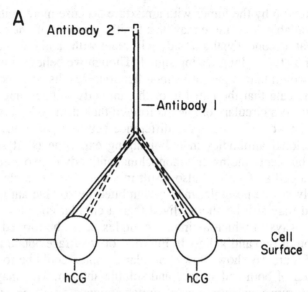

Fig. 5A.   A circular complex of surface bound antigen and two different monoclonal antibodies. The formation of the circular complex with a second monoclonal antibody may decrease the possibility of antigen molecules dissociating from the first antibody and therefore lead to a longer lifetime of the first antibody–antigen complex (even when compared with bivalent antibody–antigen complexes).

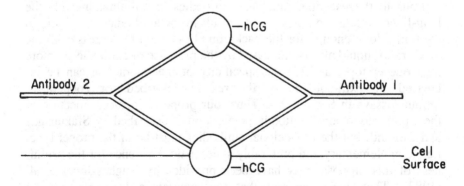

Fig. 5B.   A circular complex composed of one surface-bound antigen molecule, one soluble antigen molecule, and two monoclonal antibodies. This complex should be much more stable than one antibody molecule bound to one soluble antigen molecule and one surface-bound antigen molecule.

Primus and Goldenberg (1980) have indicated that immune complexes may enhance tumor localization. It may be that the optimal image would be generated not by the formation of a circular complex, but by a highly crosslinked antibody–antigen complex. This should also be possible with the judicious choice of monoclonal antibodies. Milstein et al. (1980) have concluded that four different monoclonal antibodies are necessary for antigen precipitation. Therefore, this number may be the minimum that are necessary to utilize the advantages of monoclonal antibodies while not giving up the advantages of antisera. Lightfoot et al. (1970) reported that four dinitrophenyl groups conjugated to each protein molecule were required for precipitation with dinitrophenyl antisera. Steensgaard et al. (1980) have detected precipitation with only two monoclonal antibodies to an antigen. However, the antigen had two epitopes for each monoclonal antibody (so that even the individual monoclonal antibodies could form immune complexes; Steensgaard et al., 1982) and, therefore, four epitopes were required for precipitation. In addition, some pairs of antibodies were better at precipitating antigen than other pairs. Stahli et al. (1981) have reported that two monoclonal antibodies directed against hCG are sufficient to precipitate the hormone. These experiments were performed by double-diffusion in agar, which may differ from a homogeneous medium. Not all pairs of monoclonal antibodies that could bind simultaneously to hCG caused the formation of a precipitin line.

5. Immunocytochemistry with Monoclonal Antibodies to hCG

The immunocytochemical localization of tumor-associated antigens has become extremely relevant in recent years, not only as a source of confirmatory evidence for other immunoassays, but also as a means of establishing clinically significant morphofunctional relationships that frequently contribute to the correct pathologic diagnosis of the tumor and clinical management of the patient. At the same time, the clinical importance of hCG as a tumor marker as been underscored by numerous reports of considerably elevated hCG serum or plasma levels not only in patients with tumors of germ or trophoblastic cell origin, but also in those with a variety of other tumors (Hussa, 1982; Braunstein, 1979; Vaitukaitis, 1979). The list of tumors with reported inappropriate or "ectopic" hCG production is quite long, and includes gynecologic carcinomas (ovary, cervix, vagina, endometrium, and vulva), breast carcinoma, gastrointestinal carcinomas (pancreas, stomach, liver, large and small intestine, esophagus, and biliary tract), and carcinomas of the lung, prostate, and kidney. Melanomas, sarcomas, and even lymphoproliferative malignancies have also been associated with serum or plasma hCG. Circulating hCG subunits have also been reported in patients with endocrine pancreatic tumors (β) and carcinoids (α) (Oberg and Wide, 1981).

Although there is sufficient evidence to accept the fact that many of these tumors do produce hCG, a major difficulty in the interpretation of elevated hCG levels in these patients is the variablity of hCG immunoassays performed with polyclonal antisera (Fowler et al., 1982). As mentioned in the introduction to this chapter, the specificity of such antisera can vary considerably, even among antisera raised against hCGβ because of this molecule's extensive structural similarity with the β subunit of hLH. Compounding this problem of undesirable cross-reactivities is the finding of immunoreactive hCG in the plasma, sera, and tissues of normal, nonpregnant subjects (Chen et al., 1976; Yoshimoto et al., 1979; Borkowski and Muquardt, 1979; Hussa, 1982).

It is evident, therefore, that the issue of hCG production by nontrophoblastic cell malignancies, and its possible clinical value, can only be clarified by the use of standardized immunoassays employing antibodies with identical, precisely defined specificity and sensitivity, an utopian situation recently made possible by monoclonal antibodies. Furthermore, the detection of circulating hCG must be correlated with the presence of the hormone in the tumor itself, either by analysis of the wet tissue or by immunocytochemistry. Reports of such correlations with carcinoembryonic antigen (Puri et al., 1977) have shown that it is not always possible to demonstrate a causal relationship between a tumor and a circulating antigen. Kurman and Scardino (1981), however, have demonstrated good correlation between serum hCG and tissue localization in testicular germ-cell tumors, although such was not always the case with alphafetoprotein.

The immunocytochemical localization of hCG with polyclonal antisera has previously been reported in placental tissues and trophoblastic disease (Hoshina et al., 1979; Tubbs et al., 1979; Tanaka, 1982) and in germ-cell tumors of the ovary and testis with trophoblastic elements (Kurman and Scardino, 1981), but less frequently in other tumors (Hustin, 1978; Case Records MGH, 1983). More recently Wahlstrom et al. (1981) reported a monoclonal antibody to hCG that immunocytochemically localized the hormone in the syncitiotrophoblast of normal plaoenta, but did not react with human pituitary gonadotrophs, indicating lack of cross-reactivity with hLH. This is a fortunate development since the immunocytochemical localization of such evolutionarily conserved hormones is particularly plagued by cross-reactivities (Swaab et al., 1977; Jagiello and Mesa-Tejada, 1979; Halmi, 1981) and obviously hCG is no exception (Mesa-Tejada and Jagiello, 1979).

The monoclonal antibodies described in this chapter, recognizing different epitopes of hCG molecule, provided a unique opportunity to study the immunocytochemical localization of the α and β subunits of hCG. Since sections of paraffin embedded tissues are most convenient for immunocytochemistry, particularly since they facilitate the use of adjacent serial sections to compare different antibodies, it was gratifying to find that all of the eight antibodies chosen for study (A102, 103, 109 and B101, 102, 103, 105, 107) were capable of staining sections of Bouin's-fixed paraffin-embedded immature first trimester placental villi (Fig. 6). Thus, the epitopes defined by each of these antibodies appears to survive such fixation and processing of tissue. Immature placental tissue was therefore used to titrate each of the antibodies and determine optimal staining concentrations, which were found to correlate well with each antibody's previously determined affinity (Table 1): the lower the affinity the higher the concentration of antibody required for optimal (most intense) staining. These concentrations were around 1:100 (culture supernatants) or 0.25–1 μg/mL (purified IgG) for the various antibodies.

The cellular distribution of the immunocytochemical reaction product using the same indirect immunoperoxidase procedure (Mesa-Tejada et al., 1978) was similar to that previously observed with polyclonal antisera (Mesa-Tejada and Jagiello, 1979). The only distinction is the quality of the intense and crisp staining reaction (Fig. 6) that is limited to the cytoplasm of the syncitiotrophoblast, in the total absence of nonspecific or background stain, with all but two of these antibodies (A109 and B105). A109 also localizes lesser amounts of hCGα in the cytotrophoblast, in agreement with previously reported immunofluorescence (Hoshina et al., 1979), immunoperoxidase (Tanaka, 1982) and *in situ* hybridization (Hoshina et al., 1982) studies, further supporting the hypothesis that some synthesis of hCG occurs in the cytotrophoblast before or during its transition to syncitiotrophoblast.

A109 and B105 also produce a weak but definite stain in the villous mesenchymal fibers as well as in some of the cells (Hofbauer cells?) found in this area. Since both of these antibodies are monoclonal and recognize individual epitopes of the hCG molecule, such localization cannot be called nonspecific and the significance of such "background" stain deserves further study.

The degree of cross-reactivity of some of these antibodies with other glycoprotein hormones, previously determined by double antibody radioimmunoassay (Table 1), was also confirmed immunocytochemically. As illustrated in Fig. 7, B103, with a 90% cross-reactivity with hLH, stains gonadotrophs in the human pituitary whereas B101 (2% cross-reactivity with hLH) and B107 (< 0.5% cross-reactivity; not illustrated) do not. A109, however, as expected from its cross-reactivity with other α subunits, stains numerous cells in the same section of human pituitary. Thus, for immunocytochemical specificity for hCG, the monoclonal antibodies of choice are B101 and B107.

Preliminary results of further immunocytochemical studies with these antibodies have raised intriguing questions that are presently under investigation. A look at several cases of trophoblastic disease, including

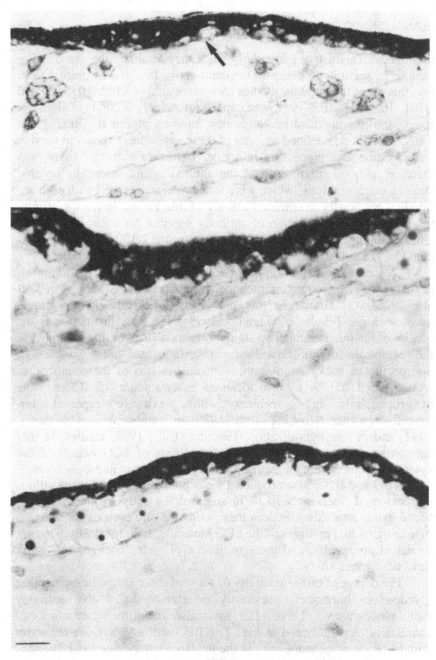

Fig. 6. Immunocytochemical stain of paraffin-embedded sections of first trimester placental villus with A109 (A), B101 (B), and B103 (C). Note discrete distribution of the reaction product limited to outer cell layer (syncitiotrophoblast) in sections stained with B101 (B) and B103 (C) whereas some reaction product is also noted in inner cell layer (cytotrophoblast) (arrow) and stromal elements in section stained with A109 (A). (Indirect immunoperoxidase; methylene blue counterstain; bar = 20 μm.)

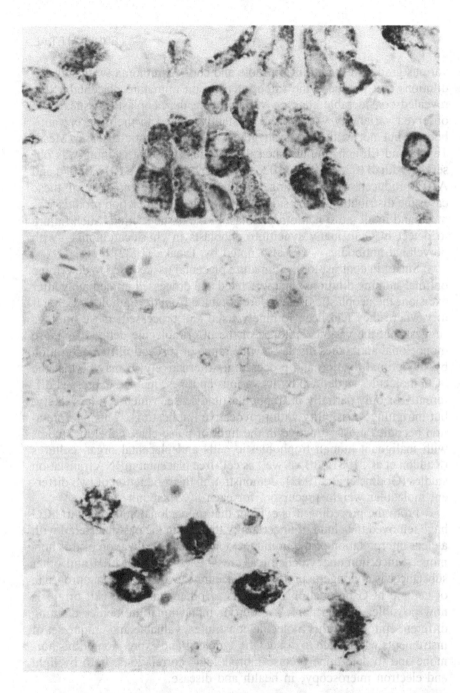

Fig. 7. Immunocytochemical stain of paraffin sections of human anterior hypophysis with A109 (A), B101 (B), and B103 (C). Because of cross-reactivity through α subunit, most cells stain with A109 (A), whereas only gonadotrophs stain with B103 (C), which has considerable cross-reactivity with LH. B101, however, is highly specific for hCGβ and does not stain any cells (B). (Indirect immunoperoxidase; methylene blue counterstain; bar = 20 μm.)

various grades of hydatidiform mole and choriocarcinoma (with staining dilutions that produced the same intensity on immature placental villi), revealed considerable staining variability in the neoplastic tissues. The observed variability was most consistently related to the different anti- bodies, but not to the different grades of trophoblastic disease (Mesa- Tejada and Ehrlich, unpublished data). Thus, the best staining was ob- served with B102, B105, A102, and A109, whereas B101, B107, and A103 produced weak staining. Furthermore, in the majority of these cases the distribution of the staining was focal, i.e., reaction product was not found in all the syncitiotrophoblast in the tissue section. Such failure to detect hCG in many syncitiotrophoblasts in choriocarcinoma—with polyclonal antibodies—was also noted by Tanaka (1982).

Since, in contrast to the immature placental tissue (used to determine optimal staining dilutions) that was fixed and processed immediately after excision, the neoplastic tissues were obtained from the Pathology Labora- tory where they had been routinely fixed and processed, these findings suggest that the various epitopes of the hCG molecule defined by these monoclonal antibodies display a wide range of susceptibility to alteration by suboptimal fixation and processing. Alternatively, it may be that the hCG molecule, as defined by its various epitopes, may be expressed dif- ferently or only partially in trophoblastic disease, which is a less likely, but intriguing, possibility with provocative implications. This interpreta- tion becomes most attractive in the light of pulse-chase labeling studies with malignant human trophoblastic cells and placental organ cultures (Ruddon et al., 1981a, b), as well as cell-free placental mRNA translation studies (Godine et al., 1982), demonstrating the production of two differ- ent molecular weight precursors for each hCG subunit.

From the preceding it is evident that monoclonal antibodies to hCG have removed the cloud of uncertainity that has in the past interfered with a clear interpretation of the immunocytochemical localization of this hor- mone. Since immunocytochemical cross-reactivity with hLH and other substances is no longer a problem, an accurate evaluation of inappropriate or ectopic hCG production by tumors of other than germ cell origin is now possible. Furthermore, a group of monoclonal antibodies defining different epitopes of this molecule constitute a valuable and unique set of instruments with which to dissect the synthesis and expression of this hor- mone and to determine precise morphologic correlations, both by light and electron microscopy, in health and disease.

6. Summary

Despite the availability of sensitive and specific antisera, monoclonal an- tibodies will be useful in detecting human chorionic gonadotropin. Indi- vidual monoclonal antibodies with similar or superior characteristics to antisera can be produced. Antibodies B107 and P_3W_{80}, to mention two that we have studied, have high affinity for hCG and low cross-reactivity with other glycoprotein hormones. The monoclonal antibodies against the COOH-terminal peptide of hCGβ isolated so far probably have a lower affinity for hormone than the antisera that have been described. However, the hybridomas can be used in differently designed assays that minimize the effect of antibody affinity. In addition, higher affinity monoclonal antibodies to the COOH-terminus of hCGβ may be isolated in the future. Therefore, in general, the characteristics of monoclonal antibodies are such that the advantages of chemical standardization and supply can be utilized. The second reason for replacing antisera with monoclonal antibodies is the ability to probe different regions of hCG, as in the studies described in Section 2.3, and, therefore, there is the potential for designing new assays. As shown in Fig. 1, antibodies are not only available that bind different regions but antibodies whose epitopes are close together can have very different properties. For example, antibodies B105 and P_3W_{80} cannot bind simultaneously to hCG but one binds hLH as well as hCG, whereas the other is specific for hCG. There may, however, be some limitation to the possibility of picking a monoclonal antibody that binds to a particular region with a set of desired characteristics. For example, we have not been able to isolate any monoclonal antibody that can bind simultaneously to hCG with B102–B103–B105 epitope region antibodies and that can bind the hCGβ subunit with a high affinity. However, immunization with different schedules or with different fragments, in addition to a more extensive screening of available colonies, may result in the isolation of even this type of monoclonal antibody.

The major advantage of monoclonal antibodies to a well-defined antigen such as hCG may be in using several antibodies in combination so that the best characteristics of both antisera and hybridoma antibodies will be apparent. This would include the use of cooperative immunoassays, the development of artificial antisera for in vivo imaging, and the design of specific and sensitive two-site "sandwich" immunoassays. However, most of this work is just beginning and the potential must still be fulfilled. One example of this is the in vivo imaging with monoclonal antibodies. If it is true that precipitation of antigen or the formation of large antibody–antigen aggregates results in the best image and that two, or probably more, specially chosen monoclonal antibodies are required for precipitation of an antigen, then a very large number of experiments must be performed before the full potential of monoclonal antibodies will be realized in only this one application.

In immunocytochemistry, the described monoclonal antibodies to hCG can totally eliminate the problem of cross-reactivities that have clouded the interpretation of the localization of hCG in tumors with suspected inappropriate or ectopic hCG production. Furthermore, since these antibodies identify specific parts of the hCG molecule, they can be used to precisely follow the synthesis of its subunits, both at the light and electron microscopic level, in normal and diseased tissues. Other evidence suggests that such precise morphofunctional relationships may produce information of considerable clinical significance.

Acknowledgments

Our studies were supported in part by grants from the National Institutes of Health (HD-15454-P.H.E., Z.A.M., A.K., and CA 32984-R.M.J.).

References

Bellet, D., J. M. Bidart, P. L. Motte, J. Lumbroso, C. Berche, M. Schlumberger, and C. Bohoun (1982), *Hybridoma*, **1**, 218.

Bellet, D., M. Ozturc, J. M. Bidart, M. C. Strugo, F. Troalen, J. M. Caillaud, J. Lumbroso, M. Jolivet, A. Tartar, J. L. Amiel, M. Assicot, and C. Bohoun (1983), in *International Symposium on Human Choriogonadotropin, Cassis, France*, Abstract.

Birken, S., and R. E. Canfield (1980), in *Chorionic Gonadotropin* (Segal, S. J., ed.), Plenum Publishing Corp., New York, p. 65.

Birken, S., R. Canfield, G. Agosto, and J. Lewis (1982), *Endocrinology*, **110**, 1555.

Borkowski, A., and C. Muquardt (1979), *New Eng. J. Med.*, **301**, 298.

Bosch, A. M. G., W. Stevens, A. Schuurs, O. Schonherr, and H. Roelofs (1981), *Protides of the Biological Fluids*, **29**, 837.

Braunstein, G. D. (1979), in *Recent Advances in Reproduction and Regulation of Fertility* (Talwar G. P., ed.), Elsevier/North-Holland Biomedical, Amsterdam, p. 389.

Canfield, R. E., E. G. Armstrong, E. S. Siris, S. Birken, and P. H. Ehrlich (1983), in *Proceedings of the International Symposium on Progress in Perinatal Medicine, Florence, Italy, May 9–12, 1983*, Excerpta Medica, Amsterdam, The Netherlands.

Case Records of the Massachusetts General Hostpital (Case 34-1983) (1983), *N. Eng. J. Med.*, **309**, 477.

Chen, H.-C., G. D. Hodgen, S. Matsuura, L. J. Lin, E. Gross, L. E. Reichert, S. Birken, R. E. Canfield, and G. T. Ross (1976), *Proc. Natl. Acad. USA*, **73**, 2885.

Ehrlich, P. H., and W. R. Moyle (1983), *Science*, **221**, 279.

Ehrlich, P. H., W. R. Moyle, Z. A. Moustafa, and R. E. Canfield (1982), *J. Immunol.* **128**, 2709.

Ehrlich, P. H., W. R. Moyle, and Z. A. Moustafa (1983a), *J. Immunol.* **131**, 1906.

Ehrlich, P. H., D. M. Anderson, and W. R. Moyle (1983b), *65th Annual Meeting of the Endocrine Society*, Abstract.

Ehrlich, P. H., W. R. Moyle, and R. E. Canfield (1984, in press), in *Methods in Enzymology, Peptide Hormone Action* (Birnbaumer, L., and O'Malley, B. W., eds.), Academic Press, New York.

Fairweather, D. S., A. R. Bradwell, and P. W. Dykes (1982), *Lancet* **2**, 660.

Fiddes, J. C., and H. M. Goodman (1980), *Nature* **286**, 648.

Fowler, J. E., G. E. Platoff, C. A. Kubrock, and R. E. Stutzman (1982), *Cancer* **49**, 136.

Godine, J. E., W. W. Chin, and J. F. Habener (1982), *Biochem. Biophys. Res. Comm.*, **104**, 463.

Goldenberg, D. M., E. E. Kim, F. H. DeLand, J. R. Van Nagell, Jr., and N. Javadpour (1980), *Science* **208**, 1284.

Gupta, S. K., and G. P. Talwar (1980), *Indian J. Exp. Biol.* **18**, 1361.

Gupta, S. K., and S. Ramakrishnan, and G. P. Talwar (1982), *J. Biosci.* **4**, 105.

Haber, E., P. Donahoe, P. Ehrlich, J. Hurrell, H. Katus, B. A. Khaw, M. N. Margolies, M. Mudgett-Hunter, and V. R. Zurawski (1981), in *Monoclonal Antibodies in Endocrine Research* (Fellows, R. E., and Eisenbarth, G., eds.) Raven Press, New York, p. 1.

Halmi, N. S. (1981), *J. Histochem. Cytochem.* **29**, 837.

Hearn, J. P. (1976), *Proc. R. Soc. Lond. B.* **195**, 149.

Holmes, N. J., and P. Parham (1983), *J. Biol. Chem.* **258**, 1580.

Hoshina, M., Y. Ashitake, and S. Tojo (1979), *Endocrinol. Japan* **26**, 175.

Hoshina, M., M. Boothby, and I. Boime (1982), *J. Cell. Biol.* **93**, 190.

Hughes-Jones, N. C., B. D. Gorick, and J. C. Howard (1983), *Eur. J. Immunol.* **13**, 635.

Hunter, W. M., and P. S. Budd (1981), *J. Immun. Methods* **45**, 255.

Hussa, R. O. (1982), *Obstet. Gynecol.* **60**, 1.

Hustin, J. (1978), *Gynecol. Obstet. Inves.* **9**, 3.

Jagiello, G., and R. Mesa-Tejada (1979), *Endocrinology* **104**, 302.

Khazaeli, M. B., B. G. England, R. C. Dieterle, G. D. Nordblom, G. A. Kabza, and W. H. Beierualtes (1981), *Endocrinology* **109**, 1290.

Kofler, R., P. Berger, and G. Wick (1982), *Am. J. Reprod. Immunol.* **2**, 212.

Kurman, R. J., and P. T. Scardino (1981), in *Diagnostic Immunohistochemistry* (DeLellis, R. A., ed.), Masson Publishing USA, Inc., New York, p. 277.

Leuvering, J. H. W., B. C. Goverde, P. J. H. M. Thal, and A. H. W. M. Schuurs (1983), *J. Immun. Methods* **60**, 9.

Levine, G., B. Ballou, J. Reiland, D. Solter, L. Gumerman, and T. Hakala (1980), *J. Nucl. Med.* **21**, 570.

Lightfoot, R. W., Jr., R. E. Drusin, and C. L. Christian (1970), *J. Immunol.* **105**, 1493.

Matsuura, S., M. Ohashi, H.-C. Chen, and G. D. Hodgen (1979), *Endocrinology*, **104**, 396.

Mesa-Tejada, R., and G. Jagiello (1979), *J. Histochem. Cytochem.* **27**, 715.

Mesa-Tejada, R., I. Keydar, M. Ramanarayanan, T. Ohno, C. Fenoglio, and S. Spiegelman (1978), *J. Histochem. Cytochem.* **26**, 532.

Miggiano, V., C. Stahli, P. Haring, J. Schmidt, M. LeDain, B. Glatthaar, and T. Staehelin (1980), *Protides of the Biological Fluids* **28**, 501.

Miles, L. E. M., and C. N. Hales (1968), *Nature* **219**, 186.

Milstein, C., M. R. Clark, G. Galfre, and A. C. Cuello (1980), in *4th Int. Congr. Immunol., Progr. Immunol. IV.* (Fougereau, M. and Dausset, J., eds.), Academic Press, London, p. 17.

Moyle, W. R., P. H. Ehrlich, and R. E. Canfield (1982), *Proc. Nat. Acad. Sci. USA,* **79,** 2245.

Moyle, W. R., D. M. Anderson, and P. H. Ehrlich (1983a), *J. Immunol.* **131,** 1900.

Moyle, W. R., C. Lin, R. L. Corson, and P. H. Ehrlich (1983b), *Mol. Immunol.* **20,** 439.

Nomura, M., M. Imai, K. Takahashi, T. Kumakura, K. Tachibana, S. Aoyagi, S. Usuda, T. Nakamura, Y. Miyakawa, and M. Mayumo (1983), *J. Immun. Methods* **58,** 293.

Oberg, K., and L. Wide (1981), *Acta Endocrinol.* **98,** 256.

Pettersson, K., H. Siitari, I. Hemmila, E. Soini, T. Lovgren, V. Hanninen, P. Tanner, and U.-H. Stenman (1983), *Clin. Chem.* **29,** 60.

Primus, F. J., and D. M. Goldenberg (1980), *Cancer Research* **40,** 2979.

Puri, S., R. Mesa-Tejada, N. Husami, S. Bennett, R. M. Richart, and C. M. Fenoglio (1977), *Gynecol. Oncol.* **5,** 331.

Ruddon, R. W., A. H. Bryan, C. A. Hanson, F. Perini, L. M. Ceccorulli, and B. P. Peters (1981a), *J. Biol. Chem.* **256,** 5189.

Ruddon, R. W., R. J. Hartle, B. P. Peters, C. Anderson, R. I. Huot, and K. Stromberg (1981b), *J. Biol. Chem.* **256,** 11389.

Sell, S., and B. Wahren (eds.) (1982), *Human Cancer Markers,* Humana Press, Clifton, N.J.

Sfakianakis, G. N., and F. H. DeLand (1982), *J. Nucl. Med.* **23,** 840.

Shimizu, S. Y., W. A. Present, E. D. Sevier, R. Wang, and R. L. Saunders (1982), *Clin. Chem.* **28,** 546.

Soini, E., and H. Kojola (1983), *Clin. Chem.* **29,** 65.

Stahli, C., V. Miggiano, M. LeDain, D. Ianelli, R. Fessler, P. Haring, J. Schmidt, and T. Staehelin (1981), in *Monoclonal Antibodies and T-Cell Hybridomas, Research Monographs in Immunology,* Vol. 3, (Hammerling, G. J., Hammerling, U., and Kearney, J. F., eds.), Elsevier/North-Holland Biomedical Press, N.Y., p. 201.

Stahli, C., V. Miggiano, J. Stocker, T. Staehelin, P. Haring, and B. Takacs (1983), *Methods in Enzymology* **92,** 242.

Steensgaard, J., C. Jacobsen, J. Lowe, D. Hardie, N. R. Ling, and R. Jefferis (1980), *Mol. Immun.* **17,** 1315.

Steensgaard, J., C. Jacobsen, J. Lowe, N. R. Ling, and R. Jefferis (1982), *Immunology* **46,** 751.

Stenman, U.-H., P. Tanner, T. Ranta, J. Schroder, and M. Seppala (1981), *Obstet. Gynecol.* **59,** 375.

Stevens, V. C. (1976), in *Physiological Effects of Immunity Against Reproductive Hormones* (Edwards, R. G., and Johnson, M. H., eds.), Cambridge University Press, New York, p. 249.

Strickland, T. W., and D. Puett (1980), *62nd Annual Meeting of the Endocrine Society,* abstract.

Stuart, M. C., P. A. Underwood, D. F. Harman, K. L. Payne, D. A. Rathjen, S. Razziudin, S. R. Von Sturmer, and K. Vines (1983), *J. Endocr.* **98,** 323.

Swaab, D. F., C. W. Pool, and F. W. van Leeuwen (1977), *J. Histochem. Cytochem.* **25**, 388.

Talwar, G. P., S. Ramakrishnan, C. Das, S. K. Dubey, M. Salahuddin, N. Shastri, A. Tandon, and Om. Singh (1979), in *Recent Advances in Reproduction and Regulation of Fertility* (Talwar, G. P. ed.), Elsevier/North Holland Biomedical Press, Amsterdam, p. 453.

Tanaka, A. (1982), *Acta Obst. Gynaec. Jpn.* **34**, 579.

Tosi, R., N. Tanigaki, R. Sorrentino, R. Accolla, and G. Corte (1981), *Eur. J. Immunol.* **11**, 721.

Tubbs, R. R., M. E. Velasco, and S. P. Benjamin (1979), *Arch. Pathol. Lab. Med.* **103**, 534.

Vaitukaitis, J. L. (1979), in *Carcino-Embryonic Proteins: Chemistry, Biology, Clinical Applications,* Vol. 1 (Lehmann, F. G., ed.), Elsevier/North-Holland, New York, p. 447.

Vaitukaitis, J. L., G. D. Braunstein, G. T. Ross (1972), *Am. J. Obstet. Gynecol.* **113**, 751.

Wada, H.-G., R. J. Danisch, S. R. Baxter, M. M. Federici, R. C. Fraser, L. J. Brownmiller, and J. C. Lankford (1982), *Clin. Chem.* **28**, 1962.

Wahlstrom, T., U. H. Stenman, C. Lundqvist, P. Tanner, J. Schroder, and M. Seppala (1981), *J. Histochem. Cytochem.* **29**, 864.

Weintraub, B. D., S. W. Rosen, J. A. McCammon, and R. L. Perlman (1973), *Endocrinology* **92**, 1250.

Yoshimoto, Y., A. R. Wolfsen, F. Hirose, and W. D. Odell (1979), *Am. J. Obstet. Gynecol.* **134**, 729.

Chapter 5

Products of the Major Histocompatibility Complex on Tumor Cells

GERALD N. CALLAHAN

*Department of Pathology, Colorado State University, Fort Collins,
Colorado*

1. Introduction

The major histocompatibility complex (MHC) was originally defined as
that region of murine genome that contained the genes that determined
the fate of allografts (Gorer, 1938 and Gorer et al., 1948). A similar complex has since been identified in all mammalian species investigated. In
addition, it is now known that the MHC contains a variety of genes whose
products are intimately involved in the development and culmination of
most, if not all, immune responses.

The murine MHC is divided into four regions: K, I, S, and D, and
there is a related (but not currently included) region called Qa/Tla. The
Qa/Tla region is located telomeric to the murine MHC on chromosome
17, and contains many genes whose structures are highly homologous to
the structures of the genes coding for H-2K and D antigens. The Human
MHC also is composed of four regions: D, B, C, and A and is located on
the short arm of chromosome 6. In addition, a region corresponding to
the murine Qa/Tla has been identified in humans. Both the human and
murine MHCs occupy a sizeable portion of their respective chromosomes. However, the products of only a very few genes within the MHC
have been identified. Of these, only one gene in the K and D regions and
four genes in the I region of the murine MHC are known to generate products that are expressed on the cell surface. Similarly, only one gene in

97

each of the A, B, and C regions, and six genes in the D region of the human MHC are known to generate products that are expressed at the cell surface.

The products of these genes are glycoproteins that appear on the surface of certain populations of cells. Collectively, these molecules are called MHC antigens. This review will focus on the relationship and relevance of the expression of MHC antigens to the identification and characterization of malignant tissue, and the potential involvement of these cell surface glycoproteins in transformation and tumorigenesis.

The products of the K and D region of the murine MHC appear to be homologous to the products of the A, B, and C regions of the human MHC. Furthermore, it is known that both sets of molecules function similarly in human and murine immune responses. The products of the K and D region of the murine MHC are known as H-2 antigens, and the products of the A, B, and C region of the human MHC are known as HLA antigens. The structure and organization of human and murine MHC antigens as well as their corresponding genes has been recently reviewed by Hood et al. (1983), Kindt and Robinson (1984), Kaufman et al. (1984), Klein et al. (1983), and Klein (1982).

H-2 and HLA antigens are extremely polymorphic within their respective species and are expressed on all nucleated cells (Klein, 1979). These antigens are known to serve as primary targets for the destruction of allogeneic tissue and to perform critical functions in T cell-mediated lysis of virus-infected and tumor cells (Zinkernagel and Doherty, 1980). Both H-2 and HLA antigens are known to be composed of an invariant light chain (beta$_2$-microglobulin) of approximately 12,000 mol wt (which is not encoded within the MHC) and a heavy chain of approximately 44,000 mol wt (Coligan et al., 1981 and Strominger et al., 1980). It is the heavy chain of H-2 and HLA antigens that bears the allogeneic (variation within the species) determinants. These heavy chains are glycosylated and are noncovalently associated with the light chains on the cell surface. At present, the carbohydrate portions of the heavy chains appear to be unrelated to their alloantigenic properties. Only the heavy chains of H-2 and HLA antigens span the plasma membrane and are exposed to the cytoplasm. Collectively, antigens with these properties are known as class I MHC antigens.

The organization of the genes that encode H-2 and HLA antigens also are very similar. Genes for H-2 antigens are composed of eight exons. These exons correspond to the leader sequence, three extracellular domains, a transmembrane domain, and three cytoplasmic domains (Steinmetz et al., 1981). Genes for HLA antigens are very similar and differ only in that they contain two, rather than three, cytoplasmic exons (Malissen et al., 1982).

The genes that encode the various alleles of H-2 and HLA antigens exhibit regions with a high degree of variation (hypervariable regions) and regions of striking similarity (conserved regions) (Maloy and Coligan, 1982). It has been proposed that both allelic variation and homology among H-2 antigens result from the occurrence of gene conversion events that involve highly homologous genes located telomeric to the MHC (Qa/Tla) (Evans et al., 1982 and Lalanne et al., 1982). Recently, there have been several reports that have provided evidence for the operation of gene conversion in the generation of variability within the H-2 gene family (Evans et al., 1982; Lalanne et al., 1982; Weiss et al., 1983; and Mellor et al., 1983). At present, there is less support for the operation of gene conversion in the maintenance of H-2 gene homology.

Products coded for by genes of the I region of the murine MHC are very similar to products coded for by the genes of the D region of the human MHC. Also, both products function very similarly in the immune response. Products of the I region of the murine MHC and the D region of the human MHC are known to be essential to effective cell–cell interaction between macrophages and T cells and between T and B cells (reviewed by Schwartz, 1984). Because of this, the products of the I region of the MHC determine the range of antigens to which the individual is capable of responding.

The products of the I region of the murine MHC and the D region of the human MHC are referred to as murine Ia and human Ia antigens, respectively. In the mouse, there are at least two distinct sets of genes coding for Ia antigens, I-A and I-E (reviewed by Hood et al., 1983). In humans, there are at least three distinct sets of genes coding for Ia antigens, DR, DC (DS, MB), and SB (reviewed by Kaufman et al., 1984). Both human and murine Ia antigens are serologically polymorphic and appear only on certain populations of cells, most notably, macrophages and B lymphoid cells.

Each of the human and murine Ia antigens is encoded by two genes. Both of these genes are located within the MHC. One gene codes for a relatively invariant heavy, or alpha-chain of approximately 34,000 mol wt. The other gene codes for a polymorphic light, or beta-chain of approximately 29,000 mol wt. At the cell surface, both the alpha- and beta-chains are glycosylated and noncovalently associated. Both the alpha- and beta-chains of human and murine Ia antigens span the plasma membrane. Collectively, antigens of this type are known as class II MHC antigens (reviewed by Kaufman et al., 1984).

The genetics of Ia antigens is not currently as well defined as is the genetics of HLA and H-2 antigens. However, several important facts are currently known about the structure of the genes for human and murine Ia antigens. The genes for Ia antigen alpha- and beta-chains exhibit variable and conserved regions of structure (Kaufman et al., 1984 and Benoist et al., 1983). Beta-chain genes are composed of six exons corresponding to the leader sequence, the beta-1 and beta-2 domains, a transmembrane domain, and two cytoplasmic domains (Larhammar et al., 1983). Alpha-chain genes appear to be composed of four exons corresponding to the leader sequence, the alpha-1, alpha-2, transmembrane, and one cytoplasmic domain (Kaufman et al., 1984). The general arrangement and structure of the genes for Ia antigens are similar in mice and humans (Kindt et al., 1984 and Larhamar et al., 1983). It has been proposed that homology has been maintained and diversity generated among class II MHC antigens (like class I MHC antigens) by gene conversion events.

H-2, HLA, and Ia antigens on tumor cells will be the subject of this review. There is now clear evidence that the host animal is frequently capable of mounting an immune response against tumor cells (Hellstrom and Hellstrom, 1969). However, it is equally clear tha this immune response is most often inadequate to eliminate the transformed cells and prevent the host's eventual death. At present, there is no apparent explanation for the frequent absence or inadequacy of the host's immune response to tumor cells. However, because of the involvement of products of MHC genes in the immune response, it has been theorized that altered expression of these cell surface molecules might be the cause for some of the aspects of the abnormal host immune response to tumor cells. As a result, a great deal of attention has been focused on quantitative and qualitative aspects of MHC antigen expression by tumor cells.

In this report we will attempt to review currently available data that is relevant to possible relationships between the expression of MHC antigens (normal and abnormal) and neoplasia. However, since some aspects of this work have been recently reviewed (Callahan et al.; 1978, Forman, 1980; and Parmiani et al., 1979), we will attempt to review only those data that were not covered by others. Furthermore, the use of monoclonal antibodies for the detection, quantitation, and characterization of MHC antigens on tumor cells has only recently become a widespread practice. Therefore, we also will attempt to identify and evaluate the contribution of this technology to current understanding of the importance of MHC antigen expression to host–tumor interactions. This review is not intended to be exhaustive, but rather will focus on work carried out in the author's laboratory and related work by other researchers.

2. Variable Expression of MHC Antigens by Tumor Cells

Much of what is presently known concerning the surfaces of tumor cells is based on work carried out with tumor cells maintained in vitro. Recently, however, it has been demonstrated that the surface phenotype of some tumor cells varies significantly in response to environmental factors. Work in this area has been greatly accelerated by the availability of monoclonal antibodies. These reagents have allowed for a more precise characterization of both quantitative and qualitative changes in surface antigen expression by tumor cells. As a result, it is now evident that some tumor cells are capable of significantly altering their MHC antigen phenotype in response to environment.

2.1. Inducible MHC Antigens on Murine Tumor Cells

Variations in MHC antigen expression has been most extensively investigated in the murine system. This is because of the availability of inbred strains of mice, the opportunity to characterize the properties of murine tumor cells grown in vitro and in vivo, and the availability of very specific monoclonal reagents for the characterization of these tumor cells. As a result, much more information is currently available on MHC antigen expression by murine tumor cells. Therefore, we will first present data obtained in this system, and later we will compare it with data obtained in the human system. In the murine system, it is now known that tumor cells may exhibit reversible, quantitative variations in H-2 and/or Ia antigen expression.

2.1.1. Variable H-2 and Ia Antigen Expression by Murine Tumor Cells

There have been several recent reports demonstrating that murine tumor cells show marked increases in levels of H-2 and Ia antigen expression in response to soluble factors (particularly gamma-interferon) produced during an immune response. King and Jones (1983), as well as Walker et al. (1982) have shown that WEHI 3 cells (a cell line derived from a murine macrophage tumor that is Ia antigen-negative under normal in vitro conditions) become strongly Ia antigen-positive when cultured with supernatants derived from concanavalin A (Con A)-stimulated normal spleen cells. Following such treatment, WEHI 3 cells express high levels of both I-A and I-E antigens. In addition, exposure to supernatants from Con A-stimulated spleen cells causes WEHI 3 cells to express much higher levels of H-2 antigens. This effect, however, appears to be limited to the H-2K antigens of this cell line.

King and Jones (1983) also have demonstrated that purified gamma-interferon is capable of stimulating Ia antigen expression and increased levels of H-2 antigen expression on WEHI 3 cells. Since supernatants derived from Con A-stimulated spleen cells contain gamma-interferon (from activated T cells), it is presumably this factor alone that stimulates MHC antigen expression by WEHI 3 cells. This has not, however, been conclusively demonstrated, and there is some evidence (see below) that other factors produced during an immune response may have similar effects.

Mathis et al. (1983) have shown that gamma-interferon-induced Ia antigen expression by WEHI 3 cells results from modification of the control of translation of the genes for Ia antigens. These authors have demonstrated that detectable levels of Ia antigen-specific mRNA are absent in untreated WEHI 3 cells, but are readily apparent after exposure of these cells to gamma-interferon.

At present, the relevance of these observations to host–tumor interactions involving WEHI 3 cells, is unclear. However, Walker et al. (1982) have shown that when WEHI 3 cells become Ia antigen-positive, they also acquire the ability to function as accessory cells in antigen presentation. It is, therefore, clear that the ability of WEHI 3 cells to alter their cell-surface phenotype in response to environmental factors might have pronounced effects on the host's response to the tumor.

The ability to differentially express Ia antigens is not a property of tumor cells only. There have been several reports (Beller et al., 1980; Scher, 1980; Beller and Unanue, 1981; Steeg et al., 1980; and Beller and Unanue, 1982) demonstrating that normal macrophages (which do not ordinarily express detectable levels of Ia antigens) also express Ia antigens and much higher levels of H-2 antigens in response to gamma-interferon. In addition, these cells concomitantly acquire Ia antigens and the ability to function in antigen presentation (Calamai et al., 1982 and Steinman et al., 1980). Under normal conditions, the source of gamma-interferon in vivo is antigen-stimulated T cells, and it is believed that gamma-interferon-stimulated activation of macrophages allows for an important, if not essential, amplification of the immune response. This finding emphasizes the importance of variable Ia antigen expression by normal cells and suggests its potential relevance to the host-immune response to tumor.

The evidence that normal macrophages behave much like macrophage-derived tumor cells in relation to their Ia antigen phenotype suggests that the ability to regulate surface antigen expression is not specifically related to malignant cells. However, there are reports that demonstrate that tumor cells that are not derived from macrophages also are capable of altering their Ia antigen phenotype. Furthermore, there is no clear evidence that the normal cell counterparts of these tumors ever share the ability to regulate surface expression of Ia antigens.

Wong et al. (1983) have reported that some B lymphoid and myeloid tumors of mice show enhanced expression of Ia antigens in response to gamma-interferon, and these authors allude to data that suggest that this ability may be shared with epithelial, hematopoietic, fibroblastoid, and neuronal cell lines.

In addition, there is evidence that factors other than gamma-interferon are capable of stimulating Ia and H-2 antigen expression on some tumor cells. Such factors are not currently known to have any effect on normal cells.

We have recently reported on two such tumors, an N-ethyl-N-nitrosourea-induced alveoligenic adenocarcinoma of C3Hf mice (LT-85) and an ultraviolet light-induced fibrosarcoma of C3H mice (1053) (Callahan, 1984). Both of these tumors exhibited significant changes in their levels of MHC antigen expression in response to a soluble factor that was not gamma-interferon.

Neither LT-85 nor 1053 cells express detectable levels of Ia antigens when maintained in vitro. In addition, both cell types express relatively low levels of H-2 antigens. However, when LT-85 cells are maintained as a subcutaneous tumor in C3H mice they express I-A, I-E, and H-2K antigens in amounts comparable to normal lymphoid cells. As with WEHI 3 cells, the observed stimulation of MHC antigen expression on LT-85 cells had less effect on H-2D than H-2K antigens.

The Ia and H-2 antigens detected on these LT-85 tumors did not derive from the host animal since tumors grown in F1 animals expressed MHC antigens of the host haplotype only. Furthermore, cloned tumor cells behaved identically to uncloned tumor cells. Therefore, the appearance of Ia antigen-positive LT-85 cells in vivo did not result from selection of an antigen-positive subpopulation of tumor cells, but arose by phenotypic conversion of Ia antigen-negative tumor cells.

Phenotypic conversion of LT-85 cells could also be induced in vitro. When LT-85 cells were cocultured with spleen cells obtained from tumor-bearing mice, the tumor cells expressed high levels of Ia antigens. However, in vitro, there was no apparent increase in the levels of H-2 antigens expressed by LT-85 cells. Only spleen cells undergoing an immune response were capable of inducing phenotypic conversion of the LT-85 cells in vitro, and supernatants derived from such spleen cells were as effective as the cells themselves in inducing Ia antigen expression by the LT-85 cells. It was thus apparent that LT-85 tumor cells were induced to express Ia antigens in vitro in response to a soluble factor (or factors) produced by spleen cells undergoing an immune response.

The ability to undergo phenotypic conversion in vitro was not unique to LT-85 tumor cells. 1053 cells, derived from an ultraviolet light-induced fibrosarcoma of C3H mice, also were induced to express Ia antigens, apparently by the same factors that stimulated Ia antigen expression by LT-85 cells.

It, therefore, appeared that other tumor cells, which were not of macrophage origin, shared with WEHI 3 cells the ability to differentially express Ia antigens in response to environmental factors. Closer examination, however, revealed several significant differences in the mechanism by which LT-85 (and 1053) cells and WEHI 3 cells were induced to express Ia antigens.

Supernatants obtained from Con A-stimulated spleen cells induced Ia antigen expression and increased levels of H-2 antigen expression by WEHI 3 cells. These same supernatants induced increased levels of H-2 antigen expression by LT-85 and 1053 cells, but did not induce Ia antigen expression by these tumor cells. Similarly, purified human gamma-interferon induced Ia antigen expression and increased levels of detectable H-2 antigens on WEHI 3 cells, but stimulated only increased levels of H-2 antigens on LT-85 and 1053 cells.

In contrast, supernatants derived from cultures of spleen cells from LT-85 tumor-bearing mice induced Ia antigen expression (but had no effect on H-2 antigen expression) by LT-85 and 1053 cells, but these same supernatants had no effect on Ia antigen expression by WEHI 3 cells. Furthermore, supernatants derived from Con A-stimulated, T cell-depleted spleen cells did not induce expression of Ia antigens or increased levels of H-2 antigens on WEHI 3 cells. However, depletion of T cells from spleen cells obtained from LT-85 tumor-bearing mice did not significantly affect the ability of these cells, or supernatants derived from them, to stimulate Ia antigen expression by LT-85 and 1053 tumor cells. T cell-depleted spleen cells from tumor-bearing mice did not, however, stimulate increased levels of H-2 antigen expression by LT-85 and 1053 tumor cells.

Finally, we observed that LT-85 cells grown in vivo expressed Ia antigens and increased levels of H-2 antigens, whereas LT-85 cells co-cultured in vitro with immune spleen cells expressed Ia antigens, but did not differ significantly from untreated controls in levels of H-2 antigen expression. No similar differences have been reported between in vitro- and in vivo-stimulated WEHI 3 cells.

On the basis of these results it appears that both WEHI 3 and LT-85 tumor cells are induced to express increased levels of H-2 antigens by gamma-interferon produced by T cells during an immune response. However, the soluble factor that is responsible for the induction of Ia antigens on WEHI 3 cells (most probably gamma-interferon) is not involved in the induction of Ia antigens on LT-85 and 1053 tumor cells. Furthermore, it appears that the soluble factor that induces Ia antigen expression on LT-85 and 1053 tumor cells is not even derived from T cells.

It is, therefore, clear that tumor cells that are not derived from macrophages or lymphoid cells may be induced to express Ia antigens by factors produced by the tumor-bearing host. It is equally clear that some of these tumors do so in response to factors other than gamma-interferon. It is not at present known whether this property is unique to these tumor cells, or is also exhibited by autologous normal cells at some point during differentiation. Several recent reports have provided evidence that some epithelial cells (not previously believed capable of expressing Ia antigens) can be induced to express Ia antigens in response to soluble factors (in most cases gamma-interferon) produced during an immune response (Daynes et al., 1983; Barclay and Mason, 1982; and de Waal et al., 1983). Currently, the relationship between these observations and those made with tumor cells is unknown.

Regardless of whether the ability to differentially express Ia antigens is unique to certain tumor cells or shared with autologous normal cells, our findings demonstrate that at least two mechanisms exist for inducing Ia antigens on tumor cells.

It is not presently clear what effects the expression of Ia antigens by tumor cells may have on host–tumor interactions. As mentioned earlier, it has been clearly shown that macrophages and macrophage-derived tumor cell lines possess the ability to function in antigen presentation only when they express Ia antigens. The ability of tumor cells to function in antigen presentation could significantly affect the tumor-bearing host's ability to mount an antitumor immune response. However, it has not yet been established that any tumor cell not derived from a macrophage can function in antigen presentation, whether or not they express Ia antigens. We have recently obtained one indirect piece of evidence that suggests that LT-85 cells might be capable of functioning in antigen presentation.

It is known that macrophages have two properties that allow them to function in antigen presentation (DeFreitas et al., 1983). First, they can be stimulated to express Ia antigens by factors produced during an immune response. We have already shown that LT-85 cells share this property with macrophages. Second, effective antigen presentation requires that macrophages produce a factor (interleukin I) that stimulates T-cell division. Very recently, we have found that LT-85 cells secrete a factor that stimulates lymphoid cell growth and division. However, we do not yet know which lymphoid cell population is the target for this growth factor. Our observations suggests that in some important ways, LT-85 cells, at least superficially, resemble macrophages, and, thus, might be capable of functioning in antigen presentation.

If, in fact, the ability of some transformed cells confers on them properties similar to those reported for macrophages (especially the capacity to function in antigen presentation), then it might be predicted that such cells would be significantly less likely to develop into tumors.

In consideration of this, it is important to note that both the LT-85 (induced transplacentally) and 1053 (induced with ultraviolet light) arose in immunoincompetent mice. It might be that the immunological state of these mice allowed for the progressive growth of transformed cells that might not generate tumors in normal mice. In support of this, it has been observed that neither tumor grows well in syngeneic normal mice.

However, the possibility cannot be completely ruled out that the ability to express Ia antigens might confer some selective advantage on the tumor, and the precise relevance of tumor cell Ia antigens to the host immune response remains to be established.

There is more direct evidence for the involvement of inducible H-2 antigens in the process of tumorigenesis and the host immune response. Ostrand-Rosenberg and Cohn (1981) have shown that some teratocarcinoma cells (which are H-2 antigen negative in vitro) can be induced by host lymphoid cells to express H-2 antigens. Furthermore, these investigators have demonstrated that at least one of these cell lines, 402AX, becomes H-2 antigen-positive in resistant hosts, but remains H-2 antigen-negative in susceptible hosts. They propose that in the absence of H-2 antigens, effective T-cell-mediated lysis of tumor cells cannot occur, and, thus, H-2 antigen-negative tumors cannot be as readily controlled by the host immune system.

2.2. Inducible MHC Antigens on Human Tumors

There also have been reports of human tumor cells that are capable of differentially expressing MHC antigens. Daar et al. (1982) found that approximately 50% of the colorectal cancers they examined were Ia antigen positive, whereas they and others have been unable to demonstrate Ia antigens on normal colorectal epithelium. Also, Basham et al. (1982) have shown that HLA synthesis by melanoma cells is markedly increased by interferon.

Furthermore, Fellous et al. (1982) have shown that interferon induces increased expression of HLA antigens by human fibroblasts and lymphoblastoid cell lines. Using a cDNA probe specific for HLA-A, B, and C antigens, they found that beta- and to a lesser extent alpha-interferon induced a significant increase in HLA-specific mRNA and HLA antigen expression by several Burkitt's lymphoma-derived cell lines and normal foreskin-derived fibroblasts. The effects of exposure to inteferon varied quantitatively from cell line to cell line. This same treatment had little or no effect on the levels of Ia-specific mRNA or the cell surface expression of Ia antigens in these cell lines.

It is, therefore, apparent that some human tumor cells can alter their cell surface complement of MHC antigens in a manner that seems to resemble that described for murine tumor cells.

2.3. Implications for Human Tumor Immunology

It is clear that the relevance of variation in MHC antigen expression by murine tumor cells to the host immune response and tumorigenesis are not yet well defined. However, because of the frequency of the reported observations, and the apparent effects of tumor cell MHC antigens on the host immune response in some systems, it would seem that more extensive investigations for similar changes in human tumor cell MHC antigens are warranted.

Furthermore, it is apparent from studies carried out in the murine system that in vitro characterization by itself is inadequate to obtain an accurate picture of the tumor cell membrane *in situ*. Most characterizations of the surface properties of human tumors have been based on observations made using in vitro-maintained cell lines. In the absence of more precise information about the properties of the surfaces of these tumor cells *in situ*, it will clearly be impossible to gain a full understanding of events that occur at the primary host–tumor interface (the tumor cell plasma membrane), and these events are of major importance to the generation of an effective immune response by the host and to the process of tumorigenesis. Finally, it is essential that an accurate picture of the tumor cell membrane *in situ* be obtained before we can fully evaluate the potential of tumor cell surface structures for immunodiagnosis and immunotherapy. It is now apparent that such characterizations cannot rely solely on data generated from in vitro studies.

3. Abnormal Expression of MHC Antigens by Tumor Cells

In addition to variable MHC antigen expression, it has been reported that some tumor cells exhibit permanent quantitative and qualitative changes in their MHC antigen phenotype.

3.1. Abnormal Expression of MHC Antigens on Murine Tumor Cells

Most of the work that has been carried out on qualitative and quantitative changes in tumor cell MHC antigen expression has been performed using the murine system. Therefore, we will initially concentrate on the significance of data derived from these systems. Later, we will discuss the potential relevance of these findings to human tumor immunology.

3.1.1. Quantitative Variations in MHC Antigen Expression by Murine Tumor Cells

Class II MHC (Ia) antigens are expressed only on a limited population of normal cells. In addition, the precise mechanisms by which these molecules accomplish their immunological functions are poorly understood. Because of these facts, simple quantitative variations, or the complete absence of class II MHC antigens on tumor cells (especially those derived from cells with no established immune function), are of questionable relevance to tumor immunology.

Class I MHC antigens, on the other hand, are expressed on all normal nucleated cells. In addition, it is known that normal T cell-mediated destruction of virus-infected and tumor cells requires that the target and effector cells be syngeneic for at least one class I MHC antigen (reviewed by Sachs, 1984). This requirement derives from the necessity for activated T cells to recognize both self MHC and foreign antigens before they can effectively lyse the target cell.

Because of the implied importance of class I MHC antigens to normal cell function, and their demonstrated importance in T cell-mediated lysis of virus-infected and tumor cells, it is of considerable interest to determine the levels of class I MHC antigen expression on tumor cells.

One of the earliest reports of variations in the levels of H-2 antigens on tumor cells was by Haywood and McCahan (1971). These workers found an apparent inverse relationship between the levels of expression of tumor- or virus-associated antigens and H-2 antigens on tumor cells in culture. Since that time, there have been many additional reports of the absence or diminished expression of H-2 antigens on tumor cells. However, only recently has it become possible to correlate H-2 expression with the efficiency of T cell-mediated lysis of tumor cells and the process of tumorigenesis. In addition, the availability of monoclonal antibodies to MHC antigens has recently made it possible to much more accurately measure the levels of expression of MHC antigens on tumor cells. As a result, many of the potential problems that made much of the early data equivocal can now be entirely avoided.

We previously described (Callahan and Allison, 1978) an estrogen-induced lymphoma of C3H mice that had apparently ceased to express the H-2K^k gene product. However, careful examination of these tumor cells revealed that H-2K^k antigens were expressed at the cell surface, but, because of an apparent association with other surface molecules, they were not accessible to antibody or, presumably, the T-cell receptor.

While these observations may have been relevant to this host-tumor system, they did not result from the absence of any H-2 antigen. Therefore, it is possible that the apparent absence of H-2 antigens on some tumor cells may result from inaccessibility of the antigens rather than their actual absence.

Other investigators have clearly demonstrated that some tumor cells do not express the complement of H-2 antigens that are expressed by autologous normal cells. Schmidt and coworkers (1979, 1981, and Testorelli et al., 1980) have described several leukemias in both BALB.K and C3H mice that do not express H-2K^k antigens, whereas autologous normal tissues do. The absence of H-2K^k antigens on these tumor cells was demonstrated by the lack of reactivity of specific mono- and polyclonal antibodies with intact tumor cells and detergent extracts of the same cells. It was further shown that because of the lack of H-2K^k antigens, these leukemic cells were not susceptible to lysis by H-2K^k-restricted T cells. Similarly, Plata et al. (1981) also have demonstrated that some gross virus-induced tumors of mice showed marked quantitative variations in H-2 antigen expression, and that these variations correlated with the susceptibility of the tumor cells to lysis by antiviral T cells.

In the above-described report, the bases for the absence of cell surface H-2 antigens were not determined. It is known that the absence of either beta$_2$-microglobulin or the H-2 antigen heavy chain will prevent the cell surface expression of H-2 antigens. It is, therefore, possible that a defect in, or absence of, the translation of either gene could be responsible for the observed absence of H-2 gene products.

However, it seems unlikely in the instances mentioned above that the absence of the H-2 antigens was due to inadequate translation of the beta$_2$-microglobulin gene. In these reports, quantiative variations were apparent in the products of one H-2 locus only. In each instance the produces of other H-2 loci appeared to be expressed normally. Since translation of the beta$_2$-microglobulin gene is required for the expression of all class I MHC antigens, it seems improbable that altered expression of beta$_2$-microglobulin was responsible for the absence of certain H-2 antigens on these tumor cells. Data more directly relating to the bases for the loss of H-2 antigens by tumor cells has been obtained using SV40-transformed mouse cells.

Transformation of murine cells with SV40 has been found to generate some tumors that no longer express all of the H-2 antigens found on autologous normal cells. Using this system, Rogers et al. (1983) found that tumor cells that lacked H-2K^k antigens were more tumorigenic than tumor cells that expressed the normal complement of these antigens. Also, these authors were able to obtain evidence that strongly suggested that the absence of the H-2K locus gene product on these tumor cells was attributable to alterations in the DNA encoding the H-2K^k antigen heavy chain.

Similarly, it has been found that rat cells transformed by highly oncogenic adenovirus 12 cease to express MHC class I antigens (Schrier et al., 1983). It is not presently known how this virus exerts its effects on class I antigens.

In addition, it has been known for some time that embryonal carcinoma cells do not express H-2 antigens (Edidin et al., 1974 and Artz and Jacob, 1974). Recently, evidence has been provided that these cells do not express detectable levels of H-2 antigens because of limited translation of the genes for both the H-2 antigen heavy chain and beta$_2$-microglobulin (Morello et al., 1982). Further evidence that the defect in these cells resides at the level of translation is provided by experiments that demonstrate that under appropriate conditions some embryonal carcinoma cells can be induced to express H-2 antigens (Ostrand-Rosenberg et al., 1983). It is also interesting to note that embryonal carcinoma cells that have the ability to express H-2 antigens in response to external stimuli appear to be less tumorigenic than similar cells that lack this ability (Ostrand-Rosenberg and Cohn, 1981).

Therefore, tumor cells may cease to express H-2 antigens because of alterations in the DNA encoding the H-2 heavy chain, or because of inadequate translation of either the H-2 heavy chain or beta$_2$-microglobulin genes. It is not, at present, clear which of these (or other) mechanisms may operate most frequently to generate genetic or epigenetic changes that diminish or block the ability of tumor cells to express H-2 antigens. Regardless of the underlying mechanisms, the available evidence suggests that quantitative changes in H-2 antigen expression by tumor cells may markedly affect the ability of the host to mount an effective immune response, and, therefore, significantly enhance the tumorigenic capacity of some transformed cells.

Support for this hypothesis has been provided by the findings of Bernards et al. (1983). These authors have obtained evidence that the oncogenicity of adenovirus 12-transformed rat cells is directly related to the absence of class I MHC antigens on these cells. Furthermore, they have demonstrated that the absence of class I MHC antigens on adenovirus 12-induced tumors significantly interfered with the ability of the host to generate tumor-specific cytotoxic T cells.

All of these findings are very suggestive of a highly important role for H-2 antigens on tumor cells. However, the general relevance of these phenomena to tumor immunology is not yet established. This can be fully evaluated only after more systematic studies have been undertaken to determine frequency of reduced levels of expression or absence of Class I MHC antigens on tumor cells.

3.1.2. Biochemical Changes in MHC Antigens on Murine Tumor Cells

It has also been reported that some tumor cells express MHC antigens that are chemically and immunologically distinct from those expressed on autologous normal cells. Several laboratories have reported finding "alien" or allogeneic MHC antigens on tumor cells (for review, *see* Parmiani et al., 1979). However, much of the early work in this area suffered from the lack of specific monoclonal reagents, and therefore, the significance of much of this data is unclear.

The availability of monoclonal antibodies to MHC antigens has greatly facilitated a more precise identification and characterization of MHC antigens on tumor cells. Because of this, many of the problems encountered during earlier investigations have been avoided. There are now several reports of the expression by tumor cells of MHC antigens that are chemically distinct from those present on autologous normal tissue. However, there is presently no convincing evidence that tumor cells possess the ability to express previously defined allogenic MHC antigens, and there is evidence to the contrary.

We will confine this portion of our review to investigations that have made use of very specific reagents and genetically well-defined tumor systems. In the absence of either monoclonal reagents or genetically cha racterized tumors, it is very difficult to interpret reports of the apparent expression of altered MHC antigens by tumor cells.

Martin et al. (1977) have described several transplacentally induced lung tumors of C3HfB mice that were immunologically cross-reactive with ancestral C3H mice and immunologically distinct from parental C3HfB mice. One of these tumors, LT-85, was found to grow progressively in C3H mice, but was rapidly rejected by C3HfB mice. At the time this work was carried out, the C3H and C3HfB mouse strains were thought to be syngeneic, since they were derived from a common ancestor (Martin et al., 1977). However, Imamura et al. (1979) found that a full range of immunological response could be generated beween C3H and C3HfB mice. We have since demonstrated that the amino acid sequence of the H-2K^k antigens of these two strains of mice are different (Callahan et al., 1981 and 1982). No differences were detectable in the I-A, I-E, or H-2D antigens of C3H and C3HfB mice. It, thus appeared that a mutation had arisen in C3HfB mice which resulted in the expression of H-2K locus gene product chemically distinct from that found on ancestral C3H mice.

The immunological and growth properties of the LT-85 tumor suggested that these cells, either as the result of a genetic reversion or some other mechanism, expressed H-2K^k antigens identical to those expressed by allogeneic C3H mice. However, detailed biochemical characterization of the H-2K^k antigens of LT-85 tumor cells revealed that their H-2K^k antigens were chemically distinct from those of both C3HfB and C3H mice (Callahan et al., 1983). These differences were confined to the amino acid sequence of LT-85 H-2K antigens. Therefore, although the changes in the K locus gene of LT-85 cells generated a molecule that immunologically mimicked an alloantigen, the H-2K^k antigen of LT-85 cells was not obviously related to any previously defined alloantigen.

Closer examination of the peptide map patterns of the H-2K^k antigens of C3HfB, C3H, and LT-85 cells revealed that some portions of the H-2K molecule of LT-85 cells were identical to ancestral C3H H-2K^k antigens, whereas others were identical to the H-2K^k antigens of syngeneic C3HfB mice (Callahan et al., 1983). Extensive isoenzyme and restriction endonuclease analyses indicated that the LT-85 tumor was derived from C3HfB mice, and that it was not contaminated by allogeneic cells (Callahan et al., 1983).

The simplest explanation for these observations is that a gene conversion event had occurred concurrently with, or shortly after, malignant transformation of the cells from which the LT-85 tumor was derived. Such a gene conversion event might have made use of genetic material in the Qa/T1a region telomeric to the murine MHC (much of which appears not to be expressed by normal tissues) to alter or correct a portion of the sequence of the mutant H-2K gene, and, thus, generate a molecule which in part more nearly resembled similar molecules on ancestral C3H cells and differed from those of the mutant C3Hf mice from which the tumor was derived.

There are now several reports that suggest that similar gene conversion events, employing genetic material in the Qa/T1a region, operate to generate diversity within the H-2 family. However, our observations provide evidence that gene conversion may also operate to maintain homology between H-2 genes. The immunological similarity between LT-85 and other tumors that were similarly induced (mentioned above) suggests that this phenomenon is not unique to the LT-85 tumor.

Very recently, another report has appeared that suggests that many tumor cells may make use of DNA that is related to genes of the MHC, but is not expressed in normal tissues.

Brickell et al. (1983) recently reported that a cDNA clone that encodes a Qa/T1a class I MHC antigen could be used to detect a mRNA species that was present in elevated amounts in all tumor cells examined. They interpreted these data as evidence that genes similar to class I MHC antigens present in the Qa/T1a region of chromosome 17 (which are apparently not expressed by normal mature cells) were expressed in significant amounts by many tumor cells.

There is no evidence currently available that argues against this interpretation. However, the results that these investigators obtained could also result from gene conversion within the MHC of the tumor cells. The authors measured the appearance in the tumor cells of mRNA that hybridized with a cDNA probe derived from the Qa/T1a region of chromosome 17. They interpreted the appearance of this mRNA as evidence for expression of the gene corresponding to their cDNA probe. mRNA that would hybridize with their cDNA probe could, however, also have been generated by a gene conversion event involving DNA in the Qa/T1a region. Further experimentation will be required to fully elucidate the mechanism responsible for the generation of the mRNA observed by these investigators. However, it seems clear from our and their work that tumor cells may make use of normally untranslated DNA to generate and express MHC antigens not found on autologous normal tissue.

Although the importance of these observations to MHC antigen genetics are obvious, their relevance to tumor immunology or tumorigenesis is not completely clear. In the case of the LT-85 tumor, the available evidence suggests that it is the modified H-2K^k antigen that is responsible for rejection of the tumor by syngeneic animals. Furthermore, it is apparent that changes similar to those that have taken place in LT-85 H-2K^k antigens might be responsible for some reports of the appearance of apparently allogeneic, or "alien," antigens on tumor cells. Our data, however, demonstrate that the H-2K^k antigens on LT-85 tumor cells are not classical alloantigens, and suggest that fortuitous cross-reactions (resulting from homology among H-2 and "H-2-like" antigens) are the bases for the apparent expression of allogeneic H-2 antigens on tumor cells.

It is also possible that tumor cells expressing altered H-2 antigens are less susceptible to lysis by host T cells. This would obviously enhance the tumorigenic properties of such cells. Chapdelaine et al. (1981) have recently presented evidence that supports this hypothesis. They have shown that H-2 mutant cell lines infected with Moloney sarcoma virus are much less susceptible to lysis by nonmutant parental virus-specific T cells than are nonmutant parental virus-infected target cells. They also demonstrated that this observation was not due to inaccessibility of the H-2 antigens at the cell surface. It is, therefore, possible that transformed cells that express altered H-2 antigens might have significantly greater likelihood of developing into tumors. However, it is clear that if this is the basis of the tumorigenicity of some transformed cells, then for reasons that are not presently understood, these antigens must not be recognized by the primary host as allogeneic histocompatibility antigens.

Brickell et al. (1983) have suggested that their findings may explain the basis for the potent NK cell activity against embryonal carcinoma cells as well as SV40 and methylcholanthrene-transformed cells. It has been proposed that NK cell activity toward embryonal carcinoma cells is actually directed against the cell surface antigens Gt-1 and/or Gt-2 (Shedlovsky et al., 1981 and Stern et al., 1980). In addition, it has been reported that some degree of cross-reactivity can be demonstrated between embryonal carcinoma cells, SV40-transformed cells, and methylcholanthrene-transformed cells (Castro et al., 1974; Medawar and Hunt, 1978; Sikora et al., 1977; and Medawar, 1974).

Brickell et al. (1983) have proposed that Gt-1 and/or Gt-2 antigens are encoded by genes in the Qa/T1a region of chromosome 17, and that the cDNA probe they have prepared contains this gene. Their findings could then be interpreted as a demonstration of the expression of this gene in the varying tumors and would provide a basis for the cross-reactivity of these tumors and their susceptibility to the action of NK cells. Our findings with the LT-85 tumor also may be relevant to these considerations. However, very little is presently known about the role of NK cells in immunity to the LT-85 tumor.

3.1.3. Implications for Human Tumor Immunology

It is clear, from the above discussion, that recent observations concerning the expression of MHC antigens by tumor cells may shed some light on the bases for previous observations concerning allogeneic H-2 antigens on tumor cells and about NK cell activity against some tumors. However, the relevance of these observations to host-tumor interactions in the primary host remains unclear.

There is considerable evidence that NK cells play a major role in the immune response against certain types of human tumors (Herberman, 1980). Because of observations made with murine tumors (described above), it would seem that investigations into the MHC antigenic profiles of human tumors susceptible to NK cell activity are warranted, and might provide some insight into the bases of their susceptibility. Furthermore, the studies described above suggest that our understanding of the involvement of MHC antigens in human tumor immunology would benefit significantly from an in-depth characterization of both the quantitative and biochemical aspects of MHC antigen expression by human tumors. This is particularly true in light of the critical function of MHC antigens in several immune phenomena, including T cell-mediated destruction of tumor cells.

3.2. Abnormal Expression of MHC Antigens on Human Tumor Cells

Considerably less evidence is currently available concerning the nature of MHC antigen expression by human tumor cells. This is due in large part to the difficulties inherent in working with outbred individuals. In addition, investigations into human tumor systems have been hampered by the fact that is has only recently become possible to carry out comparative studies on cell lines established from both malignant and normal tissue derived from the same individual. Nevertheless, there are several reports which suggest that MHC antigen expression by human tumor cells may differ significantly from that observed on normal cells.

3.2.1. Quantitative and Qualitative Variation in MHC Antigen Expression by Human Tumor Cells

Lampson et al. (1983) have reported that some cell lines derived from highly malignant neuroblastomas do not express HLA antigens. Their data indicate that this absence of HLA antigens is due to lack of expression of the HLA antigen heavy chain. $Beta_2$-microglobulin appears to be synthesized normally in these cell lines. Like others, because of the involvement of HLA antigens in T cell-mediated destruction of tumor cells, they have proposed that the absence of HLA antigens on these tumor cells may facilitate their escape from the host immune system, and, thus, render these cells much more tumorigenic. Direct evidence for a relationship between HLA antigen expression and tumorigenicity in this or other systems is, however, not yet available.

There also have been several reports of the expression of apparently inappropriate MHC antigens by human tumor cells. Recently, Claas and van Stenbrugge (1983) described a cell line derived from a prostatic adenocarcinoma that apparently expressed allotypic HLA antigens that were absent from peripheral blood lymphocytes derived from the same patient. However, they presented no evidence which ruled out allogeneic contamination of their tumor cells (a problem that has been shown to be the basis for many reports of allogeneic antigens on tumor cells) (Robinson et al., 1981) and of necessity used polyclonal reagents for their analyses. As a result, the significance of their observations is unclear.

Also very recently, it has been shown that cross-reactivity between HLA antigens and viral components results in the apparent expression of inappropriate HLA antigens by some tumor cells. Mann et al. (1983) have reported that some tumor cell lines that produce human T cell lymphoma virus also expressed HLA-A and B specificities that were not found on EBV-transformed B cells or peripheral blood lymphocytes from the same patients. These authors concluded that their observations might arise from cross-reactivity between some HLA antigens and components of the human T cell lymphoma virus. This possibility was strongly supported by the findings of Clarke et al. (1983). These investigators have reported that a high degree of homology exists in the sequences of the envelope gene region of the human T cell lymphoma genome and a region of an HLA-B gene. This homology suggests that antibody directed toward either of the two molecules might cross-react with the other, and most probably explains the apparent expression of allogeneic HLA antigens by cell lines infected with and producing the human T cell lymphoma virus.

A variety of other investigations designed to characterize the HLA antigen phenotype of tumor cells have failed to reveal any differences between human tumor cells and syngeneic normal cells. However, most of this work has been based solely on serological characterization of the cells and cell lines. Recently, several investigations have demonstrated that serological identity does not imply genetic identity (Biddison et al., 1982; Arden et al., 1982; and Owerbach et al., 1983). Also, we were unable to detect any serological differences between the MHC antigens of the C3HfB-derived LT-85 tumor and C3HfB or C3H mice. Immunological and biochemical characterization (described above), however, revealed very significant differences in the H-2K locus gene product of these cells. It, therefore, appears that serological characterization alone is inadequate to fully describe the MHC antigen phenotype of tumor cells, and that significant differences might exist between normal and tumor cells that are serologically "invisible."

Very recently, we have completed a biochemical characterization of the HLA antigens of a lung adenocarcinoma (P3) and autologous EBV-transformed lymphoid cells (PL3). There is no known serological difference between these cells. Biochemical characterization of their HLA antigens, however, revealed striking differences (Callahan and Ferrell, 1984). These differences were similar to those we previously described between LT-85 tumor cells and syngeneic C3HfB lymphoid cells, which are described above. Extensive characterization of the isoenzymes of both P3 and PL3 failed to reveal any differences between these cell lines. It seems reasonable to assume, therefore, that both cell lines were derived from the same individual. These cells were, nevertheless, clearly expressing chemically distinct HLA antigens.

Similarly Newman and Graves (1982) have recently described chemical differences in the structure of Ia antigens present on autologous leukemia and EBV-transformed peripheral blood cells. These differences were apparent both in the behavior of the Ia antigens in two-dimensional gel electrophoresis and in their rates of biosynthesis.

Thus, although considerably less information is currently available concerning altered expression of MHC antigens by human tumor cells, there, nevertheless, is evidence that suggests that variations of the type seen on murine tumors also may occur with some frequency on human tumor cells. A complete understanding of the general frequency and relevance of these phenomena will require considerable additional study. However, as mentioned before, on the basis of the available data, such studies seem likely to yield valuable information.

4. Conclusions

Much of the early work on the nature of expression of MHC antigens resulted in conflicting and often confusing results. It is now clear that much of the confusion resulted from the use of polyclonal antibodies, the specificity of which was unavoidably vague. The availability of monoclonal reagents directed toward MHC antigens has resulted in significant clarification of the status of MHC antigens on tumor cells. Through the use of such monoclonal antibodies and genetically well-characterized tumors, it has recently become possible to obtain very precise information about quantitative and qualitative aspects of MHC antigen expression by tumor cell.

Currently, there is no convincing evidence for the expression of "alien" or classic allogeneic histocompatibility antigens by tumor cells. Furthermore, the information that is currently available concerning the organization and nature of genes within the MHC indicates that the potential for the expression of multiple allelic forms of class I MHC antigens does not exist within each individual. There is, however, convincing evidence that tumor cells may make use of preexisting, but normally unexpressed, DNA to generate altered or novel surface antigens. In some instances it is conceivable that such antigens might be cross-reactive with, and, thus, appear to be, allogeneic MHC antigens. Chemical and genetic studies, however, indicate that such cell surface molecules arise either through gene conversion, or from the expression of normally unexpressed, linked, nonallogeneic genes. The role of such novel or altered MHC antigens in host–tumor interactions remains unclear, but there are suggestions that these antigens may play a role in subverting the host immune response or as targets for NK cell activity.

It is also clear from existing data that some tumor cells constitutively express fewer MHC antigens than their normal cell counterparts, or quantitatively vary MHC antigen expression in response to external stimuli. The mechanisms responsible for such variations appear to operate at the level of translation of the MHC genes. The relevance of this potential for phenotypic variability to host–tumor interactions has not yet been fully explained. However, because of the intimate involvement of MHC antigens in cell–cell interaction phenomena, particularly those of the immune response, it seems very unlikely that the ability of tumor cells to differentially express MHC antigens is fortuitous.

Obviously, much of the work in these fields remains in a state of relative infancy. Nevertheless, the work that has been carried out suggests that a full understanding of the nature of MHC antigen expression by tumor cells will provide important insights into the genetics of these antigens, their role in the malignant phenotype, and their relevance to host–tumor interactions, particularly the host immune response.

References

Arden, B., E. K. Wakeland, and J. Klein (1982), *Immunogenetics* **16**, 491.

Artz, K. and F. Jacob (1974), *Transplantation* **17**, 632.

Barclay, A. N. and D. W. Mason (1982), *J. Exp. Med.* **156**, 1665.

Basham, T. Y., M. F. Bourgeade, A. A. Creasy, and T. C. Merigan (1982), *Proc. Natl. Acad. Sci. USA* **79**, 3265.

Beller, D. I. and E. R. Unanue (1981), *J. Immunol.* **126**, 263.

Beller, D. I. and E. R. Unanue (1982), *J. Immunol.* **129**, 971.

Beller, D. I., J. Kiely, and E. R. Unanue (1980), *J. Immunology* **124**, 1426.

Benoist, C. O., D. J. Mathis, M. R. Kanter, V. E. Williams, and H. O. McDevitt (1983), *Cell* **34**, 169.

Bernards, R., P. I. Schrier, A. Houweling, J. L. Bos, A. J. van der Erb, M. Zijlstra, and C. J. Melief (1983), *Nature* **305**, 776.

Biddison, W. E., D. D. Kotsyu, J. L. Strominger, and M. S. Krangel (1982), *J. Immunol.* **129**, 730.

Brickell, P. M., D. S. Latchman, D. Murphy, K. Willison, and P. J. Rigby (1983), *Nature* **306**, 756.

Calamai, E. G., D. I. Beller, and E. R. Unanue (1982), *J. Immunol.* **128**, 1692.

Callahan, G. N. (1984), *J. Immunol.*, in press.

Callahan, G. N. and J. P. Allison (1978), *Nature* **271**, 165.

Callahan, G. N. and R. E. Ferrell (1984), submitted.

Callahan, G. N., M. A. Pellegrino, R. P. McCabe, L. Frugis, J. P. Allison, and S. Ferrone (1978), *Behring Inst. Mitt.* **62**, 115.

Callahan, G. N., L. E. Walker, and W. J. Martin (1981), *Immunogenetics* **12**, 561.

Callahan, G. N., W. J. Martin, and D. Pardi (1982), *J. Immunol.* **128**, 2116.

Callahan, G. N., D. Pardi, M. A. Giedlin, J. P. Allison, D. M. Morizot, and W. J. Martin (1983), *J. Immunol.* **130,** 471.

Castro, J. E., R. Hunt, E. M. Lance, and P. B. Medawar (1974), *Cancer Res.* **34,** 2055.

Chapdelaine, J. M., T. V. Rajan, S. G. Nathenson, and F. Lilly (1981), *Immunogenetics* **14,** 429.

Claas, F. H. J. and G. van Steenbrugge (1983), *Tissue Antigens* **21,** 227.

Clarke, M. F., E. P. Gelmann, and M. S. Reitz (1983), *Nature* **305,** 60.

Coligan, J. E., T. J. Kindt, H. Uehara, J. Martinko, and S. G. Nathenson (1981), *Nature* **291,** 35.

Daar, A. S., S. V. Fuggle, A. Ting, and J. W. Fabre (1982), *J. Immunol.* **129,** 447.

Daynes, R. A., M. Emam, G. G. Kruger, and L. K. Roberts (1983), *J. Immunol.* **130,** 1536.

DeFreitas, E. C., R. W. Chestnut, H. M. Grey, and J. M. Chiller (1983), *J. Immunol.* **131,** 23.

de Waal, R. M. W., M. J. J. Bogman, C. N. Maas, and R. A. P. Koene (1983), *Nature* **303,** 426.

Edidin, M., L. R. Gooding, and M. Johnson (1974), in *Immunological Approaches to Fertility Control,* ed., E. Diezfalusz, Karoboska Institute, Stockholm.

Evans, G. A., D. H. Margulies, R. D. Camerini-Otero, K. Ozato, and J. G. Seidman (1982), *Proc. Natl. Acad. Sci. USA* **79,** 1994.

Fellous, M., U. Nir, D. Wallach, G. Merlin, M. Rubenstein, and M. Revel (1982), *Proc. Natl. Acad. Sci. USA* **79,** 3082.

Forman, J. (1980), in *Cancer Markers: Diagnostic and Developmental Significance,* ed., S. Sell, The Humana Press, Clifton, New Jersey.

Gorer, P. A. (1938), *J. Pathol. Bacteriol.* **47,** 231.

Gorer, P. A., S. Lyman, and G. D. Snell (1948), *Proc. R. Soc. London* **135,** 449.

Haywood, G. R. and C. F. McKhann (1971), *J. Exp. Med.* **133,** 1171.

Hellstrom, K. E. and I. Hellstrom (1969), *Adv. Cancer Res.* **12,** 167.

Herberman, R. B. (ed.) (1980), in *Natural Cell-Mediated Immunity Against Tumors,* Academic Press Inc., New York.

Hood, L., M. Steinmetz, and B. Malissen (1983), *Ann. Rev. Immunol.* **1,** 529.

Imamura, M., T. G. Gipson, N. Bensky, R. Justice, and W. J. Martin (1979), *J. Immunol.* **122,** 1863.

Kaufman, J. F., C. Auffray, A. J. Kornman, D. A. Shackleford, and J. Strominger (1984), *Cell* **36,** 1.

Kindt, T. J. and M. A. Robinson (1984), in *Fundamental Immunology,* ed., W. E. Paul, Raven Press, New York.

King, D. and P. P. Jones (1983), *J. Immunol.* **131,** 315.

Klein, J. (1979), *Science* **203,** 516.

Klein, J. (1982), in *Immunology, The Science of Self-Nonself Discrimination,* John Wiley and Sons, New York.

Klein, J., A. Juretic, C. M. Baxevanis, and Z. A. Nagy (1981), *Nature* **291,** 455.

Klein, J., F. Figueroa, and Z. A. Nagy (1983), *Ann. Rev. Immunol.* **1**, 119.

Lalanne, J. L., F. Bregegere, C. Delarbre, J. P. Abastado, G. Gachelin, P. Kourilsky (1982), *Nucleic Acid Res.* **10**, 1039.

Lampson, L. A., C. P. Fisher, and J. P. Whelan (1983), *J. Immunol.* **130**, 2471.

Larhammar, D., U. Hammerling, M. Denaro, T. Lund, and R. A. Flavell (1983), *Cell* **134**, 179.

Maloy, W. L., and J. E. Coligan (1982), *Immunogenetics* **16**, 11.

Malissen, M., B. Malissen, and B. R. Jordan (1982), *Proc. Natl. Acad. Sci. USA* **79**, 893.

Mann, D. L., M. Popovic, P. Sarin, C. Murray, M. S. Reitz, D. M. Strong, B. F. Haynes, R. C. Gallo, and W. A. Blatner (1983), *Nature* **305**, 58.

Martin, W. J., T. G. Gipson, and J. M. Rice (1977), *Nature* **265**, 738.

Mathis, D. J., C. O. Benoist, V. E. Williams, M. R. Kanter, and H. O. McDevitt (1983), *Cell* **32**, 745.

Medawar, P. (1974), *Cancer Res.* **34**, 2053.

Medawar, P. B. and R. Hunt (1978), *Nature* **271**, 164.

Mellor, A. L., E. H. Weiss, K. Ramachandran, and R. A. Flavell (1983), *Nature* **306**, 792.

Morello, D., F. Daniel, P. Baldacci, Y. Cayre, G. Gachelin, and M. Kourilsky (1982), *Nature* **196**, 260.

Newman, A. and M. F. Graves (1982), *Clin. Exp. Immunol.* **50**, 41.

Ostrand-Rosenberg, S. and A. Cohn (1981), *Proc. Natl. Acad. Sci. USA*, **78**, 7106.

Ostrand-Rosenberg, S., A. L. Cohn, and J. W. Sandoz (1983), *J. Immunol.* **130**, 1969.

Owerbach, D., A. Lernmark, P. Platz, L. P. Ryder, L. Rask, P. A. Peterson, and K. Ludvigsson (1983), *Nature* **303**, 815.

Parmiani, G., G. Carbone, G. Invernizzi, M. A. Pierotti, M. L. Sensi, M. J. Rogers, and E. Appella (1979), *Immunogenetics* **9**, 1.

Plata, F., A. F. Tilkin, J. P. Levy, and F. Lilly (1981), *J. Exp. Med.* **154**, 1795.

Robinson, P. J., K. Sege, P. Altevogt, P. A. Peterson, L. Lundin, F. Garrido, and V. Schirrmacher (1981), *Immunogenetics* **13**, 261.

Rogers, M. J., L. R. Gooding, D. H. Marguiles, and G. A. Evans (1983), *J. Immunol.* **130**, 2418.

Sachs, D. (1984), in *Fundamental Immunology*, ed., W. E. Paul, Raven Press, New York.

Scher, M. G., D. I. Beller, and E. R. Unanue (1980), *J. Exp. Med.* **152**, 1684.

Schmidt, W., G. Atfield, and H. Festenstein (1979), *Immunogenetics* **8**, 311.

Schmidt, W., L. Leben, G. Atfield, and H. Festenstein (1981), *Immunogenetics* **14**, 323.

Schrier, P. I., R. Bernards, R. T. M. J. Vaessen, A. Houweling, and A. J. van der Eb (1983), *Nature* **305**, 771.

Schwartz, R. H. (1984) in *Fundamental Immunology*, ed., W. E. Paul, Raven Press, New York.

Shedlovsky, A., L. J. Clipson, J. C. Vandeberg, and W. F. Dove (1981), *Immunogenetics* **13**, 413.

Sikora, K., P. Stern, and E. Lennox (1977), *Nature* **269**, 813.

Steeg, P. S., R. N. Moore, H. M. Johnson, and J. J. Oppenheim (1980), *J. Exp. Med.* **152,** 1734.

Steinman, R. M., N. Nogueira, M. D. Witmer, J. D. Tydings, and I. S. Mellman (1980), *J. Exp. Med.* **152,** 1248.

Steinmetz, M., K. W. Moore, J. G. Frelinger, B. T. Sher, F.-W. Shen, E. A. Boyse, and L. Hood (1981), *Cell* **25,** 683.

Stern, P. L., M. Gidlund, A. Orn, H. Wigzell (1980), *Nature* **285,** 341.

Strominger, J. L., H. T. Orr, P. Parham, H. L. Ploegh, D. L. Mann, H. Bilofsky, H. A. Saroff, T. T. Wu, and E. A. Kabat (1980), *Scand. J. Immunol.* **11,** 573.

Testorelli, C., O. Marelli, W. Schmidt, and H. Festenstein (1980), *J. Immunogenetics* **7,** 19.

Walker, E. B., L. L. Lanier, and N. L. Warner (1982), *J. Exp. Med.* **155,** 629.

Weiss, E. H., A. Mellor, L. Golden, K. Fahrner, E. Simpson, J. Hurst, and R. A. Flavell (1983), *Nature* **301,** 671.

Wong, G., I. Clark-Lewis, J. L. McKimm-Breschkin, A. W. Harris, and J. M. Schrader (1983), *J. Immunol.* **131,** 788.

Zinkernagel, R. M. and P. C. Doherty (1980), *Adv. Immunol.* **27,** 251.

Chapter 6

Monoclonal Antibodies
Probes for the Study of Malignant T Cells

ELIZABETH A. HARDEN, THOMAS J. PALKER, AND
BARTON F. HAYNES

*Department of Medicine, Divisions of Rheumatic and Genetic
Diseases and Hematology, Duke University, Durham, NC*

1. Introduction

The lymphoid malignancies have long been recognized as a heterogeneous group of disorders with respect to clinical presentation, course, and response to therapy (Frei and Sallan, 1978; Simone et al., 1975). The development of immunologic techniques defining lymphocyte subsets has provided insight into the cellular origin of these malignancies. Lymphocytes are commonly divided into two major groups. Bone marrow derived (B) lymphocytes are recognized by the presence of surface immunoglobulin (sIg), other lineage specific markers, and by their ability to be stimulated to produce immunoglobulin (Maino et al., 1977; Preud'homme and Seligmann, 1972). Thymus derived (T) lymphocytes are characterized by their ability to spontaneously bind sheep erythrocytes and express a number of lineage specific antigens at various stages of T-cell maturation (Reinherz et al., 1980b; Reinherz and Schlossman, 1980a; Reinherz and Schlossman, 1980b; Haynes, 1981). The distinction between malignancies derived from T or B lymphocytes has important clinical and diagnostic implications, in that patients with T-cell malignancies tend to have a more aggressive clinical course and poorer response to therapy compared to patients with B-cell malignancies (Frei and Sallan, 1978; Heideman et al., 1978). The development of heteroantisera directed against normal peripheral blood T cells further divided T cells into two functionally distinct subsets (Evans et al., 1978). The TH2+ subset defined 20% of peripheral blood lymphocytes and contained cytotoxic/suppressor cells (Reinherz et al., 1979a). The TH2-population represented 80% of PB T cells and contained a helper cell population (Reinherz et al., 1979a). This T-cell antigen system was used to phenotypically characterize malignant T cells in patients with both T-acute lymphoblastic leukemia (ALL) and T-lymphoblastic lymphoma (LL) (Nadler et al., 1980). Nadler et al. (1980) demonstrated that the majority of patients with T-LL were TH2+ whereas most T-ALL cells were TH2-, thus providing suggestive evidence for clinical relevance for subtyping the T-lymphoblastic malignancies.

Hybridoma techniques described by Kohler and Milstein (1975) for the production of monoclonal antibodies have revolutionized the study of human T-cell differentiation. A variety of human T-cell antigens have now been described that define T-cell lineage specific differentiation antigens as well as subsets of thymocytes and peripheral blood T cells (Reinherz et al., 1979d; Reinherz et al., 1980b; McMichael et al., 1979; Brodsky et al., 1979; Engleman et al., 1981; Haynes et al., 1979; Haynes, 1981; Haynes et al., 1981a; Howard et al., 1981; Kamoun et al., 1981a; Kamoun et al., 1981b; Ledbetter et al., 1981). From these data presumed schemes of normal T-cell differentiation have been proposed (Foon et al., 1980; Minowada, 1982; Reinherz et al., 1980b; Reinherz and Schlossman, 1980a). Moreover, some of these anti-T-cell monoclonal antibodies have been used in vivo as therapy for T-cell malignancies (Janossy and Prentice, 1982; Ritz and Schlossman, 1982). Finally, use of anti-T-cell monoclonal antibodies in the study of T-cell malignancies has provided insight into potential mechanisms of malignant transformation (Minowada et al., 1982). However, two broad possibilities remain regarding the interpretation of patterns of expression of cell surface differentiation antigen on malignant T cells. If malignancy is the result of maturation arrest of T cells at a specific stage of a normal differentiation pathway, then the phenotype of malignant T cells could correspond to normal stages of T cell differentiation. However, if the pattern of T-cell antigen expression by malignant T cells is the result of dedifferentiation or aberrant T-cell maturation, then the phenotype of malignant T cells may not reflect normal pathways of differentiation (Minowada et al., 1982; Reinherz et al., 1980b).

In this paper we will briefly review the use of monoclonal antibodies in the phenotypic and functional characterization of human T-cell malignancies.

2. Monoclonal Antibodies as Probes for the Study of Malignant T Cells

With the advent of monoclonal antibody technology, a number of anti-body reagents have been produced that define surface molecules on human T cells (Reinherz et al., 1980b; McMichael et al., 1979; Brodsky et al., 1979; Engleman et al., 1981; Haynes et al., 1979; Haynes, 1981; Haynes et al., 1981a; Howard et al., 1981; Kamoun et al., 1981a; Kamoun et al., 1981b; Ledbetter et al., 1981). Although a large number of monoclonal antibodies against lymphoid differentiation antigens have been produced, a limited number of lineage-specific T-cell antigens have been defined (Table 1). Whereas many of the markers listed in Table 1 are useful in the determination of T-cell lineage of malignant cells, others are not. In particular, antibodies against antigens T6, T1, transferrin receptor, T10, HLA A, B, and C, HLA Dr, and CALLA are not particularly useful regarding T-cell lineage determination, since these markers are found on a variety of non-T-cell types of tissues (Brodsky et al., 1979; Haynes et al., 1981a; McMichael et al., 1979; Metzgar et al., 1981; Judd et al., 1980; Reinherz et al., 1980b). However, though the T6 antigen is expressed on Langerhans' cells in skin epidermis, T6 positivity of a lymphoid malignancy does generally signify T-cell origin (McMichael et al., 1979). In contrast, the E-rosette receptor and antigens T3, T4, T8, 9.3, 3A1, and T12 are essentially T-lineage specific. Although the antibodies shown in Table 1 have been used in a number of studies of T-cell malignancies, data supporting the clinical relevance of phenotypic characterization of malignant T cells with such a panel are incomplete. What follows, therefore, is a summary of normal T-cell development and a brief review of the surface antigen characteristics and functional capabilities of malignant cells in various clinical types of human T-cell malignancies.

3. Normal T-Cell Maturation as Defined by Monoclonal Antibodies

Normal thymocytes originate from bone marrow precursor cells which migrate to the thymus (Stutman, 1977). T-cell precursors most likely enter the thymus, reside in the subcapsular cortex and postnatally represent a small population of large, rapidly dividing E-rosette− cells termed prothymocytes (Galili et al., 1980). It has been postulated that prothymocytes become small, E-rosette+, functionally immature, cortical thymocytes that represent 90% of all thymocytes (Haynes, 1981). At

Table 1
Lymphoid or T-Cell Antigens Defined by Monoclonal Antibodies Used in the
Study of T-Cell Malignancies

Antigen (monoclonal antibodies)	Antigen size (daltons)[a]	Reactivity	Reference
T6(NA1/34, OKT6, Leu 6)	48,000–42,000	Cortical thymocytes	McMichael et al., 1979
		Epidermal Langerhans' cells	Reinherz et al, 1980a
T1(Leu 1, 10.2, L17F12, T101, 16B2, DUSKW3-1 A-50)	65,000	Thymocytes, mature cells	Royston et. al, 1980; Wang et al, 1980; Martin et al, 1980; Haynes et al, 1981b; Engleman et al, 1981; Boumsell et al, 1980
		Subset malignant B cells	
E-rosette receptor (9.6, OKT11, Leu 5, 35.1)	50,000	Thymocytes, mature T cells	Howard et al, 1981; Kamoun et al, 1981b; Bona and Fauci, 1980
T3(OKT3, UCHT-1, Leu-4)	19,000	Subset of thymocytes, all mature T cells	Kung et al, 1970; Ledbetter et al, 1981; Beverly et al, 1981
T4(OKT4, Leu 3a)	62,000	Cortical thymocytes, inducer mature T cells	Ledbetter et al, 1981; Reinherz et al, 1979a
T8(OKT8, Leu 2a)	33,000	Cortical thymocytes, supporessor/cyto-toxic mature T cells	Ledbetter et al, 1981 Reinherz et al, 1980b
9.3(9.3)	44,000	Subset of thymocytes, indu-cer mature T cells	Hansen et al, 1980
3A1(3A1, 4A, Leu 9, 4G6, 5A12, WT-1)	40,000	Thymocytes, 85% of mature T cells	Haynes et al, 1979; Haynes 1981; Eisenbarth et al, 1980; Vodinelick et al, 1983
T12(T12, 12.1)	100,000	Mature T cells	Kamoun et al, 1981a
Transferrin receptor (5E9, OKT9, B3/25)	90,000	Antigen of cell acti-vation	Haynes, 1981a; Judd et al, 1980; Omary et al, 1980

Table 1 (*continued*)

Antigen (monoclonal antibodies)	Antigen size (daltons)[a]	Reactivity	Reference
p80(A1G3)	80,000	Mature T cells[b]	Haynes et al, 1983a
T28(T28)	28,000	Mature T cells	Beverly et al, 1980
T10	44,000	Antigen of cell activation	Reinherz et al, 1980b
CALLA(J-5)	95,000	Subset of normal B cells, mature granulocytes, kidney tubular epithelium	Ritz et al, 1980
HLA DR(Ia-like)	33,000 28,000	Monocytes, macrophages, T cells, B cells, activated T cells	Brodsky et al, 1979 Reinherz et al, 1979b
HLA A, B, C (3F10, W6/32)	44,000 12,000	Thymocytes and mature T cells[c], many normal tissue types	Brodsky et al, 1979 Eisenbarth et al, 1980
3-40	35,000–40,000	T-ALL cells, some non B, non-T ALL cells, some AML cells, thymic epithelium, many normal tissues	Naito et al, 1983
3-3	35,000–40,000	T-ALL cells, normal connective tissue	Naito et al, 1983

[a]Antigen size in daltons as reported under reducing conditions.
[b]Although p80 Antigen in the T-cell lineage is specific for mature T cells, p80 is expressed on a wide variety of non-T cells and therefore, is not T-cell specific (Haynes et al. 1983a).
[c]HLA antigens are expressed on all thymocytes, although the density of HLA antigens is low on cortical thymocytes and high in medullary thymocytes and mature T cells (Haynes, 1981).

some point during intrathymic T-cell maturation, within the thymic microenvironment, thymocytes undergo marked changes in surface antigens and gain some degree of functional maturity. Medullary thymocytes represent only 10–15% of the entire thymocyte population and share the antigenic and functional characeristics of peripheral blood T cells (Haynes et al., 1983a); these cells are thought to be subsequently exported to the peripheral lymphoid compartment to blood, spleen, and lymph nodes. Reinherz et al. (1980b) have divided human thymocytes into three developmental categories. Stage I represents the earliest stage of thymocyte development and possibly corresponds to prothymocytes or large subcapsular thymocytes. Whereas 3A1, T4, T8, T1, and the E-rosette receptor are expressed on 80–95% of thymocytes in suspension, only antigen 3A1 is thought to be expressed by prothymocytes. Stage II (common) thymocytes are found primarily in the thymic cortex. Common thymocytes simultaneously express the T6 antigen, and as well antigens T4, T8, T10, 3A1, T1, and the E-rosette receptor (Reinherz et al., 1980b; Haynes, 1981). Stage III (mature) thymocytes are T6− and express 3A1, T1, and the E-rosette receptor. At some point during the postulated transition from Stage II to Stage III, those thymocytes that are destined to mature increase expression of HLA A, B, and C and T1 antigens, and as well acquire reactivity with anti-T3 (Reinherz et al., 1980b; Haynes, 1981). Mature thymocytes, like PB T cells reciprocally express T4 and T8 antigens. In most normal human thymuses, a small population of T4+, 3A1− medullary thymocytes can be identified (Haynes, B. F., unpublished observations). In addition, the p80 antigen has been described that, unlike HLA, T1, or T3 antigens, is absolutely acquired during the proposed maturation pathways from cortical to medullary thymocytes (Haynes et al., 1983a).

Alternative pathways within the thymus as well as possible extrathymic sites of lymphoid differentiation may well exist. In this context Umiel and colleagues (1982) have recently shown that foci of functional (strongly T1+) thymocytes are present throughout the normal thymic cortex and may represent either an alternative pathway or the major site of thymocyte maturation.

4. Phenotypic Analysis of Malignant T Cells in Defined Clinical Syndromes

4.1. T-Cell Acute Lymphoblastic Leukemia

Patients with acute lymphoblastic leukemia (ALL) can be divided into four main groups on the basis of conventional B and T markers (Brouet et al., 1975); a small group with surface Ig termed B-cell ALL, a group with intracytoplasmic Ig heavy chains termed pre-B-ALL (Brouet et al., 1979), those that form spontaneous rosettes with sheep erythrocytes (ER+) termed T-cell ALL, and a large group that do not rosette with sheep E, lack sIg, and are termed "null" ALL.

T-cell acute lymphoblastic leukemia (T-ALL) represents 15–25% of cases of ALL (Catovsky, 1974; Catovsky et al., 1983). Distinct clinical features include male predominance, older age group, high initial blast count, and the presence of a mediastinal mass (Sen and Borella, 1975). T-ALL cells are usually TdT positive, acid phosphatase positive (Bradstock et al., 1980; Greaves, 1981) and have elevated levels of adenosine deaminase (Smyth, et al., 1978). The surface antigen pheno-type of the malignant cell in T-ALL is heterogeneous with respect to T-cell differentiation antigens, but in general is that of an immature thymocyte (Reinherz et al., 1980b; Haynes et al., 1981b; Catovsky et al., 1983). Reinherz et al. (1980b) studied T-cell populations from 25 patients with T-ALL diagnosed on the basis of spontaneous ER formation and re-activity with T-cell specific monoclonal and polyclonal antisera. The ma-jority (15/21) were proposed to be derived from early thymocyte or prothymocyte subpopulations (T10+ or T10+/T9+ without other mark-ers), whereas 5/21 were classed as common thymocyte derivation (T6+, T4+, T8+). Only 1/21 expressed the mature T-cell antigen T3 (Reinherz et al., 1980b). Others have confirmed these findings (Haynes et al., 1981b; Catovsky et al., 1983; Koziner et al., 1982; Schroff et al., 1982). Monoclonal antibody 3A1 (made from murine spleen cells immunized with HSB-2 T-ALL cell line) is T-cell specific and is present on 85% of E-rosette+ PBL and essentially 100% of adolescent thymocytes including the large subcapsular prothymocyte population (Haynes et al., 1979). Regarding the T-cell specific reagents that are of use in defining lymphoid cell lineage, antibody 3A1 has been shown to be the most relia-ble T-cell marker of immature T-cell leukemias (Haynes et al., 1979; Haynes et al., 1981b). All ALL T cells tested by Haynes et al. (1981b) were 3A1+ despite phenotypic diversity, and in some cases, total lack of expression of other T-cell markers. Importantly, patients with clinically typical T-cell ALL, but expressing no other B, T, or CALLA antigens, were routinely 3A1+ (Haynes et al., 1981b). Similar findings have re-cently been obtained by others using 3A1 (Catovsky et al., 1983; Minowada, 1982; Minowada et al., 1982) and another anti-3A1 reagent, monoclonal antibody WT1 (Vodinelick et al., 1983). Naito et al. (1983) described two monoclonal antibodies (3-3 and 3-40) that reacted with cell lines derived from patients with T-ALL but not with normal hematopoietic cells. Anti-3-3 reacted only with fresh T-ALL cells whereas anti-3-40 reacted with some non-T, non-B ALL cells, and a few acute lymphoblastic leukemia cells (Naito et al., 1983). Although these reagents (3-3, 3-40) react with some normal tissues, they appear to be useful in the diagnosis of T-ALL (Naito et al., 1983).

As mentioned, the majority of cases of ALL are classified as "null" on the basis of conventional B and T markers. It is in this area that monoclonal antibodies have been particularly useful in further characterizing the cellular origin. The common acute lymphoblastic leu-kemia antigen (CALLA) was originally defined by antisera produced in rabbits by immunization with sIg, ER− ALL cells (Greaves and Brown, 1975). A monoclonal antibody, J5, reacts with CALLA and is present on leukemia cells from 70% of patients with all types of ALL (Ritz et al., 1980). CALLA has been reported to be present on a small population of lymphoid B-cell precursors in normal bone marrow (Greaves and Brown, 1975). Recently, it has been shown that the majority of "null" ALL cells express CALLA (reviewed in Foon et al., 1980; Minowada, 1982). These cells also express Ia and B1 (a B-cell lineage specific) antigens and it has been proposed that these cells are committed to B-cell lineage (Korsmeyer et al., 1981). However, a small population of null ALL cells have surface antigen phenotypes suggestive of T-cell rather than B-cell origin (Koziner et al., 1982; Schroff et al., 1982).

Koziner et al. (1982) studied 134 cases of ALL. Of these, 113 were classified as null cell ALL on the basis of absent sIg and ER negativity. Eight of the 113, however, had other markers suggestive of T-cell origin, such as T6 or variable expression of T4 and T8. Schroff et al. (1982) divided null ALL into two subgroups. The majority were HLA-DR+ and CALLA+, whereas a smaller subset were T1+, HLA-DR−. Interestingly, the patients in the latter group were adolescent males with thymic masses that were postulated to be of T-cell origin (Schroff et al., 1982).

As mentioned, antigen 3A1 appears to be the most reliable T-cell lineage marker in ALL, and frequently is the only T-cell specific surface antigen expressed on leukemic cells in clinically typical T ALL (Haynes et al., 1981b). Recently, study of the in vivo and in vitro differentiating capabilities of 3A1+, T4−, T8−, T6−, T1−, and T11− T-ALL cells has suggested that in some cases this phenotype might identify malignant multipotent stem cells that are not irreversibly committed to T-cell differentiation. Hershfield et al. (1984) recently demonstrated that in vivo and in vitro treatment of cells of this type of T-ALL with deoxycoformycin can trigger apparent malignant cell differentiation, with loss of T-cell antigen 3A1 and differentiation to mature granulocytes associated with expression of normal myeloid cell surface antigens (Hershfield et al., 1984). Thus, the demonstration of the 3A1+, T4−, T8−, T6−, T1−, T11− phenotype in T-ALL may be of relevance clinically in that these cells may be immature pre-T cells or multipotent stem cells that can be triggered to myeloid differentiation by inhibitors of DNA methylation such as deoxycoformycin or 5-azacytadine (Hershfield et al., 1984). Identification of such T-ALL cells might be important, since treatment of these patients with agents that can promote malignant cell differentiation can profoundly affect the clinical course.

Functional studies of T-cell ALL cells has generally shown them to be functionally immature with regard to in vitro T-cell effector cell analysis (Reinherz and Schlossman, 1980b). However, Broder et al. (1978) have demonstrated that leukemic T cells from a child with T-ALL and hypogammaglobulinemia functioned as suppressor cells in vitro with the cooperation of a normal immunoregulatory T-cell population. These data provided evidence for the role of T–T-cell interaction in the mediation of suppressor activity and as well suggested that some T-ALL malignant cells can mediate T-cell effector function.

4.2. T-Cell Lymphoblastic Lymphoma

T-cell lymphoblastic lymphoma (T-LL) is a type of non-Hodgkins lymphoma (NHL) usually seen in children or young adults (Berard et al., 1974). T-LL characteristically is associated with an anterior mediastinal mass without leukemia at presentation (Nathwani et al., 1976). Pleural effusions are common, and any combination of supradiaphragmatic lymph nodes may be involved (Nathwani et al., 1976). A high percentage (30–50%) of patients will evolve into a leukemic phase with circulating malignant cells morphologically indistinguishable from those seen in ALL (Sullivan, 1962; Webster, 1961). Prior to the discovery of T and B markers, a relationship between LL and the thymus was suspected (Webster, 1961). Analysis of malignant cell surface markers has confirmed that the majority of these tumors are of thymic origin (Ritz et al., 1981; Bernard et al., 1981). The tumor cells are E-rosette+ and lack sIg or reactivity with anti-Ia or anti-B cell antibodies (Bernard et al., 1981; Bernard et al., 1982). Further characterization with monoclonal antibodies has suggested that the phenotype of malignant cells in LL is heterogeneous. Bernard et al. (1981), using the OK series of T-cell reagents and the Reinherz et al. (1980b) classification of stages of T-cell differentiation, reported 29% of LL to be early thymocyte in type (ER+, T10+); 43% were related to the common thymocyte stage (T6+, T4+, T8+); and 29% expressed mature thymocyte antigens (T3 and reciprocally expressed T4 and T8). Certainly considerable overlap exists between the phenotypic characterization of T-ALL and T-LL, such that no clear malignant T-cell surface phenotypic distinction can be made between the two syndromes (Bernard et al., 1981; Bernard et al., 1982; Ritz et al., 1981). However, the common acute lymphoblastic leukemia antigen (CALLA) has been reported to help distinguish T-ALL and LL, in that 40% of LL cells express CALLA whereas less than 10% of T-ALL cells express CALLA (Ritz et al., 1980). Additionally, monoclonal antibody A-50 (which recognizes an epitope of the T1 antigen on majority of PB T cells and a subpopulation of thymocytes) was reactive with cells from five of eight patients with LL but unreactive with 12 patients with T-ALL (Bernard et al., 1981). Interestingly, Bernard et al. (1982) studied the change in surface antigens in patients with LL in leukemia relapse and found a shift in the surface antigen pattern towards dedifferentiation and expression of immature T-cell antigens.

4.3. T-Cell Prolymphocytic Leukemia

Prolymphocytic leukemia (PLL) was first described by Galton et al. in 1974. The prolymphocyte has a characteristic morphology and most cases have a B-cell membrane phenotype. However, approximately 20% of cases of T-PLL are ER+ and are thought to be of T-cell lineage (Catovsky et al., 1983). Catovsky et al. (1983) reported a detailed surface antigen and nuclear TdT analysis of 13 cases of T-PLL. Malignant T cells in all cases were negative for nuclear TdT activity. Malignant T cells in most cases had a mature helper T-cell phenotype: T3+, T4+, T8−, whereas a smaller proportion had mature cytotoxic/suppressor phenotype: T3+, T4−, T8+; 2 patients had circulating malignant cells that co-expressed T4, T8, and T3 antigens. These data suggest that malignant T cells in T-cell PLL, though heterogeneous in surface antigen phenotype, most often express T-cell antigens in a mature T-cell pattern.

4.4. Cutaneous T-Cell Lymphoma

Mycosis fungoides (MF) and the Sezary syndrome (SS) are lymphoid malignancies that are part of the spectrum of cutaneous T-cell lymphoma (CTCL) (Broder and Bunn, 1980). Classic MF presents with a scaly eruption that progresses from a plaque stage to skin tumors. SS is manifested by generalized exfoliative erythroderma with circulating malignant (Sezary) cells.

In 1976, in an important study, Broder et al. (1976) showed that Sezary cells could mediate help, but not suppression of polyclonally driven B cells in vitro, suggesting that in many cases of MF and SS, malignant T cells were derived from functionally mature, well differentiated T cells. Subsequent phenotypic and functional characterization of CTCL cells has supported this notion (Boumsell et al., 1981; Haynes 1981b; Kung et al., 1981). Peripheral blood from five CTCL patients and two Sezary T-cell lines (Haynes et al., 1983b) were consistent for OKT4+, OKT8−, and negative for immature T-cell antigens. Interestingly, CTCL leukemic cells in contrast to T-ALL leukemic cells, were found to be 3A1−, thus providing an important phenotypic differences between the two (Haynes et al., 1981b). Whether the 3A1 antigen is lost on leukemic T4+ CTCL cells as a consequence of malignant transformation or whether 3A1− CTCL leukemic cells are derived from a mature normal 3A1− T cell subset is not known. Boumsell and colleagues (1981) and Kung et al. (1981), using the OK series of reagents, reported a similar phenotypic characterization of Sezary cells and also found them to be OKT6−, OKT4+, OKT8−. Berger et al. (1982) have recently described two monoclonal antibodies, BE-1 and BE-2, produced by immunizing mice with leukemic T cells from a patient with CTCL. These monoclonal antibodies are directed against two different cell surface antigens and regarding T cells, react selectively with CTCL lymphocytes and not normal T cells; however, BE-1 and BE-2 also react with some normal transformed cultured lymphocytes (Berger et al., 1982).

The simultaneous study of blood and skin malignant T cells in CTCL (Haynes et al., 1982b) revealed that in contrast to leukemic CTCL cells, skin infiltrating malignant T cells are Ia+ and transferrin receptor+. The expression of Ia and transferrin receptor by skin T cells in CTCL cells appears to be a normal prerequisite for, or response to, migration of T-cells to skin (Haynes et al., 1982b). Functional studies have demonstrated the capability of in vitro migration of peripheral blood lymphocytes from Sezary syndrome patients to normal allogeneic skin (Laroche et al., 1983).

In contrast to leukemic CTCL cells, skin infiltrating T cells in nonleukemic, typical MF are usually 3A1+ (Haynes et al., 1982b; Wood et al., 1982). The expression of 3A1 antigen by skin infiltrating T cells in MF without leukemia may either be a reflection of a different lineage of T cells being involved in MF without leukemia or of an effect of the skin microenvironment on T-cell differentiation leading to T-cell surface phenotypic changes and expression of 3A1 antigen (Haynes et al., 1982b). Additionally, nonmalignant, normal 3A1+ T cells may be intermixed with the malignant T-cell infiltrate (Haynes et al., 1982c). Most typical MF skin T-cell infiltrates are T4+/T8−, although occasional cases have been reported to be T8+/T4− (Haynes et al., 1982a). Wood et al. (1982) also were able to subtype nonleukemic CTCL on the basis of skin T-cell expression of Ia and T1 antigens. However, the prognostic relevance of T-cell subset antigen phenotypic analysis in CTCL remains to be demonstrated.

Unfortunately, T-cell phenotypes are not diagnostic for CTCL as the skin infiltrates of contact dermatitis, granuloma annulare, and lymphomatoid granulomatosis share similar T-cell phenotypic patterns with various clinical forms of CTCL (Haynes et al., 1982a).

4.5. T-Cell Chronic Lymphocytic Leukemia

Chronic lymphocytic leukemia (CLL) is a proliferative disorder of small, mature lymphocytes. Most cases of classic CLL are derived from B cells. However, a small percentage (2%) are malignancies of T cells as defined by T-cell specific heteroantisera and E-rosetting techniques (Reinherz et al., 1979d). Further phenotypic characterization indicates that these are proliferations of mature T cells (TdT−, T6−, T3+) and can be of either helper cell (T4+/T8−) or suppressor cell (T4−/T8+) phenotype (Foon et al., 1982; Schroff et al., 1982).

Of interest are reports of CLL with both B and T markers (ER+, sIg+) in which the malignant cells were B cells that secreted surface immunoglobulins (IgM) manifesting anti-sheep erythrocyte specificity (Brouet and Prieur, 1974; Bona and Fauci, 1980).

T CLL cells have been shown to respond to mitogens in vitro (Huhn, 1983), although the response may be blunted (Foon et al., 1982).

4.6. IgG Fc Receptor Bearing (T$_G$) Lymphoproliferative Disease

Large granular lymphocytes (LGL) constitute a morphologically distinct subgroup of lymphocytes that are ER+, bear Fc receptors for IgG (FcR), and can mediate natural killer (NK) activity and antibody-dependent cellular cytotoxicity (ADCC) (Timonen et al., 1981). The concomitant expression of E-rosette receptors and IgG FcR has given rise to the term T_G for these LGL cells. Lymphoproliferative disorders of LGL are characterized by a variety of clinical symptoms including anemia, hypogammaglobulinemia, and neutropenia with recurrent infections (Bagby, 1981; Ferrarini et al., 1982; Nagasawa et al., 1981). Although these disorders include conditions that are clearly neoplastic, there are cases that pursue a more benign course with chronic persistent lymphocytosis that does not progress even without therapy (Ferrarini et al., 1982). The surface phenotype of these cells is generally ER+, T3+, T8+, and T4− (Bagby, 1981; Ferrarini et al., 1982; Timonen et al., 1981). Some variability has been reported regarding reactivity with monoclonal antibodies 3A1 and OKM1 (Schlimok et al., 1982).

The functional activity of LGL in T_G lymphoproliferative syndromes in vitro include ADCC, NK activity, suppressor activity in in vitro assays of B-cell IgG production, and spontaneous production of gamma (immune) interferon (Hooks et al., 1982; Timonen et al., 1981; Schlimok et al., 1982; Rumke et al., 1982). The mechanisms leading to neutropenia or anemia in these patients is speculative, but LGL from some patients with neutropenia have been shown to inhibit granulopoiesis in vitro (Bagby, 1981). Additionally, Nagasawa et al. (1981) reported a patient with T_G lymphocytosis, pure red cell anemia, and hypogammaglobulinemia whose cells in vitro suppressed both erythroid colony formation and B-cell differentiation.

Proliferations of IgG FcR+, LGL (T_G) cells may be benign disorders caused by aberrant immunoregulatory mechanisms or they may be part of a spectrum of diseases of neoplastic LGL cells. Kadin et al. (1981) reported two cases of erythrophagocytic T_G lymphoma that were clearly malignant. The clinical and pathologic features of these two patients resembled malignant histiocytosis with hepatosplenomegaly and lymphadenopathy, with tissues infiltrated with ER+, IgG FcR+ (T_G) cells.

4.7. Hairy Cell Leukemia

Hairy cell leukemia (leukemic reticuloendotheliosis) is a well defined syndrome of pancytopenia, splenomegaly, and the infiltration of bone marrow and blood by characteristic mononuclear cells with "hairy" cytoplasmic projections (Lobuglio, 1976; King et al., 1975). Cells are positive for tartrate-resistant acid phosphatase (King et al., 1975). The cellular origin of hairy cell leukemia (HCL) is controversial since cells share both B-cell and monocytic properties, but, in general, it is felt to represent a proliferation of leukemic B lymphocytes. In many cases immunoglobulin synthesis by leukemic HC has been demonstrated (Golde et al., 1977; Jansen et al., 1982). In rare cases, however, HCL may express a T-cell phenotype (Hernandez et al., 1978; Saxon et al., 1978). Saxon et al. (1978) described a patient with typical HCL with tartrate-resistant acid phosphatase positive cells (both fresh and cultured) that were ER positive and reacted with anti-T-lymphocyte antiserum. Additionally, in some cases malignant cells express features of both B and T cells. Hairy cells from two patients stimulated with phytohemagglutinin in culture have been shown to switch from B to T phenotypes (Guglielmi et al., 1980).

Kalyanaraman et al. (1982) reported a patient with a T-cell variant of hairy cell leukemia whose leukemic cells exhibited the typical HC morphology and contained tartrate-resistant acid phosphatase and had a T4+, mature T-cell phenotype. The patient had serum antibodies reactive with the structural protein (p24) of human T-cell leukemia/lymphoma virus (HTLV$_I$) and a cell line (MO-1) derived from patient spleen cells expressed antigens cross-reactive with HTLV proteins. The virus particles of patient MO cells in culture were not identical to HTLV$_I$ and were felt to represent a closely related retrovirus termed HTLV$_{II}$ (Kalyanaraman et al., 1982).

4.8. HTLV-Associated Japanese, Caribbean, and American Adult T-Cell Leukemia/Lymphoma (ATL)

In 1980 Poiesz and colleagues isolated and characterized a novel human retrovirus, human T-cell leukemia/lymphoma virus (HTLV$_I$) from an American patient with the clinical syndrome of ATL. Subsequently, it has been shown that HTLV$_I$ is associated with T-cell malignancies in patients from the Southern US, Southern Japan, and the Caribbean basin (Bunn et al., 1983; Blattner et al., 1983; Robert-Guroff et al., 1982; Sarin et al., 1983; Yamada, 1983; Yoshida et al., 1982; Schupbach et al., 1983). Clinically, HTLV-associated ATL is a high-grade malignancy with skin involvement, frequently leukemia, hypercalcemia, and lytic bone lesions (Uchiyana et al., 1977; Yamada, 1983). An arthritis–vasculitis syndrome has been reported with Japanese ATL (Haynes et al., 1983b). Hattori demonstrated in 1981 that most Japanese ATL malignant T cells expressed mature T-cell markers and were T4+ and T8−. Haynes et al. (1983b) have phenotypically characterized HTLV-infected fresh Japanese ATL patient PBL and infiltrating skin T cells and found them to be 3A1−, T4+ T8−. Popovic et al. (1983) and Mann et al. (1983) phenotypically characterized malignant PBL from HTLV+ ATL patients and HTLV-infected normal cord blood T cells using a panel of anti-T cell and anti-HLA reagents. It was found that HTLV fresh malignant T cells were predominantly T4+, T8−, whereas the expression of antigen 3A1 was variable (Popovic et al., 1983). However, an occasional HTLV-transformed cord blood T-cell line was seen that was HTLV+ and yet was T4−, T8+ (Popovic et al., 1983).

Using alloantisera and a monoclonal antibody (4D12) reactive with HLA antigens within the B5 cross-reactive group (Haynes et al., 1982c), Mann et al. (1983) demonstrated anomalous expression of Class I HLA antigens to be common on HTLV-infected cells and to be those of the HLA B5 group of antigens. Recent data by Clark et al. (1983) suggested that sequence homology existed between the envelope protein of HTLV and the heavy chain of HLA B molecule. Mann et al. (1983) and Clark et al. (1983) have postulated that sequence homology and thus antigenic cross-reactivity between HLA Class I antigens and HTLV envelope protein may be responsible for the observed anomalous expression of HLA B antigens on HTLV-infected cells. Whatever the explanation for this phenomenon, the availability of a monoclonal antibody (4D12) against HTLV-induced HLA-like determinants may prove useful in the identification of HTLV-infected T cells in tissue or uncultured PBL from HLA B5 group negative (4D12−) HTLV-associated ATL patients.

Although no monoclonal antibodies for HTLV specific surface proteins are as yet available for identifying HTLV-infected leukemic cells, several monoclonal reagents are available for HTLV internal core proteins that are of use in the diagnosis of HTLV-associated ATL (Haynes et al., 1984; Robert-Guroff et al., 1981). Monoclonal antibody 12/1-2 reacts with the p19 internal core protein of HTLV and with normal HTLV− thymic epithelium and basal layer of squamous keratinocytes, and therefore is not strictly HTLV specific (Robert-Guroff, 1981; Haynes et al., 1983c). We have produced four murine monoclonal antibodies, HTLV 6, 7, 8, and 9, that react with the p24 core protein of HTLV in Western blot and SDS polyacrylamide gel analysis (Palker et al., 1984a). Preclearing of ^{125}I labeled HTLV proteins with HTLV+ ATL patient serum or with goat anti-HTLV p24 serum followed by precipitation with antibodies HTLV 6, 7, 8, and 9 demonstrated that patient and goat serum as well as antibodies HTLV 6–9 all recognized the same p24 of HTLV. In competitive binding studies, antibodies HTLV 6, 7, and 8 bound to the same antigenic site on p24 (site A) whereas HTLV 9 bound to a second distinct antigenic site (site B). In similar competitive binding assays to HTLV p24, HTLV+ ATL patient sera inhibited the binding of antibodies HTLV 6, 7, 8, and 9 to HTLV p24 by 23–69%. Using indirect immunofluorescence in a wide tissue screen, antibodies HTLV 6–9 reacted only with acetone-fixed T cells infected with HTLV$_I$ or HTLV$_{II}$. Anti-p24 reactivity was localized in discrete patches at or near the cell surface (Fig. 1). Monoclonal antibodies HTLV 6–9 should be useful diagnostic probes for the identification of HTLV$_I$- and HTLV$_{II}$-infected cells, and in the study of diseases that may be associated with subtypes of HTLV, such as the acquired immunodeficiency syndrome.

As mentioned, monoclonal antibody 12/1-2 reacts with a 19 kilodalton (kd) core protein (p19) of HTLV and with HTLV− normal hu-

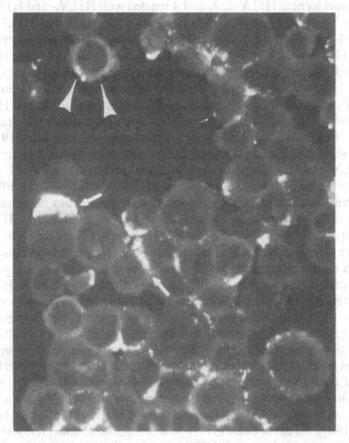

Fig. 1.   Immune fluorescence of HTLV+ acetone-fixed HUT 102 cells using anti-HTLV p24 monoclonal antibody HTLV-6. HTLV p24 was localized in discrete polar patches at or near the cell surface and between adjacent cells (arrows). Also, 5% of cells had intracytoplasmic anti-p24 fluorescence (arrow heads). Similar fluorescent staining of HUT 102 cells was also seen with HTLV 7, 8, and 9 (not shown) (× 400).

man thymic epithelium (Haynes et al., 1983). To study the antigenic relationship between HTLV p19 and thymic epithelium, Palker et al. (1984b) made three monoclonal antibodies, HTLV 2, 3, and 4, that react with HTLV p19. With isoelectric focusing of HTLV proteins followed by SDS polyacrylamide gel electrophoresis and Western blotting, antibody 12/1-2 identified a set of 19-kd proteins also recognized by 12/1-2. Using N-chlorosuccinimide to cleave proteins at tryptophan, degradation of precipitates obtained with all four anti-p19 antibodies resulted in a 17-kd fragment, in good agreement with the 16.5-kd fragment of p19 predicted from sequence analysis of the HTLV provirus. By indirect immunofluorescence, HTLV 2, 3, and 4 reacted with HTLV$_I$- and HTLV$_{II}$- infected T cells. In competitive inhibition assays, antibodies HTLV 2–4 and 12/1-2 recognize different antigenic sites on HTLV p19. Moreover, only HTLV 3 was exclusively specific for HTLV-infected T cells. HTLV 2 reacted with an intracellular antigen in all normal human tissues, and HTLV 4 reacted with human kidney and some non-HTLV associated tumors. Palker et al. (1984b) concluded that antibodies 12/1-2 and HTLV 2, 3, and 4 define different sites on a set of p19 molecules that are very similar in structure, but heterogeneous in charge. All four anti-p19 antibodies should be useful in defining the host immune response to antigens on HTLV p19 also shared by normal tissue, and in the study of HTLV-host interactions. The identification of HTLV proteins in fresh PBL or tissue has been complicated by the fact that complete virus particles, and therefore HTLV core proteins, are not expressed in uncultured HTLV-infected T cells (Poiesz et al., 1980). Only when T cells are cultured in vitro are complete budding virus particles seen by electron microscopy, and can the presence of the HTLV internal core proteins p19 and p24 be demonstrated (Poiesz et al., 1980). However, when PBL from HTLV-associated ATL are placed in culture for 5–7 d, either in the presence or absence of IL-2, the presence of virus can be easily demonstrated by staining acetone-fixed cytocentrifuge preparations of cultured T cells with monoclonal antibodies against HTLV p19 and p24 internal core proteins (Haynes et al., 1984; Robert-Guroff et al., 1981). P19 and p24 HTLV internal core proteins appear to be membrane-associated, either located on the inner surface of the T-cell membrane or inside HTLV virus located in caps on theinfected T-cell surface (Haynes et al., 1984; Robert-Guroff et al., 1981). Thus, because HTLV is an exogenous human retrovirus associated with a subtype of ATL, use of monoclonal reagents against HTLV-specific proteins has provided the ability to assay for leukemia cell specific antigens.

Regarding malignant T-cell immunoregulatory functional capabilities, in contrast to HTLV− CTCL leukemic cells that mediate T-cell help for B-cell Ig production in vitro, HTLV+ ATL T4+ cells generally function as suppressor T cells in similar in vitro B cell differentiation assays (Yamada, 1983).

4.9. Diffuse Lymphomas

Diffuse lymphomas composed of large- or medium-sized cells or a mixture of the two have been classified morphologically as "histiocytic," undifferentiated pleomorphic, or mixed lymphocytic–histiocytic. These neoplasms show considerable phenotypic heterogeneity: 50–60% of cases have B-cell features, 5–10% have markers consistent with T cells whereas approximately one-third have no detectable markers (Berard et al., 1978). Even within the T-cell subgroup there is clinical and histologic heterogeneity.

Waldron et al. (1977) described six adult patients with malignant lymphoma of peripheral T-cell origin whose disease had a predilection for lung and lymph node involvement. Pinkus et al. (1978) described four cases of a cytologically distinctive variant of T-cell lymphoma of large multilobulated lymphoid cell type. Palutke et al. (1980) described seven T-cell lymphomas of the large cell type with both regular and irregular nuclei. Lennert et al. (1982) reviewed the morphology and immunohistology of T-cell lymphomas with regards to expression of T4 and T8 antigens. Of 12 cases of pleomorphic T-cell lymphoma, most (7/12) expressed T4 only, one expressed T8 only, whereas 4 of 12 contained both T4+ and T8+ cells. Specific lymphocyte surface marker phenotype in five non-Hodgkin's lymphomas, including one Lennert's lymphoma, was reported by Borowitz et al. (1981). The five T-cell lymphomas described were morphologically heterogeneous and varied in their expression of T-cell antigens including T1, T3, T4, T8, and 3A1. Four of five, however, expressed T-cell antigens in the pattern of mature T cells (Borowitz et al., 1981).

4.10. T-Cell "Premalignant" Proliferative Diseases

Lymphomatoid granulomatosis (LyG) and parapsoriasis are T-cell proliferative disorders that are usually considered benign, but may progress to malignant states and thus could be considered "premalignant" conditions.

Lymphomatoid granulomatosis is an unusual form of granulomatous vasculitis characterized by infiltration of various organs with a lymphoreticular infiltrate (Fauci et al., 1982). The disease involves primarily the lungs, but skin, renal, and central nervous system may be involved. The disease is generally considered a benign inflammatory granulomatous process; however, LyG has been reported to progress to lymphoma in 50% of patients (Fauci et al., 1982). Phenotypic characterization of the skin infiltrates of LyG indicate that they are mature T cells (T11+, OKT4+, OKT8−, and 3A1−) (Fauci et al., 1982; Olsen et al., 1982). The lymphomas that develop have been reported as diffuse, large cell, or mixed type. Immunologic studies in one patient revealed a peripheral T-cell lymphoma (Fauci et al., 1982).

Parapsoriasis en plaques (PEP) is a heterogeneous group of cutaneous disorders characterized by plaques and a dermal lymphohistiocytic infiltrate. A subgroup of PEP, large plaque parapsoriasis, poses a major clinical problem in that is resembles mycosis fungoides both clinically and histologically and has the potential for transformation to cutaneous T-cell lymphoma (Olsen et al., 1982). Phenotypic characterization indicated that the lymphoid infiltrates were mature T cells (T1+ and T11+) and that all large plaque parapsoriasis patients had an T4+/T8− phenotype similar to the malignant T-cell infiltrates in CTCL. In contrast to large plaque parapsoriasis, which are T4+/T8−, two of five small plaque psoriasis (a more benign form of parapsoriasis) patients were found to have T8+/T4− skin T-cell infiltrates (Olsen et al., 1982).

The phenotypic characterization of human malignant T cells with respect to clinical and histologic diagnoses is summarized in Table 2.

4.11. Thymoma

Thymomas are a heterogeneous group of malignancies that arise in the anterior mediastinum and are composed of both epithelial cells and lymphocytes. Although the nature of the neoplastic cell is not known, it is thought to be derived from normal thymic epithelium. The lymphoid component of both primary mediastinal and metastatic thymoma is composed entirely of T cells. In mediastinal thymoma tissue, the epithelial component is either arrested or dedifferentiated at the stage of fetal thymus, and most thymocytes are immature and have the phenotype of cortical thymocytes (T6+, p80-) (Harden et al., 1983; Haynes et al., 1984). Mature T cells, when present, are rare and exist in small clusters or as single cells with no evidence of the normal cortical-medullary thymocyte organization (Harden et al., 1983).

5. Summary and Conclusions

Malignancies of thymus-derived (T) lymphocytes can be divided into two major groups: diseases of T cells expressing immature T-cell markers (T-ALL, T-cell lymphoblastic lymphoma) and diseases of malignant T-cells expressing markers in a pattern similar to normal mature T cells (T-cell CLL, ATL, various forms of CTCL, and T-PLL).

Until specific pathways of normal T-cell maturation are known, the relationship of phenotypic expression of various T-cell markers by malignant T cells to a particular stage of normal T-cell differentiation must remain speculative. However, phenotypic characterization of malignant T cells is an important first step in the study of events that transpire in the development of T-cell malignancies. Future parallel study into the mechanisms of normal and aberrant T-cell maturation will undoubtedly lead to greater understanding of the pathogenesis of the T-cell malignancies, and therefore pave the way for specific therapies for these difficult-to-treat syndromes.

Acknowledgments

The authors thank Ms. Joyce Lowery for expert secretarial assistance in the preparation of this manuscript.

Portions of this chapter have been previously published in *Seminars of Hematology*, 1984, and are reproduced here with permission of Grune and Stratton, Inc., New York, NY.

Table 2

Summary of Phenotypic Characterization of Clinical Types of T-Cell Malignancies[a]

Clinical or histologic diagnosis	Phenotypic characterization	References
T-acute lymphoblastic leukemia	Heterogeneous antigen profile; most express immature T-cell phenotype	Haynes et al., 1981b Catovsky et al., 1983 Koziner et al., 1982 Reinherz et al., 1980b Schroff et al., 1982 Foon et al., 1982
T-lymphoblastic lymphoma	Heterogeneous antigen profile; most express immature T-cell phenotype	Bernard et al., 1981 Bernard et al., 1982 Ritz et al., 1981
T-prolymphocytic leukemia	Most express mature T cell phenotype (T4$^+$ or T8$^+$)	Catvosky et al., 1982
T-chronic lymphocytic leukemia	Mature T-cell phenotype (T4$^+$ or T8$^+$)	Foon et al., 1982 Schroff et al, 1982
IgG Fc receptor positive (T$_G$) lymphoproliferative disease	Mature T-cell phenotype 3A1$^+$ or $-$, T4$^-$, T6$^-$	Bagby, 1981, Ferrarini et al., 1982, Schlimok et al., 1982
Cutaneous T cell lymphoma	PBL[b]: mature helper phenotype (3A1$^-$, T4$^+$, T8$^-$, T6$^-$)	Wood et al., 1982; Boumsell et al., 1981; Haynes et al., 1981b Kung et al., 1981
Mycosis fungoides/Sezary syndrome	Skin: mature helper phenotype (3A1$^+$, T4$^+$, T8$^-$, T6$^-$)	Haynes et al., 1982a Haynes et al., 1982b
T-cell type of hairy cell-leukemia	T4$^+$, T8$^-$, mature T-cell phenotype	Hernandez et al., 1978 Saxon et al., 1978
HTLV-associated Japanese Caribbean and American adult T-Cell leukemia/lymphoma	Skin and PBL: mature helper phenotype (3A1$-$, T4$^+$, T8$^-$, T6$^-$)	Yamada, 1983 Haynes et al., 1983b
Non-Hodgkins lymphoma	Mature T-cell phenotype	Berard et al., 1978 Borowitz et al., 1981
T-cell premalignant lymphoproliferative diseases		
Lymphomatoid granulomatosis	Mature helper phenotype (3A1$^-$, T4$^+$, T8$^-$)	Fauci et al., 1982 Haynes et al., 1982a
Parapsoriasis en plaque	Mature helper phenotype (3A1$^-$, T4$^+$, T8$^-$)	Olsen et al., 1982

[a]Phenotypes in this table, when given, are the usual phenotype for the clinical/histologic syndrome. In most cases, minor variations or alternative phenotypes have been reported.
[b]PBL = Peripheral blood lymphocytes.

References

Bagby, G. (1981), *J. Clin. Invest.* **68,** 1597.

Berard, C. S., and R. D. Dorfman (1974), *Clinics in Hematology,* Vol. 3 (Rosenberg, S. A., ed.), Saunders, Philadelphia.

Berard, C., E. Jaffe, R. Braylan, R. Mann, and K. Nanba (1978), *Cancer* **42,** 911.

Berger, C., S. Morrison, A. Chu, J. Patterson, A. Estabrook, S. Takezaki, J. Sharon, D. Warburton, O. Irigoyen, and R. Edelson (1982), *J. Clin. Invest.* **70,** 1205.

Bernard, A., L. Boumsell, E. L. Reinherz, L. Nadler, J. Ritz, H. Coppin, Y. Richard, F. Valensi, J. Dausset, G. Flandrin, J. Lemerle, and S. Schlossman (1981), *Blood* **57,** 1105.

Bernard, A., B. Raynal, J. Lemerle, L., and L. Boumsell (1982), *Blood* **59,** 809.

Beverly, P. C. L., D. Linch, and D. Delia (1980), *Nature* **287,** 332.

Beverly, P. C. L., and R. E. Collard (1981), in *XXIX Ann. Coll. Protides of the Biological Fluids.*

Blattner, W. A., D. W. Blayney, M. Robert-Guroff, M. Sarngadharan, V. Kalyanaraman, P. Sarin, E. Jaffe, and R. Gallo (1983), *J. Infect. Dis.* **147,** 406.

Bona, C. and A. Fauci (1980), *J. Clin. Invest.* **65,** 761.

Borowitz, M. J., B. P. Croker, and R. S. Metzgar (1981), *Am. J. Pathol.* **105,** 97.

Boumsell, L., H. Coppin, and D. Pham (1980), *J. Exp. Med.* **152,** 229

Boumsell, L., A. Bernard, E. Reinherz, L. Nadler, J. Ritz, H. Coppin, Y. Richard, L. Dubertret, F. Valensi, L. Degos, J. Lemerle, G. Flaudrin, J. Dausset, and S. Schlossman (1981), *Blood* **57,** 526.

Bradstock, K. F., G. Janossy, G. Pizzolo, A. Hoffbrad, A. McMichael, J. Pilch, C. Milstein, P. Beverly, and F. Bollum (1980), *J. Natl. Ca. Inst.* **65,** 33.

Broder, S., R. L. Edelson, M. A. Lutzner, D. Nelson, R. MacDermott, M. Drum, C. Goldman, B. Meade, and T. Waldmann (1976), *J. Clin. Invest.* **58,** 1297.

Broder, S., D. Poplack, J. Whang-Peng, M. Drum, C. Goldman, T. Muul, and T. Waldmann (1978), *New Engl. J. Med.* **298,** 66.

Broder, S., and P. A. Bunn (1980), *Semin. Oncol.* **7,** 310.

Brodsky, S., P. Parham, C. J. Barnstable, M. Crumpton, and W. Bodner (1979), *Immunol. Rev.* **47,** 3.

Brouet, J., and A. Prieur (1974), *Clin. Immunol. Immunopathol.* **2,** 481.

Brouet, J. C., J. L. Preud'homme, and U. Seligmann (1975), *Blood Cell* **1,** 81.

Brouet, J. C., J. L. Preud'homme, C. Pevit, F. Valensi, P. Rouget, and M. Seligmann (1979), *Blood* **54,** 269.

Bunn, P. A., G. Schechter, E. Jaffe, D. Blayney, R. Young, M. Mathews, W. Blattner, S. Broder, M. Robert-Guroff, and R. Gallo (1983), *New Engl. J. Med.* **309,** 257.

Catovsky, D. (1974) *Lancet* **2,** 327.

Catovsky, D., A. Wechsler, E. Matutes, R. Gomez, G. Bourchas, M. Cherchi, E. Pepys, M. Pepys, T. Kitani, A. Hoffbrand, and M. Greaves (1982), *Scand. J. Haematol.* **29,** 398.

Catovsky, D., J. F. San Miguel, J. Soler, E. Matutes, J. Meid, G. Bourikas, and B. Haynes (1983), *J. Exp. Clin. Ca. Res.,* in press.

Clark, M., E. Gelmann, and M. Reitz (1983), *Nature* **305,** 60.

Costello, C., D. Catovsky, M. Obrien, R. Moulla, and S. Varadi (1980), *Leuk. Res.* **4,** 463.

Eisenbarth, G. S., B. F. Haynes, J. A. Schroer, and A. S. Fauci (1980), *J. Immunol.* **124,** 1237.

Engleman, E. G., R. Warnke, R. I. Fox, and R. Levy (1981), *Proc. Nat'l Acad. Sci. (USA)* **78,** 1791.

Evans, R. L., H. Lazarus, A. C. Penta, and S. Schlossman (1978), *J. Immunol.* **120,** 1423.

Fauci, A., B. Haynes, J. Costa, P. Katz, and S. Wolfe (1982), *New Engl. J. Med.* **306,** 68.

Ferrarini, M., S. Romagnani, E. Montesoro, A. Zicca, G. Del Prete, A. Nocera, E. Maggi, A. Leprini, and C. Grossi (1982), *J. Clin. Immunol.* **3,** 30.

Foon, K. A., R. J. Billing, P. Terasaki, and M. Cline (1980), *Blood* **11,** 20.

Foon, K., R. Schroff, and R. Gale (1982), *Blood* **60,** 1.

Frei, E., and S. Sallan (1978), *Cancer* **42,** 828.

Galili, U., A. Polliack, E. Okon, R. Leizerovitz, H. Gamliel, A. Korkesh, J. Schenkar, and G. Izah (1980), *J. Exp. Med.* **152,** 1423.

Galton, D. A. G., J. M. Goldman, E. Wiltshaw, D. Catovsky, K. Henry, and G. Goldenberg (1974), *Br. J. Haematol.* **27,** 7.

Golde, D. W., R. H. Stevens, S. G. Quan, and A. Saxon (1977), *Br. J. Haematol.* **35,** 359.

Greaves, M. F. and G. Brown (1975), *Clin. Immunol. Immunopathol.* **4,** 67.

Greaves, M. C. (1981), *Canc. Res.* **41,** 4752.

Greaves, M., J. Rao, G. Hariri, W. Verbi, D. Catovsky, P. Kung, and G. Goldstein (1981), *Leuk. Res.* **5,** 281.

Guglielmi, P., J. Preud'homme, and G. Flandrin (1980), *Nature* **286,** 166.

Hansen, J. A., P. J. Martin, and R. C. Nowinski (1980), *Immunogenetics* **10,** 247.

Harden, E. A., K. H. Singer, E. J. McFarland, A. S. Wechsler, and B. F. Haynes (1983), *Blood* **62,** 286.

Hattori, T., T. Uchiyama, T. Toibana, K. Takatsuki, and H. Uchino (1981), *Blood* **58,** 645.

Haynes, B. F., G. S. Eisenbarth, and A. S. Fauci (1979), *Proc. Natl. Acad. Sci. (USA)* **76,** 5829.

Haynes, B. F. (1981), *Immunol. Rev.* **57,** 127.

Haynes, B. F., M. Hemler, T. Cotner, D. Mann, G. Eisenbarth, J. Strominger, and A. Fauci (1981a), *J. Immunol.* **127,** 347.

Haynes, B. F., R. S. Metzgar, J. D. Minna, and P. A. Bunn (1981b), *New Engl. J. Med.* **304,** 1319.

Haynes, B. F., L. L. Hensley, and B. V. Jegasothy (1982a), *Blood* **60,** 463.

Haynes, B. F., L. L. Hensley, and B. V. Jegasothy (1982b), *J. Invest. Dermatol.* **78**, 323.

Haynes, B. F., E. Reisner, M. Hemler, J. Strominger, and G. Eisenbarth (1982c), *Human Immunol.* **4**, 273.

Haynes, B. F., E. A. Harden, M. J. Telen, M. E. Hemler, J. Strominger, T. Palker, R. Scearce, and G. Eisenbarth (1983a), *J. Immunol.* **131**, 1195.

Haynes, B. F., S. E. Miller, T. J. Palker, J. O. Moore, P. Dunn, D. Bolognesi, and R. Metzgar (1983b), *Proc. Natl. Acad. Sci. (USA)* **80**, 2054.

Haynes, B. F., M. Robert-Guroff, R. S. Metzgar, G. Franchini, V. Kalyanaraman, T. Palker, and R. Gallo (1983c), *J. Exp. Med.* **157**, 907.

Haynes, B. F., T. J. Palker, and R. M. Scearce (1984), in *Cancer Cells*, Vol. 3, *Human T-Cell Leukemia Viruses* (R. Gallo and M. Essex, eds.), Cold Spring Harbor Press, New York, in press.

Heideman, R., J. Falletta, N. Mukhopadhyay, and O. Fernbach (1978), *J. Ped.* **92**, 540.

Hernandez, D., C. Cruz, J. Carnot, E. Dortrios, and E. Espinosa (1978), *Br. J. Haematol.* **40**, 504.

Hershfield, M., J. Kurtzberg, E. Harden, J. Moore, J. Whang-Peng, and B. Haynes (1984), *Proc. Natl. Acad. Sci. (USA)*, in press.

Hooks, J., B. Haynes, B. Detrich-Hooks, L. Diehl, L. Gerrard, T. Gerrard and A. Fauci (1982), *Blood* **59**, 198.

Howard, F. D., J. A. Ledbetter, J. Wong, C. Beiber, E. Stinson, and L. Herzenberg (1981), *J. Immunol.* **126**, 2117.

Huhn, D., E. Thiel, H. Rodt, G. Schlimok, H. Theml, and P. Rieber (1983), *Cancer* **51**, 1434.

Janossy, G. and H. G. Prentice (1982), *Clinics in Haematol.* **11**, 631.

Jansen, J., T. LeBien, and J. Kersey (1982), *Blood* **59**, 609.

Judd, W., C. A. Poodry, and J. A. Strominger (1980), *J. Exp. Med.* **152**, 1430.

Kadin, M., M. Kamoun, and J. Lamberg (1981), *New Engl. J. Med.* **304**, 648.

Kalyanaraman, V., M. Sarngadharan, M. Robert-Guroff, I. Miyoshi, D. Blayney, D. Golde, and R. Gallo (1982), *Science* **218**, 571.

Kamoun, M., M. E. Kadin, P. J. Martin, J. Nettleton, and J. Hansen (1981a), *J. Immunol.* **127**, 987.

Kamoun, M., P. J. Martin, J. A. Hansen, M. Brown, A. Siddak, and R. Nowsinki (1981b), *J. Exp. Med.* **153**, 207.

King, G. W., P. E. Hurtubise, A. L. Sagone, Jr., A. Lobuglio, and E. Metz (1975), *Am. J. Med.* **59**, 411.

Kohler, G., and C. Milstein (1975), *Nature* **256**, 495.

Korsmeyer, S. J., P. A. Hieter, J. V. Ravetch, D. Poplack, T. Waldmann, and P. Leder (1981), *Proc. Natl. Acad. Sci.* **78**, 7096.

Koziner, B., A. Gebhard, T. Denny, S. McKenzie, B. Clarkson, D. Miller, and R. Evans (1982), *Blood* **60**, 752.

Kung, P. C., G. Goldstein, E. L. Reinherz, and S. Schlossman (1979), *Science* **206**, 347.

Kung, P., C. Berter, G. Goldstein, P. Olgerfo, and R. Edelson (1981), *Blood* **57**, 261.

Laroche, L., M. Papiernek, and J. Bach (1983), *J. Immunol.* **130**, 2467.

Ledbetter, S. A., R. L. Evans, M. Lipinski, C. Cunningham-Rundles, R. Good, and L. Herzenberg (1981), *J. Exp. Med.* **153**, 310.

Lennert, K., H. Stein, A. Feller, and J. Gerdes (1982), *B and T Cell Tumors*, Academic Press.

Lobuglio, A. F. (1976), *New Engl. J. Med.* **295**, 219.

Maino, V., J. Kurnick, R. Hubo, and H. Grey (1977), *J. Immunol.* **118**, 743.

Mann, D. L., M. Popovic, P. Sarin, C. Murray, M. Reizt, D. Strong, B. Haynes, R. Gallo, and W. Blattner (1983), *Nature* **305**, 58.

Martin, P. J., J. A. Hansen, R. C. Nowinski, and M. Brown (1980), *Immunogenetics* **11**, 429.

McMichael, A. J., J. R. Pilch, G. Galfre, D. Mason, J. Fabre, and C. Milstein (1979), *Eur. J. Immunol.* **9**, 205.

Metzgar, R., M. Borowitz, N. Jones, and B. Dowell (1981), *J. Exp. Med.* **154**, 1249.

Minowada, J. (1982), in *Membrane and Other Phenotypes of Leukemia Cells*, 13th International Cancer Congress, Alan R. Liss, Inc. New York.

Minowada, J., K., Minato, B. Srivastava, S. Nakazawa, I, Kubonishi, E. Tatsumi, T. Ohnuma, H. Ozer, A. Freeman, E. Henderson, and R. Gallo (1982), *Current Concepts in Huamn Immunology and Cancer Immunomodulation*, Elsevier Biomed. Press.

Nadler, L. M., E. L. Reinherz, H. J. Weinstein, C. D'orzi, and S. Schlossman (1980), *Blood* **55**, 806.

Nagasawa, T., T. Abe, and T. Nakagawa (1981), *Blood* **57**, 1025.

Naito, K., R. Knowles, F. Real, Y. Moushima, and B. Dupont (1983), *Blood*, in press.

Nathwani, B. N., H. Kim, and H. Rappaport (1976), *Cancer* **38**, 964.

Olsen, E., B. Jegasothy, and B. F. Haynes (1982), *Clin. Res.* **30**, 600A.

Omary, M. D., I. S. Trowbridge, and J. Minowada (1980), *Nature* **286**, 888.

Palker, T. J., R. M. Scearce, M. Popovic, R. C. Gallo, D. P. Bolognesi, and B. F. Haynes (1984a), *Clinical Res.*, in press.

Palker, T. J., R. M. Scearce, W. Ho., D. P. Bolognesi, and B. F. Haynes (1984b), *Clinical Res.*, in press.

Palutke, M., P. Tabaczka, R. Weiss, A. Axelrod, C. Palacas, H. Margolis, P. Khilanan, V. Ratanathrarathor, J. Piligian, R. Pollard, and M. Husain (1980), *Cancer* **46**, 87.

Pinkus, G., J. Said, and H. Hargreaves (1978), *Am. J. Clin. Pathol.* **72**, 540.

Poiesz, B., F. Ruscetti, A. Gazdar, P. Bunn, J. Minna, and R. Gallo (1980), *Proc. Natl. Acad. Sci. (USA)* **77**, 7415.

Popovic, M., P. S. Sarin, M. Robert-Guroff, V. Kalyanaraman, D. Mann, J. Minowada, and R. Gallo (1983), *Science* **219**, 856.

Preud'homme, J. L., and M. Seligmann (1972), *Blood* **40**, 774.

Reinherz, E. L., P. C. Kung, G. Goldstein, and S. Schlossman (1979a), *J. Immunol.* **123**, 2894.

Reinherz, E. L., P. C. Kung, J. M. Pesandro, J. Ritz, G. Goldstein, and S. Schlossman (1979b), *J. Exp. Med.* **150**, 147.

Reinherz, E. L., L. Nadler, D. Rosenthal, W. Moloney, and S. Schlossman (1979c), *Blood* **53**, 1066.

Reinherz, E. L., L. M. Nadler, S. E. Sallan, and S. Schlossman (1979d), *J. Clin. Invest.* **64**, 392.

Reinherz, E. L., R. E. Hussey, and S. F. Schlossman (1980a), *Eur. J. Immunol.* **10**, 758.

Reinherz, E. L., P. C. Kung, G. Goldstein, R. Levy, and S. Schlossman (1980b), *Proc. Natl. Acad. Sci. (USA)* **77**, 1588.

Reinherz, E. L. and S. F. Schlossman (1980a), *Cell* **19**, 821.

Reinherz, E. L. and S. F. Schlossman (1980b), *New Engl. J. Med.* **303**, 370.

Ritz, J., J. M. Pesandro, J. Notis-McConarty, H. Lazarus, and S. Schlossman (1980), *Nature* **283**, 583.

Ritz, J., L. M. Nadler, A. K. Bhan, J. Notis-McConarty, J. Pesandro, and S. Schlossman (1981), *Blood* **58**, 648.

Ritz, J., and S. F. Schlossman (1982), *Blood* **59**, 1.

Robert-Guroff, M., F. W. Ruscetti, L. E. Posner, B. Poiesz, and R. Gallo (1981), *J. Exp. Med.* **154**, 1957.

Robert-Guroff, M., Y. Nakao, K. Notake, Y. Ito, A. Sliski, and R. Gallo (1982), *Science* **215**, 975.

Royston, I., J. A. Majda, S. M. Baiad, B. Meserve, and J. Griffiths (1980), *J. Immunol.* **125**, 725.

Rumke, H., F. Miedema, J. Ten Berge, F. Terpstra, H. vander Reijden, R. vandeGriend, H. deBruin, A. Von demBorne, J. Smit, W. Ziejlemaker, and C. Melief (1982), *J. Immunol.* **129**, 419.

Sarin, P. S., T. Aoki, A. Shibata, Y. Ohnishi, Y. Aonagi, H. Miyakoshi, I. Emura, V. Kalyanaraman, M. Robert-Guroff, M. Popovic, M. Sarngadharan, P. Nowell, and R. Gallo (1983), *Proc. Natl. Acad. Sci. (USA)* **80**, 2370.

Saxon, A., R. Stevens, and D. Golde (1978), *Ann. Int. Med.* **88**, 323.

Schlimok, G., E. Thiel, E. Rieber, D. Huhn, H. Feucht, I. Lohneyer, and G. Reithmuller (1982), *Blood* **59**, 1157.

Schroff, R. W., K. A. Foon, R. J. Billing, and J. Fahey (1982), *Blood* **59**, 207.

Schupbach, J., V. S. Kalyanaraman, M. G. Sarngadharan, W. Blattner, and R. Gallo (1983), *Cancer Res.* **43**, 886.

Sen, L. and L. Borella (1975), *New Engl. J. Med.* **292**, 828.

Simone, J., M. Versoza, and J. Rudy (1975), *Cancer* **36**, 2099.

Smyth, J. F., D. G. Poplack, and B. J. Holeman (1978), *J. Clin. Invest.* **67**, 710.

Stutman, O. (1977), *Contemp. Top. Immunobiol.* **7**, 1.

Sullivan, M. P. (1962), *Peds.* **29**, 589.

Timonen, T., J. Outaldo, and R. Herberman (1981), *J. Exp. Med.* **153**, 569.

Uchiyama, T., J. Yodoi, K. Sagawa, K. Takatsuki, and H. Uchino (1977), *Blood* **50**, 581.

Umiel, T., J. F. Daley, A. K. Bhan, R. Levy, S. Schlossman, and E. Reinherz (1982), *J. Immunol.* **129**, 1054.

Verbi, W., M. F. Greaves, K. Koubek, G. Janossy, P. Kung, and G. Goldstein (1982), *Eur. J. Immunol.* **12**, 81.

Vodinelick, L., W. Tax, Y. Bai, S. Pegram, P. Capel, and M. Greaves (1983), *Blood*, in press.

Waldron, J., J. Leech, A. Glock, J. Flexner, and R. Collins (1977), *Cancer* **40,** 1604.

Wang, C. Y., R. A. Good, P. Ammirati, G. Dymbort, and R. Evans (1980), *J. Exp. Med.* **151,** 1539.

Webster, R. (1961), *Med. J. Aust.* **48,** 582.

Wood, G., D. Deneau, R. Miller, R. Levy, R. Hoppe, and R. Warnke (1982), *Blood* **59,** 876.

Yamada, Y. (1983), *Blood* **61,** 192.

Yoshida, M., I. Miyoshi, and Y. Hinuma (1982), *Proc. Natl. Acad. Sci. (USA)* **79,** 2031.

Chapter 7

Antigenic Markers on Normal and Malignant B Cells

STEPHEN BAIRD

Laboratory Service, VA Medical Center, San Diego, and Department of Pathology, University of California, San Diego

1. Introduction

Monoclonal antibodies and appropriately absorbed antisera have defined a large number of surface markers on B cells. The distribution of these markers has been studied both in the normal maturation of B cells and in B cell malignancies. It is now possible to give rather detailed descriptions of the markers expressed by normal cells at any given stage of differentiation and to do the same for B cell lymphomas and leukemias in each of the morphological categories of commonly used classification systems. As might be expected, some old concepts of the pathogenesis of lymphomas and leukemias have been shown to be in need of revision.

Today there are probably two basic questions about human B cell lymphomas that can be at least partially answered by studies of surface markers. They are: Do B cell lymphomas mimic normal B cells that have been transformed and "frozen" at a particular stage of differentiation? And, in the case of nodular lymphomas, do the cells comprising the nodules mimic the cells of germinal centers (follicular-center cells of Lukes and Collins)? The first question is a general one and is of interest to everyone studying cancer. It is commonly believed that cancer cells are transformed and frozen at various stages of normal differentiation. Whether or not such a concept will aide medical scientists in finding cures for neoplasms is an open question. The second question relates specifically to B

cell lymphomas. The follicular center cell concept of lymphomas postulates that the cells of all nodular and some diffuse lymphomas morphologically resemble the cells of germinal centers. By implication one can also
postulate that such malignant cells might mimic many biological properties of germinal center cells. One may, possibly, gain insight into both the
process of lymphomagenesis and the migratory behavior of the transformed cells by exploring the implications of this hypothesis.

To approach these questions and their more obvious corollaries, we
shall first review the orderly change of surface markers during normal B
cell differentiation, then examine the same markers on B cell lymphomas
and leukemias. There are still a number of gaps in our knowledge in both
fields, but a coherent picture is beginning to emerge.

2. Antigenic Markers on Normal B Cells

One of the earliest discovered and therefore most extensively studied surface markers on B cells is immunoglobulin, SIg. SIg serves as an antigen
receptor and can receive signals that cause cell division as well as specific
inhibition of reactivity or tolerance. Early studies of the distribution of
SIg on lymphocytes were done with antisera. More recently, monoclonal
antibodies specific for various heavy and light chains have been used.
These studies have produced a reasonable consensus concerning the expression of various types of Ig in and on B cells during normal maturation. Some of the studies have been done in mice and others in humans.
Obviously, the techniques have not been identical but the findings are
similar enough to warrant the conclusion that B cell maturation in mice
and men procedes along the same general lines. The following is the current view of B cell maturation in mice and men as reflected by changes in
cytoplasmic and surface Ig.

Figure 1 shows a scheme of B cell maturation in which IgM, IgD,
IgG, and IgA are followed. The figure represents a compilation of data
generated both in mice and men by several different techniques.

In the bone marrow B cells first express cytoplasmic μ chains. During the process of B cell differentiation, DNA is rearranged to bring appropriate heavy and light chain constant regions into alignment with
specific variable regions. A unique nucleic acid sequence is thus generated in each B cell coding for heavy and light immunoglobulin chains
with specific antigen binding activity. The protein product of this rearrangement is first detected by immunofluorescence as cytoplasmic μ
chains. Such cells are commonly called "pre-B cells."

The cell next goes on to express IgM on its surface. At this point, it
is still in the marrow and initially is probably not antigen-sensitive. As
the B cell begins to leave the marrow, it expresses an Fc receptor for solu-

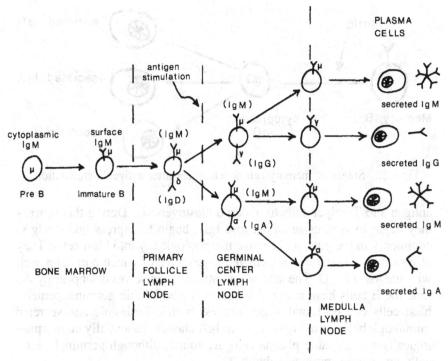

Fig. 1.   Stages of B cell maturation correlated with immunoglobulin expression and location in the lymphoid system.

ble Ig and gains anitgen sensitivity at about the same time. Thus, the bloodstream contains some B cells that express only cell surface IgM and Fc receptors. Though these cells can respond to antigen, their response is probably not induction of Ig synthesis and secretion, but specific antigenic tolerance.

B cells from the marrow circulate to the lymph nodes, spleen, and gut-associated lymphoid tissues (tonsils, adenoids, Peyer's patches). In lymph nodes and spleen, they home to primary follicles (described in more detail below). By the time the B cells have arrived in primary follicles, they express surface IgM and IgD. They still express Fc receptors and have added Ia antigens and complement (C'3) receptors. These cells are antigen responsive and mitogen responsive: They respond to the binding of specific antigen or B cell mitogens by cell division and further maturation. Before this point, B cell maturation proceeded in the absence of specific antigenic stimulation. Further maturational events are thought to require the presence of antigen and usually T cell help. In the absence of antigen the cells merely wait in follicles or recirculate slowly.

After antigenic stimulation germinal centers form in all peripheral lymphoid tissues. The lymph node has been best studied and will serve as our model. The IgM$^+$, IgD$^+$ B cells of primary follicles are stimulated by

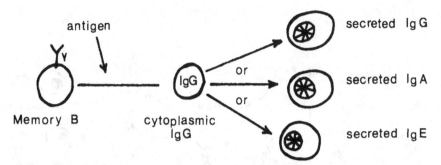

Fig. 2.   Stages of memory cell development after antigenic stimulation.

antigen and T helper cells to undergo blastogenesis. During this process they begin to synthesize DNA, lose IgD, begin to express IgG (or IgA, commonly in the gut), and change morphologically into blast cells. They also express activiation antigens the appearance of which correlates well with the loss of IgD. The activation antigens themselves disappear by the time the B cells have matured to plasma cells. Within germinal centers, blast cells can be found which express both cytoplasmic and secreted immunoglobulin of the IgM, IgG, or IgA classes. Essentially no morphologically recognizable plasma cells are found, although germinal center cells do secrete immunoglobulin.

After germinal centers have formed, plasma cells begin to accumulate in the medulla of the lymph nodes. These cells are easily recognized by their characteristic morphology. They express large amounts of cytoplasmic immunoglobulin and secreted immunoglobulin, but do not display significant amounts of Ig on their surfaces. These cells also lose the Ia antigen. Plasma cells of the IgM, IgG, or IgA type may be found in the medulla of any reactive lymph node. They are presumably derived from emigrants from germinal centers because a few plasma cells can also be found in the cortex, between the follicles and medulla.

The foregoing represents an outline of the sequence of events in normal B cell maturation. Part of the sequence is antigen-dependent and part apparently antigen-independent. There is an orderly acquisition and loss of expression of specific heavy chains in the cytoplasm and on the cell surface, coupled with an equally orderly expression and loss of other cell surface markers and activation antigens.

Memory B cells have not been studied as well, but in the case of the γ-bearing memory B cell the following sequence has been worked out.

At least one class of memory B cell expresses surface IgG. It apparently arises by asymmetric division as a byproduct of the primary immune response. Upon secondary antigenic stimulation, the memory cell divides, expresses cytoplasmic IgG, then goes on to secrete either IgG, IgA, or IgE. Other antigens expressed by B memory cells have not been as well-characterized.

The structure of lymph nodes in which the preceding events take place has been well described. Antisera and monoclonal antibodies have been used in immunofluorescent or immunoperoxidase studies to define the location of cells expressing different surface antigens. The results for surface immunoglobulin, Ia, and a B cell activation antigen (B532) are shown in Fig. 3(a). Figure 3(b) shows the distribution of T cells and is included for reference.

IgM is found on the cells of primary follicles (an aggregation of B cells which contains no germinal center), within germinal centers both in blast cells and in the intercellular space, on reticular cells in germinal centers, and in plasma cells in the medulla. IgD is found on the cells of primary follicles but not in germinal centers. When a follicle contains a germinal center the IgD bearing cells are found only on the mantle cells, the residual cells of the primary follicle in which the germinal center formed. IgD is also not found in plasma cells of the medulla. These anatomic locations of IgM and IgD bearing cells indicate that the cell which expresses both IgM and IgD homes to and resides in the primary follicles of lymph nodes. This same cell is also the most common type of B cell to be found in the bloodstream. B cells expressing IgM only (early B) or IgG only (memory B) are very rare in the circulation.

IgG is not found on the cells of primary follicles. Instead it is found in germinal centers where it is in blast cells, secreted into the intercellular space, and on reticular cells. Reticular cells have been demonstrated to have Fc receptors and therefore probably acquire both surface IgM and IgG by Fc binding. There is no evidence that reticular cells synthesize antibody. IgG is also found in plasma cells in the medulla. Note that some plasma cells secrete IgM and others secrete IgG. There is no evidence that individual IgM secreting plasma cells change to IgG secreting cells even though there is a switch from IgM secretion to IgG secretion during the immune responses. (See Fig. 1.) Often reactive lymph nodes which contain many germinal centers and many plasma cells have large quantities of IgG secreted into the intercellular space throughout the node. When this occurs, it makes interpretation of the distribution of other heavy chain types more difficult, but not impossible if one's reagents are truly specific.

The distribution of K and λ chains in normal lymph nodes is what one might expect considering the preceding description of heavy chain expression. The light chains are found on primary follicle cells, in germinal centers, and in plasma cells in the medulla. When one labels anti-K or anti-λ antibodies with fluorescein and rhodamine respectively, one finds that the individual cells of primary follicles express either K or λ, but not both. Within a single follicle, one finds both K and λ expressing cells, but each cell appears restricted, at least with respect to light chain expression. Primary follicles are therefore polyclonal aggregates of individual B cells and presumably contain cells capable of reacting with a large number of

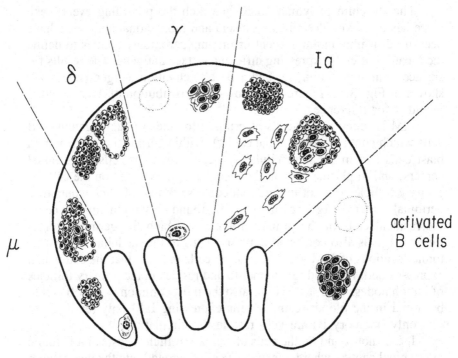

Fig. 3(a).   Surface markers on B cells within a lymph node. The lymph node is schematically divided into five parts. The cells detected by antibodies to the indicated antigens are drawn in each segment. The circles formed of small dots in the γ and activated B cell segments indicate that primary follicles are not recognized by antibodies directed against the antigens.

different antigens. Germinal centers are also polyclonal proliferations made up of K expressing blast cells and λ expressing blast cells. Both light chains are also secreted and bound to reticular cells. Individual K-secreting or λ-secreting plasma cells are found throughout the medulla. Again a single cell expresses only one light chain.

The Ia antigen is found on all B cells in lymph nodes except at the plasma cell stage. It is also present on the reticular cells of lymph nodes both in germinal centers and throughout the cortex. Recognition of antigen in combination with Ia has been shown to be a requirement for activation of T helper cells. The reticular cells of lymph nodes are therefore candidates for antigen presenting cells. They can fix antigen–antibody complexes to their surfaces by means of Fc receptors and they express surface Ia. T helper cells encountering antigen in such an environment can be stimulated to further differentiation and to secrete products that stimulate B cell differentiation.

The B cell activation antigen detected by B532 antibody is found only in germinal centers and occasionally on the adjacent mantle cells. It

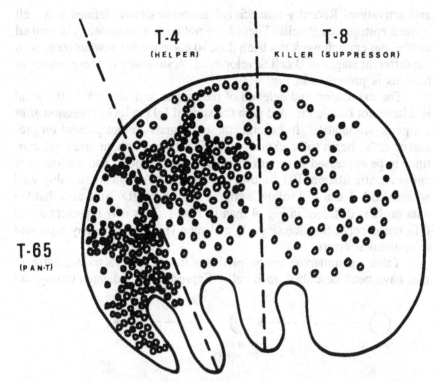

T-4
(HELPER)

T-8
KILLER (SUPPRESSOR)

T-65
(PAN-T)

Fig. 3(b). Surface markers on T cells within a lymph node. T cells of both helper and suppressor type are distributed randomly throughout the diffuse cortex. A few T cells, mostly of helper phenotype, are always present in primary follicles and in germinal centers.

is not found on primary follicle cells nor on plasma cells. Its expression correlates well with the loss of IgD and the expression of IgG after antigenic stimulation. This same correlation holds true after stimulation in vitro with B cell mitogens. In the mouse, peanut agglutinin binds to germinal center cells but not to IgD bearing cells. Recirculating B cells in the blood, most of which express IgM and D on each cell, do not bind peanut agglutinin. If one separates the peanut agglutinin-binding cells out of lymph nodes and reinjects them into mice, they do not home back to the lymph nodes, whereas IgD-bearing cells do. These observations indicate that the cells of primary follicles are capable of circulation and homing but that the cells of germinal centers are not. It is most reasonable therefore to consider germinal centers as a local response to antigenic stimulation. This concept will become more significant when we discuss nodular lymphomas.

The changing expression of Ig, Ia, and activation antigens in B cells in the lymphoid organs and in vitro after antigenic or mitogenic stimulation has produced an internally consistent description of B cell maturation and activation. Recently monoclonal antibodies have defined new cell surface epitopes on B cells. These have not been as completely described as SIg, but enough work has been done to correlate the new antigens with the different stages of B cell development. A summary of these studies in humans is presented in Fig. 4.

The expression and deletion of the human antigens BA-1, B-1, and B-2 have not been correlated with the shift of IgD to IgG expression after antigenic stimulation. In general, these antigens are not present on precursor cells, begin to be expressed on B cells in the bone marrow, continue to be expressed on mature B cells in lymph nodes, and are lost after antigenic stimulation. B-1 follows the expression of IgM reasonably well whereas BA-1 and B-2 follow a course similar to IgD. Note also that the data on Ia is different in Fig. 4 than in Fig. 1. This may represent a real difference between mice (Fig. 1) and men (Fig. 4) or it may represent experimental errors.

Table 1 summarizes the properties of the well-characterized antigens that have been described on B cells. Expression is indicated throughout

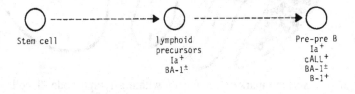

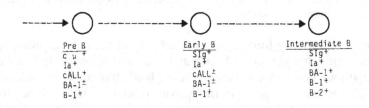

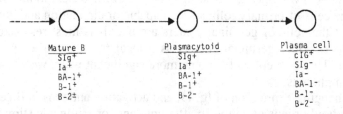

Fig. 4. Correlation of surface markers with B cell maturation.

Table 1
Molecular Weights and Distribution of Surface Markers on B Cells

Marker	Mol wt × 10^{-3}	Stem	Pre B	Early B	Mature B	Blast[a]	Plasma cell
cµ	70	−	+	−	−	+	+
cIgM	190	−	+	−	−	+	+
sIgM	190	−	−	+	+	+	−
IgD	190	−	−	+	+	−	−
cIgG	150	−	−	−	−	+	+
sIgG	150	−	−	−	+[b]	−	−
IgA	170	−	−	−	−	+	+
Ia	28±33	−	+	+	+	+	−
Fc	?	−	+	+	+	?	−
C	?	−	−	+	+	?	−
B532	45	−	−	−	−	+	−
BA-1	?	−	−	+	+	+	−
B-1	30	−	+	+	+	+	−
B-2	120						
	140	−	−	−	+	−	−
J-5(cALL)	?	+	+	−	−	−	−

[a]Blast transformation due to antigen or mitogen
[b]These are memory cells, which are apparently rare. They are recorded in this column for convenience.

the cell cycle, as is the molecular weight of the marker, if known. This information makes it possible to define a series of normal B cell phenotypes and compare them to the phenotype of cells in B cell lymphomas.

3. Antigenic Markers on Malignant B Cells

To understand the significance of cell surface markers on B lymphoma cells, one should examine them in the context of the biologic behavior of lymphomas. There are two major areas in which lymphoma biology has been investigated: animal models and clinical studies in humans. The information generated in these two systems has been of a significantly different nature. In animal models, essentially all lymphomas are caused by RNA retroviruses although some of the herpes viruses are lymphomagenic in primates. Virally induced lymphomas in a given animal tend to be uniform with regard to the target cell and disease process. Thus, retroviruses cause B cell lymphomas in chickens and T cell lymphomas in mice. Most lymphomas in humans appear to be of B cell origin, so man resembles the chicken more than the mouse at least in this respect. Somewhat ironically, a human T cell lymphoma virus has recently been described in humans, but no B cell retrovirus has yet been discovered. The Epstein-Barr virus, which is associated with Burkitt's lymphoma, does not appear to cause the majority of human B cell neoplasms.

In spite of the current gaps in our knowledge and lack of complete consistency between animal models and human disease, the course of retrovirus induced lymphomas should be kept in mind when studying the human diseases. In susceptible strains of chicken when an appropriate retrovirus is injected into chicks, the Bursa of Fabricius (the site of B cell maturation), becomes infected. A generalized polyclonal proliferative response ensues during which a polyclonal IgM gammopathy can also be demonstrated. The B cell proliferative reaction remains confined to the bursa until sexual maturity is reached, when, mostly in females, the proliferating cells break out and spread to the lymph nodes, spleen, liver, and the rest of the body. At this point one clone of B cells has usually become dominant. The involved cells express IgM on their surfaces and usually produce infectious virus. Certain strains of chicken spontaneously develop lymphomas that follow the same pattern, and are also associated with virus production. Recent experiments suggest that the role of the virus in transformation is to integrate itself in the host DNA upstream from genes that are important in regulating cell growth. Constitutive synthesis of the products of such genes, in this case *C myc,* is associated with B cell transformation by an as yet undefined mechanism. As far as anyone knows, the products of the *myc* gene or other transforming genes are not expressed as cell surface markers. Instead many such genes function as enzymes which catalyze the phosphorylation of tyrosine. The event which leads to B cell transformation by retroviruses may, therefore, not be reflected by any consistent cell surface marker change. This is even true in the case of virus production by the tumor cells, for continuous production of infectious virus is not always necessary to induce lymphomagenesis. The relevance of this for human B cell lymphomas remains to be seen. It is important to remember that a tumor may be initiated by a virus even though the tumor no longer produces the virus by the time the disease is clinically apparent.

The process of viral induction of T cell lymphomas in mice is also worth reviewing because it helps to illustrate a general point. When a lymphoma virus is injected into mice, the thymus becomes infected. After an initial period of involution, the thymus repopulates with cells, all of which are replicating viral antigens, but not necessarily whole virus.

After several months a transformed clone emerges, breaks out of the thymus, and invades the lymph nodes, spleen, liver, bone marrow, and other organs. The tumor cells may or may not produce infectious virus particles although they always continue to produce some viral antigens, usually the envelope glycoprotein. Again, gene rearrangements similar to those in the chicken can be demonstrated in many of the lymphomas. By surface marker analysis, lymphomas of "immature" T cells, helper cells, and suppressor cells can all emerge from this process. The tumor in one animal is usually monoclonal when it becomes clinically apparent, but it can be polyclonal. The initial proliferative response in the thymus is usually multicentric.

Both the chicken and mouse models show that lymphomas usually begin in a central lymphoid organ, the bursa or thymus, and then spread peripherally.

When they are clinically apparent they are always Stage IV according to human criteria. Human B cell lymphomas seem to follow this rule for they, in contrast to Hodgkin's disease, almost never present at a low stage. If future experiments identify a human B cell lymphoma virus, one would predict that its mode of action would be similar to the chicken virus and that human B lymphomas would usually *originate* in the bone marrow (the bursa equivalent?) and spread peripherally rather late in the disease process.

Clinical studies on human B lymphomas have produced little evidence on what causes the disease, but have instead concentrated on how the diseases behave. The type of data which has been generated is mostly due to the nature of B lymphoma classification systems and the studies that have been done on patients classified according to these systems. The first useful system was published by Rappaport and Gall in the 1950s. These authors divided non-Hodgkin's lymphomas into two large categories, nodular and diffuse. Nodular lymphomas replaced lymph nodes with grossly obvious nodules of cells while diffuse lymphomas replaced lymph nodes with uniform sheets of cells. Within these two broad categories, the diseases could be further categorized by describing the predominant cell type as assessed by microscopy. Four categories were used. These were small round cells, small wrinkled cells, large cells, and mixtures of large and small cells. Such a system was easy to use and was shown to be prognostically significant. In general nodular lymphomas had a more favorable prognosis than diffuse lymphomas, and small cells behaved better than large cells. The Rappaport and Gall system made no attempts to determine whether the lymphoma cells were of T or B cell origin. These studies came later:

Non-Hodgkin's Lymphoma Classification
(Rappaport and Gall)
Nodular or diffuse
Well-differentiated lymphocytic
Poorly differentiated lymphocytic
Lymphocytic and histiocytic
Histiocytic
Undifferentiated
Unclassifiable

In the 1970s, Lukes and Collins proposed a major reorganization of lymphoma classification systems. By that time analysis of surface markers had shown that T and B cells were distinguishable and had different functions. Most human non-Hodgkin's lymphomas, whether they were nodular or diffuse, or of large or small cell type could be shown to be of B cell origin. In an extensive reorganization of the classification system, Lukes and Collins proposed that T and B cells could be distinguished morphologically and that nodular, as well as many diffuse lymphomas, were composed of cell types that were normally found in germinal centers. They divided the cells of germinal centers into four classes: small noncleaved, small cleaved, large cleaved, and large noncleaved. Comparing the distribution of B cells in normal reactive lymph nodes to the histological patterns of lymphomas, they proposed that the nodules of lymphomas mimicked the "follicular centers" (germinal centers) of lymph nodes and that, "nodular lymphomas involve follicular center cells (B cells) and as such are best considered as lymphomatous follicles."

Further studies confirmed that most human non-Hodgkins lymphomas expressed surface Ig and were therefore of B cell origin. As more markers became available many attempts were made to find lymphomas, the markers for which were the same as those of normal B cells at various stages of differentiation. Such studies represented a direct test of the hypothesis that B cell lymphomas are composed of transformed cells that are frozen at certain specific states of normal differentiation. If this hypothesis is correct, one should be able to draw a path of B cell differentiation in which each normal cell stage has a malignant counterpart. Figure 5, which is derived from Figure 4, is an example of such an attempt. Many other similar attempts have been published.

This figure shows that one can indeed find examples of B cell lymphomas whose surface marker distribution closely mimics normal cells at various stages of normal differentiation. It is next important to ask whether the examples of tumors that fit the model will represent the average case or are exceptions to the general rule. Unfortunately, as one looks more closely at individual lymphoma categories, the system of Fig. 5 breaks down. This is illustrated in Table 2, which shows the results of surface marker analysis of eleven patients with the "syndrome" of chronic lymphocyte leukemia (CLL).

In this study, the lymphocytes of patients with CLL were analyzed for Ig heavy and light chains, T-65 (a pan T lymphocyte marker), and B-532 (a B cell activation antigen). The Ig type was determined on populations purified by the cell sorter if the CLL cells were a minority population of the blood lymphocytes. A number of observations can be made. First with regard to Ig heavy chain type, the cells of individual patients seem to mimic immature B cells (IgM only), mature B cells (IgM and D),

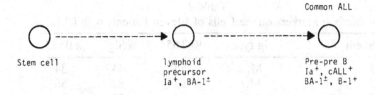

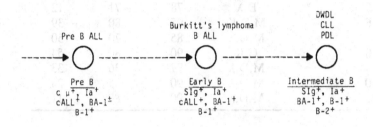

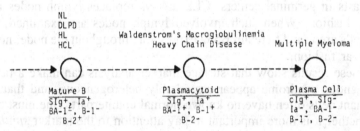

Fig. 5.   Correlation of B cell maturation stages and B cell malignancies. The diseases listed above the cells are putative examples of a transformed cell that mimics the normal counterpart that is listed below the cell. The most common antigenic phenotype for both benign and malignant cell types is summarized below each cell.

ALL = acute lymphoblastic leukemia, DWDL = diffuse well differentiated lymphocytic, CLL = chronic lymphocytic leukemia, PDL = poorly differentiated lymphocytic, NL = nodular lymphoma, DLPD = diffuse poorly differentiated lymphocytic, HL = histiocytic lymphoma, HCL = hairy cell leukemia

or antigen-stimulated, possibly even memory cells (IgG). In addition, one case displayed only light chains and one only IgD. Neither of these types represents a significant normal population; at least a normal counterpart has not yet been described.

Most of the CLL cells were found to express the pan T cell antigen T-65 as detected by the monoclonal antibody T-101. This observation has now been confirmed in many other studies and is occasionally seen on other B lymphomas. The expression and retention of a pan T cell antigen on B cells of all stages has not been described for normal B cells. The CLL cells also frequently express the B532 antigen, which is never nor-

Table 2
Surface Markers on the Cells of Eleven Patients with CLL

Patient #	Ig type	% T65$^+$	%SIg$^+$	%B532$^+$
1	M,K	53	44	34
2	M,λ	93	82	56
3	M,D,λ	67	72	68
4	?,λ	97	45	55
5	D,λ	78	71	12
6	M,D,K	95	80	39
7	M,D,λ	85	70	50
8	G,K	90	80	54
9	M,D,λ	77	36	33
10	M,D,λ	90	35	25
11	M,D,λ	90	80	11

mally seen on B cells in the blood. It is essentially always confined to B cell blasts in germinal centers. CLL always replaces lymph nodes in a diffuse fashion. When such involved lymph nodes are examined, the CLL cells are found to retain B532 expression throughout the node, not in a nodular fashion.

These results show that surface marker analysis can make a rather homogenous syndrome appear remarkably heterogeneous, and that the malignant cells often have no known normal counterpart. One must then ask whether it is more important to pay attention to the marker *similarities* between normal and malignant cells or whether the key to understanding lymphomas lies in the differences. It is possible that certain markers may have prognostic significance by themselves regardless of other diagnostic features such as nodularity, diffuseness, cell size, or expression of other surface markers. Studies asking this question have been done and are summarized in Table 3.

This study confirms that the expression of cell surface immunoglobulin is an important prognostic feature of non-Hodgkin's lymphomas. It also shows that the specific heavy chain type of immunoglobulin is itself prognostically significant. Referring back to Fig. 1, it is tempting to infer that B lymphoma cells do in fact mimic the properties of their normal counterparts. For example, cells that express both IgM and D are normally in a resting phase either in the circulation or in primary follicles. Lymphomas expressing both IgM and D have the best prognosis. This phenotype is the most common phenotype for CLL and for diffuse, well-differentiated lymphocytic lymphoma (DWDL), both rather indolent diseases. Unfortunately, both these lymphomas infiltrate lymph nodes in a diffuse fashion whereas their normal B cell counterparts form primary follicles, so the analogy cannot be made complete.

Table 3
Prognosis in Non-Hodgkin's Lymphomas[a]

Grouped according to T, B, or null cell		
Cell type	# pts	% 50-month survival[c]
B (Ig$^+$E$^-$)[b]	85	58
T (Ig$^-$E$^+$)	8	0
null (Ig$^-$E$^-$)	32	30

Grouped according to heavy chain type (85 pts)	
Ig type	% 50-month survival
IgM only	32
IgM+D$^+$	92
IgM$^+$G$^+$ or A$^+$	0
IgG$^+$ or A$^+$ only	59

Light chain type was found to have no significance.

[a]These data represent 250 lymphoma patients of whom 130 were consecutive and untreated at the time of entry into the study. From Rudders, R. A. *Hosp. Pract.* **18** (1), 161 (Jan. 1983).

[b]Ig = surface Ig, E = sheep erythrocyte receptor

[c]Survivors with B cell disease were essentially never disease-free, while survivors with null cell disease were often apparently disease-free.

Lymphomas that express IgM only, or IgM and IgG, or IgM and IgA, have poorer prognoses than those that express IgM and IgD. Normal B cells expressing IgM only are active cells in the bone marrow, presumably dividing as well as differentiating. Cells expressing IgM and G, or IgM and A, are normally rapidly dividing cells in germinal centers. To the extent that rapid cell division implies a poorer prognosis, then lymphomas expressing IgM only, or IgM and G or A, do mimic their normal counterparts. The same can be said for cells expressing IgG or IgA only. At least one class of memory B cell expresses IgG only. This is normally a resting cell so its malignant counterpart should be rather slow growing, which appears to be the case.

The preceding data can also be combined with data on cell size, cleaved versus noncleaved status, and nodular versus diffuse pattern, to see if good and bad prognoses can be further separated. The number of diagnostic categories will increase exponentially as one makes all the possible combinations. Given enough markers, and the proven tendency for malignant cells to express unusual combinations of antigens, one might eventually arrive at a diagnostic quagmire in which each patient is in a unique category.

Besides prognostic studies, cell surface markers have been used in studies of the architecture of lymph nodes involved by lymphoma. These studies have delineated the composition of malignant nodules, and the internodular cortex, the composition of diffuse lymphomas, and the relationships of cells of different sizes and shapes. Figure 6 presents a summary of the findings.

Basically, there are two types of nodular lymphoma and two types of diffuse lymphoma. In the first type of nodular lymphoma the nodules are composed of a monoclonal aggregation of B cells. The cells usually express IgM only or IgM and IgD although other combinations can be seen. All the cells express either K or λ chains, but not both. In most of the nodules a majority of cells express the B532 activation antigen, but in some nodules the quantity of this antigen is low or even absent. This implies different states of activation in morphologically similar cells. All the cells in the nodules are also Ia⁺. A few T cells are also present. These surface marker features can be seen in nodular lymphomas composed of small or large cells but the most common cell types, using Rappaport's terminology, are small, poorly differentiated lymphocytic, or mixed

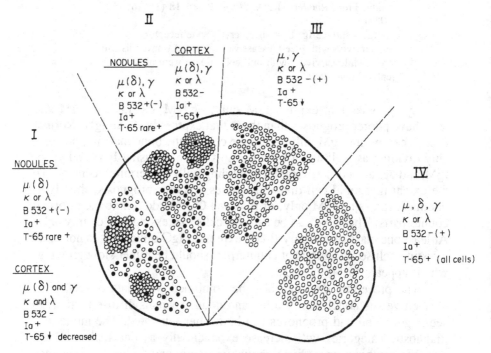

Fig. 6. Surface markers and lymph node architecture in B cell lymphomas. The lymph node has been schematically divided into four segments, each with a different form of B cell lymphoma. Two are nodular and two diffuse. Open circles represent B cells and closed circles represent T cells. The antigens detected on the cells in various locations are summarized in the figure.

cellularity. The uniform expression of a single light chain on cells of different sizes in mixed cellularity lymphomas indicates that all the cells are of the same clonal derivation. Size differences presumably represent only cell cycle differences. It is tempting to presume that lymphomas composed only of small cells are merely dividing more slowly than lymphomas composed of large cells. Rapidly dividing cells would be more likely to be seen in S phase and therefore be larger than cells in G_o, the resting phase.

The internodular cortex of the first type of nodular lymphoma is not similar to the cortex of normal lymph nodes. First, the number of T cells is significantly decreased. These cells are partially replaced by a polyclonal infiltrate of apparently normal B cells. Some express IgM and D, whereas others express IgG. Some cells express K chains and others λ. All of the B cells express Ia, but none express B532. The internodular cortex therefore appears to contain a reactive population of T and B cells. The tumor cells either confine themselves to the nodules or are confined by the reactive process.

Throughout the body of a given patient, all the nodules of the lymphoma are composed of the same cell type. This is evidence that the malignant cells recirculate and home to or form nodules in lymph nodes throughout the body. The malignant cells behave in this respect as primary follicle B cells, not "follicular center" cells.

In the second type of nodular lymphoma, the nodules are again composed of a monoclonal aggregation of B cells that express a wide variety of surface heavy chains. One can find cells expressing IgM only, IgM and D, IgM and G, or IgG only. Only one light chain is expressed. The cells are also uniformly Ia^+ but the expression of B532 is variable. As in the first type of nodular lymphoma, most nodules are $B532^+$ but some are $B532^-$ even within the same lymph node.

The major difference between the two types of nodular lymphoma lies in the internodular cortex. In the second type the cells between the nodules express identical markers to the cells within the nodules. This pattern suggests progression from a previous nodular lymphoma in which the cortex contained benign, reactive cells. Invasion of the cortex by the malignant cells was recognized on morphological grounds before it was confirmed by marker studies. It is natural to suppose that this form represents progression of disease, but it is possible that some B lymphomas are both nodular and diffuse from the beginning. Such a pattern could be due to the inability of recirculating cells to completely organize themselves into nodules rather than invasion outward from preexisting nodules. Either mechanism would result in a lesser tendency of the malignant cells to aggregate.

In a given patient, one can see both the strictly nodular and the combination of nodular and diffuse patterns. The idea that nodular lymphomas can evolve into diffuse lymphomas was presented in the 1950s by

Rappaport. The cell marker evidence is consistent with this idea but a specific marker that differentiates cells that form nodules from those that do not has not been identified.

The two types of diffuse lymphomas are also quite different from one another when analyzed for surface markers. The first kind is composed of a monoclonal proliferation of cells that can express different types of heavy chains. Expression of IgM only, IgM and G, or IgG only have been described. Cells expressing IgM and D are usually not seen in this type of diffuse lymphoma. Essentially all cells are Ia$^+$ but their reactivity with B532 varies. In some cases all cells are B532$^+$ and in others they are B532$^-$. The markers expressed by the cells in this type of diffuse lymphoma suggest that it derives from a previous nodular lymphoma. Such a progression has certainly been reported in older morphologic studies of lymphomas. The cell types (size, cleaved, or noncleaved) of this form of diffuse lymphoma show the same range as the nodular lymphomas and have led Lukes and Collins to refer to them as "diffuse, follicular-center-cell" lymphomas because of their morphology.

The accumulated evidence from marker studies on normal lymph nodes and on lymphomas calls this concept into question. First, nodular lymphomas mimic primary follicles rather than germinal centers. The cells of germinal centers arise peripherally and do not recirculate. Animal models suggest that most lymphomas arise centrally (i.e., the bone marrow) and invade the lymph nodes from the bloodstream. A recent piece of evidence generated with the fluorescence-activated cell sorter is consistent with this concept. Patients with lymphomas apparently confined to lymph nodes can be shown to have circulating malignant cells, even when they have a normal absolute lymphocyte count. Considered together, all the evidence suggests that some B lymphomas do mimic the normal cells that form primary follicles but that lymphomas do not mimic germinal center cells, except morphologically. The importance of this distinction is specifically that the cells of primary follicles are known to come from the marrow and to circulate to lymph nodes. The cells of germinal centers develop *in situ*. One would therefore presume that a lymphoma mimicking primary follicle cells was in the bone marrow from the beginning. If a lymphoma mimicked germinal center cells, one might presume that the disease had a good chance of being confined to peripheral lymphoid organs, or even a local group of lymph nodes. Clinical studies on the staging of non-Hodgkin's lymphomas indicate that over 80% are Stage IV at the time of diagnosis, so the prediction of the primary follicle model is upheld.

The second type of diffuse lymphoma has no apparent relationship to the first. It is the pattern represented by diffuse well-differentiated lymphocytic lymphoma and by chronic lymphocytic leukemia in lymph nodes. The cells are monoclonal and express the range of heavy chains indicated in Table 2. The most common phenotype is IgM^+D^+. All the cells are Ia^+ and are usually $B532^+$ as well, although some cases are completely $B532^-$. A major difference from all other B cell lymphomas is that most of the malignant cells are $T-65^+$. The expression of the pan T cell antigen on these "B" cells shows that some types of lymphoma routinely express combinations of normal antigens that are not seen on normal cells at any stage of their differentiation. CLL cells do not express helper or suppressor T cell markers or the E receptor, but they consistently express the T65 antigen. Perhaps this indicates something about the gene rearrangement which is characteristic of CLL.

The cells of DLWD and CLL resemble each other morphologically and by marker analysis. They differ only in their tendency to home to lymph nodes or to remain in the circulation. So far the surface marker(s) associated with this difference have not been described.

Despite having many of the surface markers of the B cells that make primary follicles, the cells of CLL and DLWD never make nodules in lymph nodes. They do grow in a rather indolent fashion (although they can convert to a rapidly growing lymphoblastic disease), and they appear to be in the bone marrow from the beginning. Because these cells do not have any known normal counterpart, the significance of these correlations is unclear.

In the acute leukemias the distinction between B cells, T cells, and "null cells" is of proven clinical relevance. In general, "null cell" leukemias have the best prognosis, B cell leukemias have an intermediate prognosis, and T cell leukemias have the worst prognosis. Most of the data from which these conclusions are drawn was generated simply by looking for SIg or sheep red cell rosette formation. Cells expressing SIg were defined as B cells. Additional information is now available for the prognosis of leukemias expressing various Ig classes, Ia, B-1, B-2, and BA-1. In general, the more a leukemic cell mimics the "mature" B cell phenotype, the better the prognosis. In contrast to null cell leukemias, in which (apparently) indefinite disease-free survivals can sometimes be achieved, survivors with B cell leukemias are usually not disease free. This most clearly seen in the syndrome of chronic lymphocytic leukemia. The so-called "null" cell, a cell without SIg that also does not make E rosettes has been redefined with monoclonal antibodies. Referring to Fig. 4, one can see that cells which express the CALLA (common acute lymphocytic leukemia antigen) marker may usually be classified as pre B cells by their reactions with B-1 and BA-1 antibodies. This observation therefore contradicts the general observation that the more mature the B cell phenotype of a malignant cell, the better the prognosis for the patient.

4. Conclusions

In summary, cell surface markers are just that: markers. As ongoing research defines the functions of molecules recognized by monoclonal antibodies, new ways of taking advantage of the presence or absence of these molecules on malignant cells will be developed. The hypothesis that malignant cells mimic normal cells frozen at a specific stage of differentiation may or may not stand the test of time. After this question is settled, we may then be able to move on to an exploration of the function of marker molecules and use that knowledge to institute radical new therapeutic modalities.

Bibliography for Further Reading

Lymphoma Classification

Lukes, R. J., and Collins, R. D., *Br. J. Cancer* **31,** Suppl. II, 1–28 (1975).
Rappaport, H., Tumors of the Hematopoietic System, in *Atlas of Tumor Pathology,* Sect. III, Fasc. 8, Washington, D.C., Armed Forces Institute of Pathology (1966).

Maturation of B Cells

Bhan, A., Nadler, L., Stashenko, P., McCluskey, R., and Schlossman, S., *J. Exp. Med.* **154,** 737 (1981).
Frisman, D., Slovin, S., Royston, I., and Baird, S., *Blood* **62,** 1224 (1983).
Raschke, W. C., *Biochem. Biophys. Acta* **605,** 113 (1980).
Reichert, R., Gallatin, W., Weissman, I., and Butcher, E., *J. Expt. Med.* **157,** 813 (1983).
Robertson, S. M., Clayton, L., Dev, V. G., Wall, R., Capra, J. D., and Kettman, J. R., *Fed. Proc.* **41,** 2502 (1982).
V., Jerabek, L., Stevens, S. K., Scollay, R. G., and Butcher, E. C., *J. Supramol. Struct. Cell Biochem.* **15(3),** 303 (1981).

Surface Markers on B Cell Malignancies

Aisenberg, A. C., *N. Engl. J. Med.* **304(6),** 331 (Feb. 5, 1981).
Borowitz, M. J., Croker, B. P., and Metzgar, R. S., *Am. J. Pathol.* **105(2),** 97 (Nov. 1981).
Bowman, W. P., Melvin, S., and Mauer, A. M., *Adv. Intern. Med.* **25,** 391 (1980).
Foon, K. A., Schroff, R. W., and Gale, R. P., *Blood* **60(1),** 1 (Jul. 1982).
Watanabe, S., Shimosato, Y., Shimoyama, M., and Minato, K., *Cancer* **50(11),** 2372 (Dec. 1, 1982).

Prognosis Correlated with Surface Markers

Rudders, R. A., *Hosp. Pract.* **18(1),** 161 (Jan. 1983).

Chapter 8

Nonlymphoblastic Leukemia-Associated Antigens Identified by Monoclonal Antibodies

ROBERT G. ANDREWS AND IRWIN D. BERNSTEIN

Pediatric Oncology Program, Fred Hutchinson Cancer Research Center, and the Department of Pediatrics, University of Washington School of Medicine, Seattle, WA

1. Introduction

In recent years leukemia-associated markers potentially useful for diagnostic and therapeutic purposes have been defined by monoclonal antibodies. The initial and perhaps most significant advance was the development of antibodies that defined stages of differentiation of T (Bradstock et al., 1980; Hansen et al., 1980; Kung et al., 1979; Levy et al., 1979; McMichael et al., 1979; Reinherz et al., 1980) and B (Nadler et al., 1981, 1983, 1984; Stashenko et al., 1980; Thorley-Dawson et al., 1982) lymphocytes and functionally discrete subsets of T lymphocytes (Reinherz et al., 1979; Reinherz and Schlossman, 1980). These antibodies, many of which were raised against leukemia cells, also delineated immunologically distinct subsets of acute lymphoblastic leukemia (ALL) (Chen et al., 1983; Kersey et al., 1982; LeBien et al., 1982; Sallan et al., 1980). More recently the monoclonal antibody–hybridoma technology has been extended to the study of the myeloid leukemias. Numerous antigens associated with normal and malignant hematopoietic stem cells and their progeny have now been defined and their biological and clinical significance is currently under evaluation.

This chapter will focus on the development of monoclonal antibodies that recognize antigens expressed at specific stages of normal myeloid differentiation, and will examine the potential of these antibodies for defining the differentiative states within the heterogenous group of disorders that comprise the myeloid leukemias. We will emphasize the acute nonlymphoblastic leukemias (ANL) since these disorders have been the most extensively studied.

Myeloid leukemias, and in specific ANL, represent a unique situation in which the relationship of normal and malignant myeloid stem cells can be assessed. Leukemic as well as normal proliferative subpopulations can be assayed in vitro (Bradley and Metcalf, 1966; Buick et al., 1977; Harris and Freireich, 1970; Minden et al., 1978; Pluznik and Sachs, 1966; Robinson et al., 1971; Senn et al., 1967) and thus provide model systems for the development of therapeutic approaches aimed at depleting malignant stem cells. Rendering these studies more challenging is the knowledge of the heterogeneity of this group of disorders.

The heterogeneity of ANL has classically been defined on the basis of morphological and histochemical characteristics. The French, American, British (FAB) schema for classification is a recent refinement of this approach (Bennett et al., 1976; van Rhenen et al., 1980; Whittaker et al., 1979). Further evidence of the diverse nature of ANL has come from the identification of numerous chromosomal abnormalities in leukemic cell populations from patients with ANL (Berger et al., 1982; Golomb et al., 1982; Kamada et al., 1968; Kaneko et al., 1982; Rowley, 1973, 1977, 1983, Rowley et al., 1982; Yunis et al., 1981). Certain of these abnormalities appear to be associated with specific morphologic and histochemical phenotypes (Berger et al., 1982; Kamada et al., 1986; Kaneko et al., 1982; Rowley, 1977, 1983; Rowley et al., 1982). Evidence of the heterogeneous origin has come from studies of patients with myeloid leukemia who are heterozygous at the X-linked locus for glucose-6-phosphate dehydrogenase (G6PD) that have demonstrated that, in morphologically similar leukemias, the malignant clone may be expressed in single or multiple hematopoietic lineages (Fialkow, 1982; Fialkow et al., 1977, 1978, 1979, 1981). Thus, myeloid leukemias may arise in different stem cell populations that have different maturational capacities, or they may arise from similar stem cells that have different lesions resulting in variable patterns of malignant differentiation.

Early attempts to identify myeloid leukemia-associated antigens required extensive absorption of polyclonal heteroantisera with nonmyeloid cells before specific reactivity with myeloid cells could be detected. Frequently the results of such studies were inconclusive since the antiserum often was available in insufficient amounts or titer for extensive studies. However several investigators have reported the development of antisera with high degrees of specificity for myeloid leukemia cells. Metzgar et al. (1972, 1974), Mohanakumar et al. (1974, 1976), and Baker et al. (1981) reported a simian antiserum that reacted with leukemic cells from most patients with ANL and apparently lacked reactivity with normal mature and immature hematopoietic elements. Baker and Taub (1973) and Baker et al. (1974, 1976, 1979, 1981, 1982) generated a mouse antiserum that precipitated an antigen with relative molecular weight (M_r) of 75–80 kilodaltons (kD) shed by leukemic cells cultured in vitro. This antiserum reacted with leukemic cells from most patients with ANL. Also of interest were reports by Al-Rammahy et al. (1980) and Malcolm et al. (1982, 1983) of a rabbit antiserum that precipitated a M_r 68 kD antigen from leukemic cells and reacted with leukemic cells from most patients with ANL and a small proportion with ALL. Both Baker et al. and Malcolm et al. have reported expression of these leukemia-associated antigens on morphologically normal hematopoietic cells in patients with ANL. Whether these cells represented elements derived from the leukemic clone that were capable of undergoing maturation or whether antigen was adsorbed onto the surface of nonleukemic cells is not known. For each of these antisera the possibility that a minor subpopulation of normal marrow cells, in particular progenitor cells, express the identified antigens has not been rigorously excluded.

The development of hybridoma technology (Köhler and Milstein, 1975) has now made it possible to overcome many problems inherent in the use of polyclonal antisera. Thus it has been possible to generate monoclonal antibodies of defined specificity that can be produced in virtually unlimited amounts. In the following sections we will review what has been a virtual explosion of efforts to prepare monoclonal antibodies against antigens expressed by both normal and malignant myeloid cells. For the most part the antibodies appear to define normal differentiation antigens rather than leukemia-specific antigens regardless of whether normal or malignant cells were used for immunization.

The recently released report of the First International Workshop on Human Leukocyte Differentiation Antigens (Bernard et al., 1984) includes studies on 50 of such antibodies and has established a nomenclature in which antibodies are grouped in Differentiation Clusters. For the granulocyte and monocyte associated antigens 5 CD's (Differentiation Clusters CD11, CDw12, CDw13, CDw14, and CDw15) were defined based primarily on serologic studies. For CD11 a specific molecule was identified, whereas for the other four groups antigens were either not defined or less well characterized and thus the provisional workshop designation CDw was given. Antibodies in the CD11 group recognize the C3bi receptor. Antibodies grouped in CDw12 and CDw13 recognize antigens expressed on granulocytes and monocytes, those in CDw14 are primarily monocyte-associated and those in CDw15 are primarily granulocyte-associated. For purposes of comparison in this review we will group many previously described antibodies, many of which were not studied in the First International Workshop, on the basis of patterns of reactivity. The antigens identified by most of these antimyeloid antibodies have not been biochemically characterized; thus the basis for comparison is frequently limited to serologic data for which there is presently no uniform reporting method. Moreover, it is important to note that antibodies with similar reactivities may identify different epitopes of the same molecule or may identify an epitope shared by different molecular species.

We will therefore first discuss the expression of these antigens by normal myeloid stem cells and their progeny and then examine their expression by malignant myeloid cells. Following this, the utility of these markers in defining subsets of ANL and distinguishing ANL from ALL, and their potential therapeutic applications will be considered.

2. Myeloid-Associated Antigens Expressed by Normal Hematopoietic Cells and Cell Lines

Myeloid-associated antigens identified by monoclonal antibodies on normal mature and immature hematopoietic elements can be used as markers for specific myeloid lineages as well as for levels of maturation within a lineage. Initially, we will group antibodies to these antigens based upon their described reactivities with normal peripheral blood elements. Antigens that are most highly expressed by (1) granulocytes, (2) monocytes, (3) granulocytes and monocytes, or (4) platelets or red cells will be described separately as well as (5) certain antigens that are not expressed by mature peripheral blood elements.

2.1. Monoclonal Antibodies to Antigens Expressed Primarily on Granulocytes

Whereas numerous antibodies that react primarily with granulocytes have been reported, a major proportion of these recognize the same highly immunogenic epitope that is the trisaccharide X-hapten Galβ1-4[Fuc α 1-3]GlcNAcβ1-R (also known as Le^x). Antibodies recognizing the X-hapten were grouped in CDw15 [i.e., CDw15 (granulocyte, CHO) 1G10] by the First International Workshop. Since antibodies against this structure point out certain of the potential pitfalls as well as the advantages of monoclonal antibodies, we will discuss this group of antibodies at greater length. Following that will be a brief description of other antigranulocyte antibodies.

2.1.1. Antibodies Against the X-hapten

More than 25 monoclonal antibodies have been reported that are known to bind the X-hapten (Table 1) (Bernstein et al., 1982a; Brockhaus et al., 1982; Civin et al., 1981; Cuttita et al., 1981; Ferrero et al., 1983a,

Fukuchi et al., 1984; Girardet et al., 1983; Gooi et al. 1983; Hakomori et al., 1981; Hansson et al., 1983; Huang et al., 1983a, 1983b; Knapp et al., 1981; Majdic et al., 1981; Mannoni et al., 1982; Stockinger et al., 1984; Urdal et al., 1983). Many of these were derived by immunizing mice with cells from nonhematopoietic malignancies including tumors of the colon (Brockhaus et al., 1982), lung (Cuttita et al., 1981; Huang et al., 1983), and stomach (Brockhaus et al., 1982). This determinant is expressed on cell surface glycolipids (Girardet et al., 1983; Gooi et al., 1983; Hakomori et al., 1981; Hakomori and Kanagi, 1983; Urdal et al., 1983), serum glycoproteins (Fournet et al,. 1978), in human milk (Kobata and Ginsburg, 1969), and on certain normal tissues and their secretions (Hakomori and Kanagi, 1983; Metzgar et al., 1984; Yamashita et al., 1980; Yurewicz et al., 1982). Moreover, the murine stage specific embryonic antigen identified by the SSEA-1 monoclonal antibody has been identified as the X-hapten (Hakomori et al., 1981; Knowles, et al., 1982; Solter and Knowles, 1978). More than 20 other antibodies have been described that may also bind to the X-hapten (Ferrero et al., 1983a; Kemshead et al., 1981; Perussia et al., 1982; Skubitz et al., 1983a, 1983b; Tetteroo et al., 1984). Some of these antibodies inhibit antigen-specific binding of one or more of the known X-hapten reactive antibodies (Perussia et al., 1982; Skubitz et al., 1983a, 1983b, Tetteroo et al., 1984). Other antibodies immunoprecipitate glycoproteins (gp's) with relative molecular weights similar to those precipitated by known X-hapten reactive antibodies (Ferrero et al., 1983a; Skubitz et al., 1983a, 1983b; Tetteroo et al., 1984).

The X-hapten is expressed on both glycolipids and glycoproteins on the cell surface of normal and malignant myeloid cells (Girardet et al., 1983; Gooi et al., 1983; Huang et al., 1983; Skubitz et al., 1983a; Urdal et al., 1983).

From granulocytes two glycoproteins with M_rs of 100 and 150 kD have been precipitated (Skubitz et al., 1983a), whereas from the HL-60 cell line the dominant species precipitated have M_rs of 200 to 240 kD (Urdal et al., 1983).

Within the hematopoietic system the X-hapten is highly expressed on mature and immature granulocytes as early as the myeloblast to promyelocyte stage and is expressed at very low levels by a small subset of mature monocytes (Bernstein et al., 1982a; Bettleheim et al., 1982; Mannoni et al., 1982). It is not expressed to any measurable extent on the surface of cells of the megakaryocytic, erythrocytic, or lymphoid lineages.

There are many similarities in the patterns of reactivity of anti-X-hapten antibodies with normal hematopoietic elements and cell lines. However it is also apparent that there are distinct but subtle differences between some of these antibodies. Although all of these antibodies react

TABLE 1
Monoclonal Antibodies Reactive Primarily with Granulocytes

Antibody	Cell type				
	Granulocyte	Monocyte	Lymphocyte	Platelets	Red blood cells
Anti-X-hapten 1G10[a] (Bernstein et al., 1982, Urdal et al., 1983), VIMD5[a] (Knapp et al., 1981; Stockinger et al., 1984) VEP8,VEP9 (Gooi et al., 1983), HL-C5 (Girardet et al., 1983) MY-1,-6,-8,-25 (Civin et al., 1981; Huang et al., 1983; Strauss et al., 1983) SSEA-1 (Hakomori et al., 1981; Solter and Knowles, 1978), WGHS29.1 (Brockhaus et al., 1982) D1-56-22 (Hansson et al., 1983; Skubitz et al., 1983a) 81H1[b],80H5[b] (Manonni et al., 1982) 525A5,534F8,538F12 (Huang et al., 1983)	+	±	−	−	−
Probable anti-X-hapten R1B19 (Perussia et al., 1982), AHN-1,-2,-3,-4,-5,-6 (Skubitz et al., 1983a, 1983b), D51-1 (Skubitz et al., 1983a), B4.3[a] (Tetteroo et al., 1984), MI/N1 (Kemshead et al., 1981; Tetteroo et al., 1984), UJ308 (Tetteroo et al., 1984), FMC-10[a], -11, -12[a] (Tetteroo et al., 1984; Zola et al., 1981), S5-22,S5-28 (Skubitz et al., 1984; Zola et al., 1981),	+	±	−	−	−

al., 1983a), B37.2,B40.1,B40.4,B40.8,
B40.9,B43.5,L8.1,L11.1 (Perussia et al., 1982), S4-7
(Ferrero et al., 1983)

Other anti-
granulocyte an-
tibodies

B13.9[a] (Tetterro et al., 1984), 82H7[a] (Manonni et al.,
1984), Tü-5[a] (Bernard et al., 1984), DUHL60.1[a]
(McKolanis et al., 1984), 75B10[a] (Bernard et al.,
1984), TG-1 (Beverley et al., 1980, Mulder et al.,
1981), 3C4[a] (Bernard et al., 1984), G1120[a] (Bernard et
al., 1984), TG-8[a] (Bernard et al., 1984), MCCH36.71[a]
(Bernard et al., 1984), DUHL60.3[a] (McKolonis et al.,
1984), G2[a] (Martin et al., 1984), Tü-9[a] (Bernard et al.,
1984), MCS-1[a] (Tatsumi et al., 1981), FMC-11[c] (Zola
et al., 1981), PMN-6,-29 (Ball et al., 1982; Ball and
Fanger, 1983), 4D1, 1B5 (Clement et al., 1983), 1F10
(Yamada et al., 1983)

AHN-8,L12.2,L13.1 (Skubitz et al., 1983a)

52/10,52/40,53/40,54/16 (Papayannopoulou et al.,
1984)

[a]Clustered in CDw15 by First International Workshop
[b]Mannoni, P., personal communication
[c]Not clustered by First International Workshop

with granulocytes, four also were reported to react with eosinophils (Bernstein et al., 1982a; Gooi et al., 1983; Mannoni et al., 1982), whereas at least two other antibodies did not (Girardet et al., 1983; Gooi et al., 1983). Reported reactivities with specific myeloid and lymphoid cell lines differ, although some of these differences might be accounted for by antigenic variants arising in cell lines as demonstrated by differences in reactivity of antibody ViMD5 with populations of the K562 cell line grown in different laboratories (Knapp et al., 1981). Further, many antibodies have been shown to react with a portion of marrow-derived committed granulocyte/monocyte progenitors (CFU-GM) (Andrews et al., 1983; Ferrero et al., 1983a; Mannoni et al., 1982; Skubitz et al., 1983a) whereas at least two others (Knapp et al., 1981; Strauss et al., 1983) have been reported not to do so, although such differences could result from differences in sources of complement and how they were used in the cytolytic assays. Finally, phenotyping studies with multiple antibodies reactive with X-hapten show differences in the reactivities of these antibodies with leukemic cells (van der Reijden et al., 1983). It is very likely that different antibodies may recognize the X-hapten only when presented in the context of other specific structures. However all of the antibodies appear to require a terminal X-hapten structure on type 2 carbohydrate chains for reactivity (Hakomori and Kanagi, 1983).

The X-hapten may be expressed on carbohydrate chains of differing lengths and branching points. In preliminary studies comparing X-hapten reactive monoclonal antibodies, several findings have appeared (Symington, F., Hakomori, S.-I., personal communication). First, all antibodies capable of binding the pentasaccharide glycolipid shown as Structure 1 (*see* Fig. 1) could also bind the longer monofucosylated chain glycolipids as shown as Structure 2, although there may be affinity differences (Hakomori and Kanagi, 1983). Secondly, some X-hapten reactive antibodies seem able to recognize the internally alpha 1-3 fucosylated structure to some extent (Structure 3) while at least one antibody appears unable to do so in competitive binding inhibition studies. Thirdly, antibodies may prefer more than one α 1-3 fucosyl residue for binding, for example the FH4 antibody readily binds Structure 3, but is only weakly cross reactive with Structure 2 (Fukuchi et al., 1984). Extensive binding studies using purified carbohydrate haptens of known structure and purified monoclonal antibodies will be necessary to elucidate potential differences in affinity and antigen recognition sites, which may account for published differences in reactivities of X-hapten binding antibodies.

2.1.2. Other Antibodies to Granulocyte-Associated Antigens

The antigens identified by most of these antibodies have yet to be determined although five of these, AHN-8 (Skubitz et al., 1983a), PMN-6 (Ball et al., 1982; Ball and Fanger, 1983), PMN-29 (Ball et al., 1982;

(1) Galβl→4GlcNAcβl→3Galβl→4Glcβl→1 Ceramide
          3
          ↑
       Fucαl

(2) Galβl→4GlcNAcβl→3Galβl→4GlcNAcβl→3Galβl→4Glcβl→1
          3   Ceramide
          ↑
       Fucαl

(3) Galβl→4GlcNAcβl→3Galβl→4GlcNAcβl→3Galβl→4Glcβl→1
          3   3   Ceramide
          ↑   ↑
       Fucαl   Fucαl

Fig. 1. Structure 1, Lacto-N-fucopentaosyl (III) ceramides (III^3 FucLcOse$_4$Cer); structure 2, Y$_2$ glycolipid (V^{3}FucLcOse$_6$Cer); structure 3, Difucosyllacto-N-norhexaosylceramide (difucosyl Y$_2$ glycolipid, III^{3}FucV^{3}Fuc-LcOse$_6$Cer).

Ball and Fanger, 1983), L12.2 (Skubitz et al., 1983a), and L13.1 (Skubitz et al., 1983a), recognize determinants present in lipid extracts of granulocytes. In contrast to most of the antibodies that react with virtually all normal mature granulocytes, antibodies 4D1, which immuno-precipitates a M_r 59 kD antigen from granulocytes, and 1B5, which recognizes an undefined antigen, appear to react with distinct subpopulations of mature granulocytes (Clement et al., 1983). The biological significance of these findings is unclear, but it may be that, as with monocytes and lymphocytes, there are functionally distinct granulocyte subsets.

2.2. Monoclonal Antibodies to Antigens Primarily Expressed by Monocytes

Monoclonal antibodies that react primarily with peripheral blood monocytes (Table 2) have been described. A group of these react primarily with the monocyte population in peripheral blood (Andrews et al., 1983; Brooks et al., 1981; Dimitriu-Bona et al., 1983; Griffin et al., 1981, 1984; Hogg et al., 1981; Linker-Israeli et al., 1981; Perussia et al., 1982; Raff et al., 1980; Todd et al., 1981, 1984; Todd and Schlossman, 1982; Ugolini et al., 1980; Van Voorhis et al., 1983) and at least two of these antibodies, L4F3 (Andrews et al., 1983) and MY-9 (Griffin et al., 1984),

TABLE 2
Monoclonal Antibodies Reactive Primarily with Monocytes

Antibody	Cell type				
	Granulocyte	Monocyte	Lymphocyte	Platelets	Red blood cells
D5D6, C10H5 (Linker-Israeli et al., 1981), UC-45 (Hogg et al., 1981) Mac-120 (Raff et al., 1980), MoP-15[a] (Dimitriu-Bona et al., 1983, 1984), B44.1 (Perussia et al., 1982), Mo-2[a] (Todd et al., 1981), Mo-3 (Todd and Schlossman, 1982), MY-9 (Griffin et al., 1984), FMC-17[a] (Brooks et al., 1981), TM-18[a] (Bernard et al., 1984), 1D9, 3C10, 1E8 (Van Voorhis et al., 1983)	−	+	−	−	−

L4F3 (Andrews et al., 1983), MY-3,-4[a] (Griffin et al., 1981) MoP-9[a], MoS-1[a],-39[a] (Dimitriu-Bona et al., 1983, 1984), Mo-6 (Todd et al., 1984)

5F1[a] (Andrews et al., 1983; Bernstein et al., 1982), F13 (Andrews et al., 1984), 20.3[a] (Kamoun et al., 1983), MPA (Burckhardt et al., 1982), Mo4 (Todd and Schlossman, 1982),

OKM-3,-5,-6,-8 (Talle et al., 1983), 63D3 (Ugolini et al., 1980), 4F2 (Eisenbarth et al., 1980), 3A1 (Levine et al., 1981), TA-1 (LeBien and Kersey, 1980), S3-13, S17-15 (Ferrero et al., 1983), MOP-7, MOR-17 (Dimitriu-Bona et al., 1983, 1984)

[a]Clustered in CDw14 by First International Workshop

appear to react with the same molecule (Andrews and Griffin, unpublished observations). Although the L4F3/MY-9 antigen is expressed primarily by monocytes in peripheral blood, it is expressed by both immature granulocytes and monocytes in marrow.

Deserving mention is a subset of antibodies that recognize antigens on both monocytes and platelets (Bernstein et al., 1982a; Burckhardt et al., 1982; Dimitriu-Bona et al., 1983; Talle et al., 1983; Todd and Schlossmann, 1982). At least three of these antibodies appear directed to a common antigen and two were grouped in CDw14 of the First International Workshop [CDw14 (monocyte-platelet, gp85) 5F1]. Antibodies 5F1 and F13 both precipitate an M_r 85 kD glycoprotein from platelets under reducing conditions (Andrews et al., 1984) and 5F1, F13, and 20.3 (Kamoun et al., 1983) competitively inhibit binding of each other to the HEL cell line (unpublished observation). This antigen is interesting because of its unusual distribution on immature monocytes, megakaryocytes, and nucleated erythrocytes in marrow. As can be seen in Table 2, a number of other antibodies to monocyte-associated antigens also react weakly with all or a subset of granulocytes (Dimitriu-Bona et al., 1983; Griffin et al., 1981; Todd et al., 1984) or a subset of lymphocytes (Dimitriu-Bona et al., 1983; Eisenbarth et al., 1980; Ferrero et al., 1983a; Haynes et al., 1981; LeBien and Kersey, 1981; Levine et al., 1981; Ugolini et al., 1980). It is important to note that antigens identified by certain of these antibodies are also expressed by progenitor cells committed to granulocyte/monocyte pathways (Ferrero et al., 1983a; Levine et al., 1981).

Although the monocytic cells that express some of these antigens function as antigen-presenting (Raff et al., 1980; Rosenberg et al., 1981) and phagocytic cells, the functions of the antigens themselves have yet to be determined. The expression of some of these antigens is altered with in vitro culture of monocytes (Dimitriu-Bona et al., 1984; Todd and Schlossmann, 1982). Of particular interest has been the Mac 120 antibody that recognizes an M_r 120 kD gp selectively expressed by a subset of peripheral blood monocytes capable of antigen presentation (Raff et al., 1980). Thus, it may be possible to define subsets of monocytes with distinct immune functions.

2.3. Monoclonal Antibodies to Antigens Associated with Granulocytes and Monocytes

A significant proportion of antibodies reactive with both granulocytes and monocytes (Table 3) recognize epitopes expressed by leukocyte function antigens (LFA), a family of heterodimeric molecules found on granulocytes, monocytes, some T lymphocytes, and NK cells (Arnaout et al., 1983; Ault and Springer, 1981; Beatty et al., 1983; Breard et al., 1980; Davignon et al., 1981; Hildreth et al., 1983; Krensky et al., 1983;

Kurzinger et al., 1983; Lohmeyer et al., 1981; McMichael et al., 1982; Sanchez-Madrid et al., 1982; Springer et al., 1978, 1982; Wright et al., 1983; Zarling and Kung, 1980). Several antibodies inhibit C3bi binding to monocytes and granulocytes (Arnaout et al., 1983; Beatty et al., 1983; Wright et al., 1983), whereas others inhibit the lytic function of alloreactive cytotoxic T cells (Beatty et al., 1983; Davignon et al., 1981; Hildreth et al., 1983; Krensky et al., 1983; McMichael et al., 1982; Sanchez-Madrid et al., 1982), and NK cells (Beatty et al., 1983; Hildreth et al., 1983; Lohmeyer et al., 1981) or inhibit granulocyte migration in response to chemotactic stimuli (Beatty et al., 1983). The absence of structures identified by one of these antibodies is associated with abnormal leukocyte function and an immunodeficiency syndrome (Beatty et al., 1984). The CD11 group of the First International Workshop is defined by the Mo-1 antibody, a member of this LFA family, which identifies the C3bi receptor (Arnaout et al., 1983) [CD11 (monocyte-granulocyte, gp100-155) Mo-1]. The C3bi receptor as identified by Mo-1 antibody is expressed as early as the myeloblast to promyelocyte stage in granulocytic development, but does not appear to be expressed on earlier myeloid progenitor cells (Griffin and Schlossman, 1984).

Other antibodies reactive with both granulocytes and monocytes have been extensively characterized for reactivity with hematopoietic elements (Andrews et al., 1983; Ball et al., 1982, 1983; Ball and Fanger, 1983; Griffin et al., 1981; Hanjan et al., 1982; Kamoun et al., 1983; Mannoni et al., 1982, 1984; Nauseef et al., 1983; Todd et al., 1984); yet, in most cases, the target antigen has not been defined and the functional roles are unknown. Antibody T5A7 reacts with lactosylceramide (Symington et al., 1984) that is highly expressed only at very late stages of granulocytic and monocytic differentiation (Andrews et al., 1983). As with the Mo-1 antigen, the MY-8 (Griffin et al., 1981), PM-81 (Ball et al., 1983), and AML-2-23 (Ball and Fanger, 1983) antigens first appear at the promyelocytic stage in granulocyte maturation.

2.4. Monoclonal Antibodies to Antigens Primarily Expressed on Immature Granulocytes and Monocytes

There is a group of antibodies that react only with immature, but not mature myeloid elements (Andrews et al., 1983; Bodger et al., 1981; Chiao and Wang, 1984; Civin et al., 1982). Certain antibodies identify determinants primarily expressed by immature myeloid elements, including MY-10 (Civin et al., 1982, 1983, 1984) that recognizes a M_r 95 kD protein, Pro Im-1 (Chiao and Wang, 1984) that identifies a M_r 85 kD antigen, and L1B2 (Andrews et al., 1983) that recognizes the same antigen as L4F3 (Andrews et al., 1983) and MY-9 (Griffin et al., 1984). The reasons for lack of L1B2 reactivity with the L4F3/MY-9 antigen as expressed on mature monocytes may result from modification of the antigen

TABLE 3

Monoclonal Antibodies Reactive Primarily with Both Granulocytes and Monocytes

Antibody	Cell type				
	Granulo- cyte	Mono- cyte	Lympho- cyte	Plate- lets	Red blood cells
Anti-LFA antigens	Mo-1[a] (Arnaout et al., 1983; Todd et al., 1981), Mac-1 (Ault and Springer, 1981; Springer et al., 1978, 1982), OKM-1 (Beard et al., 1980; Wright et al., 1983; Zarling et al., 1980), OKM-9,-10 (Talle et al., 1983; Wright et al., 1983), IB4 (Wright et al., 1983), LFA-1 (Davignon et al., 1981), LFA-2, LFA-3 (Sanchez-Madrid et al., 1982), 60.3 (Beatty et al., 1983), B2.12[a] (Tetteroo et al., 1984), M522[a] (Lohmeyer et al., 1981)	+	+	+	—	—

Other antibodies

MY-7[b] (Griffin et al., 1981), MCS-2[b] (Tatsumi et al., 1981), DUHL60.4[b] (McKolanis et al., 1984)

20.2[c] (Kamoun et al., 1983), M67[c] (Bernard et al., 1984)

MY-8[d] (Griffin et al., 1981), 80H.1, 80H.3 (Mannoni et al., 1982) PM-81 (Ball et al., 1983), HL-1 (Namikawa et al., 1983), Mo-5 (Todd et al., 1984), C3, D1, I2 (Mirro et al., 1984)

T5A7[c] (Andrews et al., 1983; Symington et al., 1984), MMA[e] (Hanjan et al., 1982) AML-2-23 (Ball et al., 1982; Ball and Fanger 1983)

[a]Clustered in CD11 by First International Workshop
[b]Clustered in CDw13 by First International Workshop
[c]Clustered in CDw12 by First International Workshop
[d]Not clustered by First International Workshop
[e]React with PHA stimulated lymphoblasts

during maturation or from differences in antibody affinity and demonstrates again the need for caution in interpretation of antibody binding studies. The MY-10 determinant in marrow is expressed by monoblasts, myeloblasts, and hematopoietic progenitors (Civin et al., 1983, 1984). There are also determinants associated with immature myelocytic elements as well as lymphoid cells, including the antigen identified by antibody RFB-1 (Bodger et al., 1981, 1983), which reacts with myeloblasts and a portion of promyelocytes as well as with T cells and a subset of thymocytes.

2.5. Antibodies Against Erythroid and Megakaryocytic Lineage-Associated Antigens

In the erythroid series, antibodies against glycophorin-A (Anstee and Edwards, 1982; Edwards, 1980; Knapp et al., 1981) are reactive with mature and nucleated erythoid elements, whereas antibodies to carbohydrate blood group antigens such as B and A (Barnstable et al., 1978; Edelman et al., 1981; Sacks and Lennox, 1981; Sieff et al., 1982; Voak et al., 1980) and to transferrin receptors (Lebman et al., 1982; Sutherland et al., 1981) are reactive with erythrocytic and myelocytic elements.

Antibodies against platelet–megakaryocyte-associated antigens have been generated and shown to react with platelet glycoproteins 1b (McGregor et al., 1983; McMichael et al., 1981; Ruan et al., 1981), 1a (McGregor et al. 1983), and the IIb/IIIa complex (Bennet et al., 1983; Burckhardt et al., 1982; Collier et al., 1983; Damiani et al., 1983; McEver et al., 1980; McGregor et al., 1983; Thiagarajan et al., 1983; Vainchenker et al., 1982). Binding of antibodies to several of these determinants interferes with normal platelet activation and function (Collier et al., 1983; McGregor et al., 1983; Ruan et al., 1981), and some antibodies crossreact with glycoproteins of similar M_r on monocytes (Burkhardt et al., 1982). Vainchenker et al. (1983) have examined the expression of the platelet–megakaryocyte-associated AN-51 and J-15 antigens on marrow cells and have found rare small lymphoid appearing cells that expressed these markers and which they felt represented early stages of megakaryopoiesis because of the concomitant expression of platelet specific peroxidase activity.

2.6. Myeloid-Associated Antigens Expressed by Hematopoietic Progenitors

Monoclonal antibodies provide probes for studying the cell surface of the various hematopoietic progenitor subclasses. Although studies have demonstrated the presence of HLA-A,B,C, HLA/DR, and beta-2 microglobulin on unipotential progenitors (Fitchen et al., 1981; Robinson et al., 1981), many new antigens have now been identified using monoclonal antibodies. These antigens appear to be expressed in a hierarchical fashion by the various stem cell subclasses and their progeny. Antigens on myeloblasts that are either not expressed on or are present in very reduced amounts on mature granulocytic cells, are often found on multipotential precursor cells (CFU-GEMM or CFU-Mix). The L4F3/MY-9 (Griffin et al., 1984), MY-10 (Civin et al., 1983, 1984), and RFB-1 (Bodger et al., 1983) antigens are expressed on CFU-Mix, early erythroid progenitors (BFU-E), and virtually all marrow derived CFU-GM. However, the L4F3/MY-9 antigen is not on erythroid colony-forming cells (CFU-E), whereas RFB-1 is on CFU-E as well as CFU-Meg (megakaryocyte colony-forming cells).

Antigens that are weakly expressed on myeloblasts and more highly by mature myelomonocytic elements including the X-hapten (Andrews et al., 1983; Ferrero et al., 1983; Mannoni et al., 1982; Subitz et al., 1983a), MY-7 (Griffin and Schlossman, 1984), D5D6 (Linker-Israeli et al., 1982), and MMA (Hanjan et al., 1982) antigens are also on CFU-GM. However, the X-hapten and MY-7 antigen are not on erythroid progenitors (Andrews et al., 1983; Griffin and Schlossman, 1984). Additionally, the X-hapten is virtually absent from circulating CFU-GM, although its expression can be induced with culture in vitro (Ferrero et al., 1983a). Other antigens expressed as early as the promyelocyte stage during granulocytic maturation are either very weakly expressed by CFU-GM or are not on committed progenitors of either the erythroid or granulocyte/monocyte lineages, including T5A7 (anti-lactosylceramide) (Andrews et al., 1983), Mo-1 (anti-C3bi) (Griffin and Schlossman, 1984), MY8 (Griffin and Schlossman, 1984), MY-4 (Griffin and Schlossman, 1984), PM-81 (Ball et al., 1983), PMN-29 (Ball and Fanger, 1983), and AML-2-23 (Ball and Fanger, 1983). Of interest is the 5F1 antigen that is expressed by CFU-E, but not by BFU-E or CFU-GM (Andrews et al., 1983) in contrast to glycophorin A that is expressed on mature and nucleated RBCs, but is absent from CFU-E and BFU-E (Robinson et al., 1981).

Monoclonal antibodies can serve as tools to isolate various subgroups of hematopoietic progenitors and their progeny based on cell surface antigen differences. Beverley et al. (1980) used anti-HLe-1 to highly enrich CFU-GM, BFU-E and CFU-E. Griffin et al. (1982) have recently purified CFU-GM from the peripheral blood of patients with chronic myelogenous leukemia (CML) to the point that one of every three cells separated gave rise to a colony or cluster in vitro. Linch et al. (1983) have been able to isolate normal BFU-E with a cloning efficiency of up to 25%. Whether these were the only progenitors enriched in each of these last two cases was not studied. The ability to specifically isolate purified populations of normal and malignant progenitor cells will be important for elucidating specific mechanisms regulating stem cell proliferation and maturation.

2.7. Expression of Myeloid-Associated Antigens During Ontogeny and Phylogeny

Few studies have examined ontogenetic or phylogenetic aspects of myeloid differentiation using monoclonal antibodies to differentiation antigens. It is possible that there are hematopoietic oncofetal antigens that are expressed by myeloid leukemias, but none has been as yet identified.

Rosenthal et al. (1983) examined fetal liver and bone marrow cells and observed that at 11–14 wk gestation, liver-derived cells reacted with MY-7, MY-8 and Mo-1. Further, at 15-17 wk, gestation, bone marrow cells that expressed these determinants were identified as belonging to the myelocytic lineage. We have examined two fetal livers at 9 ½ and 10 wk gestation (unpublished observations) when morphologically the vast majority of hematopoietic elements are erythroid and megakaryocytic. The 5F1 antigen was expressed by the majority of cells whereas the X-hapten identified by 1G10 as well as the L4F3/MY-9 antigen were not expressed as determined by flow microfluorimetry. In contrast, CFU-GM present in the fetal liver reacted with L4F3, determined by a cytolytic assay, as do CFU-GM in normal marrow.

Granulocytes from closely related species also express determinants reactive with monoclonal antibodies to human myeloid differentiation antigens. Antigenic determinants associated with important cellular housekeeping or general recognition functions might be expected to be conserved phylogenetically as has been observed for certain T lymphocyte differentiation antigens (Hansen et al., 1984; Ledbetter et al., 1980). In studies of granulocytes from several primate and nonprimate species, Letvin et al. (1983) found that the Mo-1 antibody (anti-C3bi receptor) and two other antibodies probably against the same antigen all reacted with granulocytes from dogs as well as all primate species tested. In contrast, antibody MY-7 reacted only with human and chimpanzee granulocytes. Antibody MY-8 and MY-3 reactivity was limited to human, chimpanzee and gibbon granulocytes, whereas MY-4 reacted with all of these as well as granulocytes from several other primate species. Whether the molecules that express the target epitopes on cells of these other species are similar to those from human myeloid cells, and whether these antigens are expressed at the same stages of differentiation and serve the same function as they do in humans remains to be determined.

2.8. Myeloid-Associated Antigens on Human Myeloid Cell Lines

The aim of this paper is not to characterize the reactivity of monoclonal antibodies with known cell lines as has been recently studied in some detail (Minowada et al., 1984). Deserving mention however is the use of cell lines in the study of antigenic modulation and induction. Myeloid leukemia cell lines can be induced to undergo differentiative changes with the development of morphologic (Andersson et al., 1979; Breitman et al., 1980; Collins et al., 1978, 1980, Koeffler et al., 1980; Koeffler and Golde, 1980) and functional (Breitman et al., 1981; Collins et al., 1979; Newberger et al., 1979) properties similar to those of normal mature myeloid cells, accompanied by loss of proliferative ability (Rovera et al., 1980). These morphologic and funtional changes occur concomitantly with alterations in cell surface antigen expression by either acquisition of new markers or changes in density of markers already expressed. For example, induction of monocytic characteristics in the HL-60 cell line is associated with Mo-3 expression (Todd and Schlossman, 1982) as well as increased expression of other antigens (Ferrero et al., 1983a; Stockbauer et al., 1983), whereas induction of more mature granulocytic features is associated with expression of the AML-2-23 (Graziano et al., 1983), 63D3 (Graziano et al., 1983), B9.8.1 (Perussia et al., 1981), and other antigens (Ferrero et al., 1983a; Urdal et al., 1983). Studies using cell lines may also be important in decifering the functional roles of some of these antigens. Some investigators have demonstrated that leukemic cells from patients may be induced to mature by some of these same agents (Koeffler et al., 1980; Marie et al., 1981; Pigoraro et al., 1980). This has supported hypotheses that inducers of differentiation may be useful for therapy of leukemia (see Koeffler, 1983, for review).

3. Expression of Myeloid-Associated Antigens by Myeloid Leukemias

The majority of myeloid leukemic cells express normal myeloid-associated antigens as detectable by monoclonal antibodies. Certain of these antibodies that react with myeloid leukemic cells are useful for diagnostic purposes whereas others recognize subgroups of this heterogeneous group of diseases. Below we review the extent to which these antibodies are useful in discriminating acute nonlymphocytic from acute lymphocytic leukemia, the nature of subsets of ANL defined by these antibodies in relation to FAB classification, and the potential clinical significance of these subsets. Finally, the usefulness of antibodies to differentiation antigens as tools for studying the biology and possibly for the treatment of ANL will be discussed.

3.1. Diagnosis of Acute Nonlymphoblastic Leukemia Using Monoclonal Antibodies: Discrimination from ALL

Certain antibodies are potentially useful for diagnostic purposes as outlined in Table 4. Perhaps the most frequently expressed antigen is that identified by L4F and MY-9. Griffin et al. (1984) found the L4F3/MY-9

TABLE 4

Reactivity of Monoclonal Antibodies with Leukemic Cells from Patients with
Acute Nonlymphoblastic and Acute Lymphoblastic Leukemias[a]

		Leukemia type	
Antibody (References)		ANL[b]	ALL
Anti-L4F3/MY-9	L4F3[c]	105/115	5/62
antigen	L1B2[c]	94/116	5/62
	MY-9 (Griffin et al., 1984)	82/98	1/109
Anti-X-hapten	1G10[c]	69/117	0/63
	VIMD5 (Stockinger et al., 1984)	122/169	2/141
	MY-1 (Civin et al., 1981; Vaughn et al., 1983)	13/32	0/20
Other antibodies	5F1[c]	62/117	0/63
	MY-7 (Griffin et al., 1984)	84/98	1/109
	MY-8 (Griffin and Schlossman, 1984)	40/70	0/82
	Mo-1 (Griffin and Schlossman, 1984)	36/70	0/82
	D5D6 (Linker-Israeli et al., 1981)	44/50	0/15
	R-10 (Greaves et al., 1983)	34/246[d]	0/327
Anti-Ia	I2 (Griffin et al., 1984)	84/98	81/109

[a]Data presented as the number of patient samples reported positive for antibody reaction with leukemic cells over the number of patient samples tested as reported by authors.
[b]Acute nonlymphoblastic leukemias including FAB classes M1 through M6
[c]Dinndorf, P. A., R. G. Andrews, I. D. Bernstein, and D. Benjamin, manuscript in preparation
[d]Virtually all specimens reported as positive were M6, acute erythroleukemias

antigen on leukemic cells from 84% of 98 adult patients, whereas we have identified it on leukemic cells from 91% of 115 children and 90% of 39 adults with ANL (Dinndorf, Andrews, Bernstein, and Benjamin, manuscript in preparation). Other frequently expressed antigens have been identified by antibodies D5D6 (Herrmann et al., 1983; Linker-Israeli, 1982), MY-7 (Griffin and Schlossman, 1984; Griffin et al., 1984), and anti-HLA/DR antibodies (Griffin et al., 1984; Herrmann et al., 1983). In addition, antibodies against the X-hapten react with cells from a significant proportion of patients with ANL (Bernstein et al., 1982a; Herrmann et al., 1983; Majdic et al., 1982; Stockinger et al., 1984; van der Reijden et al., 1983).

The diagnostic importance of antibodies to these antigens lies in their ability to discriminate ANL from ALL. For this purpose, the L4F3/MY-9 antigen, while present on most ANL specimens, is expressed by less than 10% of ALL specimens. Griffin et al. (1984), using the MY-9 antibody, found only one patient out of 109 with ALL whose leukemic cells expressed the antigen, whereas Dinndorf et al. (manuscript in preparation) found L4F3 and L1B2 reacted with cells from five of 62 (8%) pediatric age patients. Also useful for this purpose are antibodies against the X-hapten that is rarely expressed by ALL cells. Stockinger et al. (1984) found that VIMD5 reacted with only two of 141 patients with ALL, whereas Dinndorf et al., using 1G10, found no positive reactions with leukemic cells from 63 children with ALL. In that study we also found that the 5F1 antigen was not expressed on the blasts of these 63 patients. Civin et al. (1981) reported that MY-1 did not react with leukemic cells from 20 patients with ALL. Also useful is the MY-7 antibody, as it reacted with only one of 109 ALL specimens studied by Griffin et al. (1984) and antibodies MY-8, Mo-1, and MY-4, none of which reacted with leukemic cells from 82 patients with ALL (Griffin and Schlossman, 1984). Such antibodies also distinguish lymphoid from myeloid blast crises in CML (Griffin et al., 1983a).

In contrast to the selective absence of certain myeloid antigens from ALL cells, Ia antigens, as well as several other determinants, appear to be expressed by a significant proportion of ALLs. A number of laboratories have reported HLA/Dr expression by 86–100% of ANL specimens and by 74–88% of ALLs (Greaves et al., 1983; Griffin et al., 1984; Herrmann et al., 1983; Pesando et al., 1979; Schlossman et al., 1976). Other antigens such as those identified by PM81 (Ball et al., 1983) and MMA (Hanjan et al., 1982) that are expressed by leukemic cells from a large proportion of patients with ANL also are found on leukemic cells from a significant proportion of ALLs tested. Three antibodies that identify determinants expressed primarily on primitive hematopoietic cells also have been shown to react with a small but significant proportion of ALLs. Civin et al. (1983) reported that antibody MY-10 reacted with leukemic cells from approximately 30% of patients with ANL or ALL. Antibody B5, described by Billings et al. (1982), reacted with leukemic cells from 66% of 50 patients with ALL tested, and antibody HL-47, described by Namikawa et al. (1983), reacted with leukemic cells from 12 of 32 patients with ALL tested.

The above findings indicate that the assessment of cell surface antigens can be used to distinguish the vast majority of acute myeloid leukemias from acute lymphoid leukemias. This is similar to the selective expression of lymphoid differentiation antigens such as CALLA by ALL cells and its virtual absence on ANL cells (Greaves et al., 1983; Pesando et al., 1979, 1980). Additionally, surface markers may be an important adjunct in discriminating ANL from ALL when standard morphologic and histochemical criteria are inconclusive. Dinndorf, Benjamin, Ridgway, and Bernstein (submitted for publication) reported two patients

diagnosed as having ALL who had a poor response to standard chemotherapy for this form of leukemia. When stored leukemic cells obtained
from these patients at diagnosis and at relapse were studied with a panel
of monoclonal antibodies against myeloid-associated determinants, it was
found that these leukemias expressed cell surface determinants compati-
ble with diagnosis of ANL. Greaves et al. (1983) described a small percentage of patients initially diagnosed as ALL whose leukemic cells expressed glycophorin A. These cases were subsequently diagnosed as
acute erythroleukemias. This is similar to findings of studies using
heteroantisera against glycophorin (Andersson et al., 1981). However,
not all patients diagnosed as having ALL whose leukemic cells expressed
myeloid antigen may necessarily represent misclassifications. Bettelheim
et al. (1982) reported two patients diagnosed as having ALL. Leukemic
cells from one of these patients were TdT positive, CALLA positive and
reacted with the anti-X-hapten antibody, VIMD5. The importance of the
small percentage of leukemias that express both myeloid- and lymphoid-
associated differentiation antigens is not yet clear. McCulloch has advanced a theory of "lineage infidelity" to explain these cases
(McCulloch, 1983; Smith et al., 1983). The possibility that a small population of normal hematopoietic cells may demonstrate coexpression of
such antigens at some point during fetal or adult hematopoietic differentiation has not been rigorously excluded.

3.2. Subsets of Acute Nonlymphoblastic Leukemia Defined
by Monoclonal Antibodies

Subsets of myeloid leukemias can now be defined based on the cell surface expression of myeloid differentiation antigens as well as by expression of cytoplasmic markers. Acute nonlymphoblastic leukemia is presently divided into subgroups based on morphology and by the expression
of specific gene products in the cytoplasm of the leukemic cells including
specific enzymes, for example, peroxidase or alpha-naphthyl acetate esterase. Monoclonal antibodies against cell surface myeloid-associated
differentiation antigens also identify the expression of other gene products in leukemic cells. As with cytoplasmic markers, it has been demonstrated that there is considerable heterogeneity in the expression of
myeloid-associated antigens by leukemic cells.

The relationship of lineage of the malignant myeloid cells as determined by conventional criteria according to the French, American, British (FAB) classification system versus using monoclonal antibodies has
been examined in a number of studies. Dinndorf, Andrews, Bernstein,
and Benjamin (manuscript in preparation) did not find concordance between FAB classification and differentiative status of leukemic cells as
defined by monoclonal antibody. Specifically 58% of 19 M1 or M2 myeloid leukemias expressed the determinant detected by 5F1 that is not

known to be expressed by normal granulocytes. Similarly all four monocytic M5 leukemias expressed the X-hapten that is predominately found on normal granulocytic cells. Moreover, a comparison between the degree of morphologic differentiation in leukemia classified as M1 or M2 and the expression of antigens associated with early granulocytic differentiation, i.e., L4F3, and late granulocytic differentiation, i.e., T5A7, failed to show a relationship. In studies by Herrmann et al. (1983) and van der Reijden et al. (1983,) there was a suggestion that leukemias within a single FAB type expressed specific clusters of cell surface markers. However, in these studies the X-hapten was also expressed by the majority of monocytic (M5) leukemias, and with the exception of glycophorin A that was expressed specifically by the M6 erythroleukemias in one study (Hermann et al., 1983), no specific FAB subgroup was identified by antibodies to a specific antigen. Leukemias classified as morphologically more mature (M2, M3, or M5A) appeared to either lack or express low levels of Ia, whereas non-Ia myeloid-associated antigens were more frequently expressed (van der Reijden et al., 1983). Nevertheless, monoclonal antibodies against myeloid-associated antigens can define subsets of ANL that are often distinct from those defined by FAB criteria.

Griffin et al. (1983b) studied the extent to which the antigenic phenotype of ANL cells are reflective of particular stages in normal myeloid differentiation. In those studies they were able to define four phenotypes that included 88% of 70 patients studied. All patients morphologically characterized as having AMoL were classified in one group based on reactivity with MY-8 and three patients with acute promyelocytic leukemia were classified in another group based on reactivity with MY-7. Most patients categorized morphologically as having AML on AMML did not express a phenotype that could be directly associated with a morphologic appearance.

3.3. Prognostic Implications of Cell Surface Phenotype

As yet it has not been possible to accurately predict the clinical outcome for patients with ANL whereas the prognosis of patients with ALL can be predicted based on clinical parameters such as age, white count, physical findings, and leukemic cell morphology and phenotype at diagnosis (Bowman et al., 1981; Greaves, 1981; Kersey et al., 1982; LeBien et al., 1981; Robinson et al., 1980; Sallan et al., 1980). Although chemotherapy and bone marrow transplantation appear to be effective therapies in ANL, particularly for the younger age groups, it cannot yet be determined whether one or the other form of treatment may be more appropriate for a given patient. The prognostic significance of age, white count at diagnosis, or FAB classification of M5 or M3 reported by some investigators have not been consistent findings (Bennett and Begg, 1981; Brandman et al., 1979; Foon et al., 1979; Gale, 1979; Mertelsmann et al., 1980; Reid and Proctor, 1982; Weinstein et al., 1980). Definitive information on the prognostic significance of subgroups of ANL defined by monoclonal antibodies is not yet available. Preliminary studies suggesting the usefulness of this approach, however, have come from Vaughn et al. (1983) who used antibodies to determinants expressed either by less mature or by more mature myelocytic cells to phenotype leukemic cells from 32 adult patients with ANL. These antibodies included the anti-X-hapten antibody MY-1, AHN-1, and AHN-2, which react with antigens most highly expressed by mature granulocytic elements, and antibody MY-10 that reacts with immature hematopoietic elements including progenitor cells and myeloblasts, but not with more mature myeloid elements. These studies suggested that patients whose leukemic cells expressed late (mature) myeloid markers and did not express markers found on immature hematopoietic cells had a significantly higher response rate to induction chemotherapy than did patients whose blast cells expressed only early markers. Of particular interest also is the study by Smith et al. (1983) where patients whose leukemic cells expressed markers of more than one lineage were less likely to respond to chemotherapy. In this study of 20 patients, myeloid markers identified by the MY-1, OKM1, AN-51, R10 antibodies and lymphoid markers defined by B1, J5 (CALLA), OKT-3, -4, -6, -8, and -11 were studied. Six patients had malignant cells that expressed markers of more than one lineage and 83% of these did not respond to induction chemotherapy. Whether the finding of multiple lineage markers on leukemic cells reflects a more abnormal differentiative program or indicates to some extent the differentiative capacity of the stem cell type in which the leukemia arose (multipotential vs. unipotential) is not clear. In the study by Griffin et al. (1983b) in which leukemia antigenic phenotype was related to stages of normal differentiation there was no significant association between phenotype and response to induction therapy. Larger prospective studies will be necessary to provide definitive evidence as to whether or not subsets of ANL can be defined that display significantly different responses to current therapeutic regimens.

4. Monoclonal Antibodies as Probes of Leukemic Stem Cell Phenotype and Differentiation

In addition to the heterogeneity of leukemias from different patients described in the previous sections, leukemic cell populations of individual patients are antigenically heterogeneous. It has been hypothesized that leukemic cell populations are derived from a small subset of leukemic cells with proliferative and self renewal potential (Buick et al., 1977; McCulloch et al., 1982; Minden et al., 1978). Thus, most leukemic cells are thought to be derived from this stem cell population through a defective maturation process, and though these cells are immature in appearance they are incapable of in vitro proliferation. Through analysis of cell surface antigens expressed by leukemic colony-forming cells and their progeny, it has been suggested that proliferative cells can be distinguished phenotypically.

Griffin et al. (1983c) have demonstrated that leukemic colony-forming cells represent a phenotypically distinct subset within leukemic populations. In their study of four patients, the leukemic colony-forming cells expressed Ia and MY-7 antigens that are normally expressed by CFU-GM, and did not express the antigen detected by MY-4 that is normally expressed on mature monocytes and weakly on granulocytic elements. Importantly, they isolated M-7 positive cells and demonstrated their capacity to form colonies and to differentiate in vitro into cells that express determinants recognized by MY-4. These studies therefore were taken to suggest that the Ia and MY-7 positive cells represented less mature proliferating cells, possibly leukemic stem cells, that presumably differentiate and give rise to the major portion of leukemic cells within each population.

Studies in our laboratory have also found that leukemic colony-forming cells may be phenotypically distinct from most of the leukemic cell population (unpublished observations). In these studies the expression of antigenic determinants by leukemic progenitors was determined by the ability of antibody and complement treatment of leukemic cell populations to inhibit leukemic colony formation. As in the study by Griffin et al. (1983c), we found that leukemic colony-forming cells express antigens also expressed on normal CFU-GM. Thus in 16 of 20 patients antibody L4F3 inhibited leukemic colony formation by greater than 90%, whereas antibody 1G10 (anti-X-hapten) inhibited greater than 50% of the colony formation in 10 of 17 patients. These determinants are expressed on all or a subpopulation of normal CFU-GM. Additionally, antibody 5F1 that does not react with normal CFU-GM was found to inhibit leukemic colony formation in vitro. These studies suggest that leukemic progenitors are phenotypically similar, though not always identical, to normal CFU-GM. Studies using markers to identify the malignant clone (i.e., G6PD or chromosomal abnormalities) will be necessary to determine whether the residual colony-forming cells remaining following antibody-mediated lysis represent leukemic or normal progenitors.

5. Therapy of Myeloid Leukemias Using Antibodies to Leukemia-Associated Antigens

The ability to distinguish the antigenic phenotype of ANL stem cells may suggest a strategy or antibody therapy of ANL. Ideally, serotherapy of leukemias would use antibodies against leukemia-specific antigens, but the status of such putative antigens is still in question. The leukemia associated antigens thus far identified by monoclonal antibodies are normally occurring antigens. Nevertheless, if antigens can be defined that are expressed by the leukemic stem cells that maintain the malignancy, but are not expressed by normal pleuripotential hematopoietic stem cells required for normal hematopoietic reconstitution, then it might be possible to achieve selective depletion of malignant stem cells while not depleting stem cells required for survival.

Are there differences in cell surface antigen expression between leukemic and normal stem cells? Studies by Griffin et al. (1983c) and in our laboratory suggest that normal and leukemic cells capable of growing in vitro under the same culture conditions have many antigenic similarities. Importantly, most malignant colony-forming cells express the L4F3/MY-9 antigen that is also expressed by nearly all normal CFU-GM. Are these cells, however, truly the stem cells that maintain the malignancy in vivo?

Insights into the nature of the leukemic stem cells have come from studies by Fialkow et al. (1977, 1978, 1979, 1981, 1982), which have determined that myeloid leukemias are clonal disorders as demonstrated by studies of patients who are heterozygous at the X-linked G6PD locus. Because of the random inactivation of a single X chromosome in somatic cells early in embryogenesis, a woman who is heterozygous for G6PD, with both the normal Gd^B and variant Gd^A genes, will effectively be a mosaic with each tissue having two cell populations, one with type B and the other with type A G6PD enzyme. These two enzymes are easily distinguishable electrophoretically. Therefore, if a neoplasm in such an individual is derived from a single cell (clonal), then all cells derived from it should express only a single G6PD enzyme phenotype, whereas normal tissue or a polyclonally derived process should express both enzymes. The clonal abnormality in myeloid leukemias may be expressed in single or multiple hematopoietic lineages. Patients with CML have clonal abnormalities involving both myeloid and lymphoid lineages, indicating the etiology of the malignancy in a pluripotent stem cell (Fialkow et al., 1977, 1978). Patients with ANL display two patterns of clonal involvement. In younger patients the clonal abnormality is restricted in expression to the malignant myelocytic cells, whereas in older patients the clonal abnormality is expressed by the erythroid and megakaryocytic lineages as well (Fialkow et al., 1979, 1981; Fialkow, 1982). Two hypotheses are possible to explain the observations. The first is that the two patterns of clonality result from malignant transformation occurring at different stem cell stages during differentiation. The second is that the malignant transformation occurs at the same stem cell stage, but that dissimilar maturational potentials result from different lesions. Using monoclonal antibodies to differentiation antigens it is now possible to directly test these hypotheses. Singer et al. (1984) have reported preliminary findings that monoclonal antibodies to antigens on committed myeloid progenitors, which react with leukemic CFC, can delete the malignant clone and leave populations of normal CFC. Whether these residual CFC represent immature stem cells capable of reestablishing normal hematopoiesis is not known. However, the demonstration of such findings provides a further rationale for proceeding to trials of therapy using monoclonal antibodies to selected antigens expressed by leukemic stem cells.

Monoclonal antibodies for therapy of myeloid leukemia may be beneficial in conjunction with bone marrow transplantation when a histocompatible donor is not available. In this setting antibodies could be used to eliminate contaminating leukemic cells from remission bone marrow used for autologous transplantation, provided they do not damage normal hematopoietic stem cells required for engraftment. Nonetheless, the antigenic heterogeneity of leukemic stem cells will undoubtedly require the use of multiple antibodies for treatment. It should be noted that it is not known whether residual leukemic cells in stored autologous marrow are capable of reestablishing the malignancy. Further, successful use of this approach will, of course, require effective eradication of leukemic cells from the patient with high dose chemotherapy and radiation therapy.

Several investigators have studied the feasibility of using monoclonal antibodies for in vivo serotherapy of leukemia (Ball et al., 1983b; Ritz et al., 1981). In an earlier study of ALL, Ritz et al. (1981) used the J-15 (CALLA) antibody to treat patients. Although there was little toxicity, the effects of treatment were minor and short-lived. However this study was important for pointing out potential difficulties of such therapy, including antigenic modulation (Pesando et al., 1983) and the inability to treat large tumor burdens. Additionally, circulating antigen, expression of antigen by vital nonhematopoietic tissues, antibody isotype, and access of antibody and effector cells (if antibody is not toxin conjugated) to sanctuary sites for elimination of disease may also limit effectiveness (Bernstein et al., 1982b). More recently Ball et al. (1983b) used several monoclonal antibodies to treat patients with ANL. It is uncertain if the failure to influence the malignant state in these patients was due to the above cited reasons or because the antibodies used were not reactive with leukemic progenitor cells that continued to maintain the malignancy.

6. Conclusions

Monoclonal antibodies that recognize myeloid leukemia-associated cell surface antigens identify normal hematopoietic differentiation antigens that are expressed in a lineage and stage-restricted fashion by normal myeloid progenitor cells and their progeny. Many of these antigens are selectively expressed by ANL and define unique subsets of this disease that may be of prognostic significance. Additionally monoclonal antibodies provide probes for studying the heterogeneity and differentiative capacity of leukemic stem cells. As a result, it may be possible to distinguish leukemic stem cells from normal pleuripotent hematopoietic stem cells, thus providing a rationale for trials of antibody therapy. Further, studies are needed to identify the biochemical and functional nature of most of these antigens and to identify antigenic determinants that distinguish major hematopoietic stem cell compartments to enable the development of technologies for manipulating normal and malignant hematopoietic stem cells for therapeutic purposes.

Acknowledgments

We thank Drs. J. Pesando, J. Griffin, F. Symington, P. Martin, and Ms. T. Gooding for their help.

This work was supported in part by Grants AM33298, CA36011, CA26828, and CA09351. R. G. A. is supported by a Junior Faculty Clinical Fellowship from the American Cancer Society and the Poncin Scholarship Fund.

References

Al-Rammahy, A. Kh., R. Shipman, A. Jackson, A. Malcolm, and J. G. Levy (1980), *Cancer Immunol. Immunother.* **9,** 181.

Andersson, L. C., M. Jokinen, and C. J. Gahmberg (1979), *Nature* **278,** 364.

Andersson, L. C., E. von Willebrand, C. J. Gahmberg, M. Siimes, and P. Vuopio (1981), in *Leukemia Markers* (Knapp, W., Ed.), Academic Press, London, p. 249.

Andrews, R. G., B. Torok-Storb, and I. D. Bernstein (1983), *Blood* **62,** 124.

Andrews, R. G., T. A. Brentnall, B. Torok-Storb, and I. D. Bernstein (1984), in *Leucocyte Typing: Human Leucocyte Differentiation Antigens Detected by Monoclonal Antibodies* (Bernard, A., L. Boumsell, J. Dausset, C. Milstein, and S. F. Schlossman, Eds.), Springer-Verlag, Berlin, p. 398.

Anstee, D. J., and P. A. W. Edwards (1982), *Eur. J. Immunol.* **12,** 228.

Arnaout, M. A., R. F. Todd, N. Dana, J. Melansel, S. F. Schlossman, and H. R. Colten (1983), *J. Clin. Invest.* **72,** 171.

Ault, K. A., and T. A. Springer (1981), *J. Immunol.* **126,** 359.

Baker, M. A., and R. N. Taub (1973), *Nature* (New Biol.) **241,** 93.

Baker, M. A., K. Ramachandar, and R. N. Taub (1974), *J. Clin. Invest.* **54,** 1273.

Baker, M. A., R. E. Falk, J. Falk, and M. F. Greaves (1976), *Br. J. Haematol.* **32,** 13.

Baker, M. A., J. A. Falk, W. H. Carter, R. N. Taub, and the Toronto Leukemia Study Group (1979), *New Engl. J. Med.* **301**, 1353.

Baker, M. A., T. Mohanakumar, D. A. K. Roncari, K. H. Shumak, J. A. Falk, M. T. Aye, and R. N. Taub (1981), in *Leukemia Markers* (Knapp, W., Ed.), Academic Press, London, P. 225.

Baker, M. A., D. A. K. Roncari, R. N. Taub, T. Mohanakumar, J. A. Falk, and S. Grant (1982), *Blood* **60**, 412.

Ball, E. D., M. W. Fanger (1983), *Blood* **61**, 456.

Ball, E. D., R. F. Graziano, L. Shen, and M. W. Fanger (1982), *Proc. Natl. Acad. Sci. USA* **79**, 5374.

Ball, E. D., R. F. Graziano, and M. W. Fanger (1983a), *J. Immunol.* **130**, 2937.

Ball, E. D., G. M. Bernier, G. C. Cornwell, O. R. McIntyre, J. F. O'Donnell, and M. W. Fanger (1983b), *Blood* **62**, 1203.

Barnstable, C. J., W. F. Bodmer, G. Brown, G. Galfre, C. Milstein, A. F. William, and A. Ziegler (1978), *Cell* **14**, 9.

Beatty, P. G., J. A. Ledbetter, P. J. Martin, T. H. Price, and J. A. Hansen (1983), *J. Immunol.* **131**, 2913.

Beatty, P. G., H. D. Ochs, J. M. Harlan, T. H. Price, H. Rosen, R. F. Taylor, J. A. Hansen, and S. J. Klebanoff (1984), *Lancet* **1**, 535.

Bennet, J. S., J. A. Hoxie, S. F. Leitman, G. Vilaire, and D. B. Cines (1983), *Proc. Natl. Acad. Sci. USA* **80**, 2417.

Bennett, J. M., and C. Begg (1981), *Cancer Res.* **41**, 4833.

Bennett, J. M., D. Catovsky, M. T. Daniel, G. Flandrin, D. A. G. Galton, H. R. Granlick, and C. Sultan (1976), *Br. J. Haematol.* **33**. 451.

Berger, R., A. Bernheim, M.-T. Daniel, F. Valensi, F. Sigaux, and G. Flandrin (1982), *Blood* **59**, 171.

Bernard, A., L. Boumsell, J. Dausset, C. Milstein, and S. F. Schlossman, Eds., (1984), *Leucocyte Typing: Human Leucocyte Differentiation Antigens Detected by Monoclonal Antibodies,* Springer-Verlag, Berlin.

Bernstein, I. D., R. G. Andrews, S. F. Cohen, and B. E. McMaster (1982a), *J. Immunol.* **128**, 876.

Bernstein, I. D., R. C. Nowinski, and P. Wright (1982b), in *Immunological Approaches to Cancer Therapeutics* (Mihich, E., Ed.), J. Wiley and Sons, New York, p. 277.

Bettelheim, P., E. Paietta, O. Majdic, H. Godmer, J. Schwarzmeier, and W. Knapp (1982), *Blood* **60**, 1392.

Beverley, P. C. L., D. Linch, and D. Delia (1980), *Nature* **287**, 332.

Billing, R., K. Lucero, B. J. Shi, and P. I. Terasaki (1982), *Blood* **59**, 1203.

Bodger, M. P., G. E. Francis, D. Delia, S. M. Granger, and G. Janossy (1981), *J. Immunol.* **127**, 2269.

Bodger, M. P., C. A. Izaguirre, H. A. Blacklock, and A. V. Hoffbrand (1983), *Blood* **61**, 1006.

Bowman, W. P., S. L. Melvin, R. J. A. Aur, and A. M. Mauer (1981), *Cancer Res.* **41**, 4794.

Bradley, T. R., and D. Metcalf (1966), *Aust. J. Exp. Biol. Med. Sci.* **44**, 287.

Bradstock, K. F., G. Janossy, G. Pizzolo, V. A. Hoffbrand, A. McMichael, J. R. Pilch, C. Milstein, P. Beverley, and F. J. Bollum (1980), *J. Natl. Cancer Inst.* **65**, 33.

Brandman, J., R. M. Bukowski, R. Greenstreet, J. S. Hewlett, and G. C. Hoffman (1979), *Cancer* **44**, 1062.

Breard, J., E. L. Reinherz, P. C. Kung, G. Goldstein, and S. F. Schlossman (1980), *J. Immunol.* **124**, 1943.

Breitman, T. R., S. E. Selonick, and S. J. Collins (1980), *Proc. Natl. Acad. Sci. USA* **77**, 2936.

Breitman, T. R., S. J. Collins, and B. R. Keene (1981), *Blood* **57**, 1000.

Brockhaus, M., J. L. Magnani, M. Herlyn, M. Blaszczyk, Z. Steplewski, H. Koprowski, and V. Ginsburg (1982), *Arch. Biochem. Biophys.* **217**, 647.

Brooks, D. A., J. Bradley, and H. Zola (1981), *Clin. Exp. Pharmacol. Physiol.* **8**, 415.

Buick, R. N., J. E. Till, and E. A. McCulloch (1977), *Lancet* **1**, 862.

Burckhardt, J. J., W. A. K. Anderson, J. F. Kearney, and M. D. Cooper (1982), *Blood* **60**, 767.

Chen, P. M., H. Chiang, C. K. Chou, T.-S. Hwang, B. N. Chiang, and M. F. Greaves (1983), *Leuk. Res.* **7**, 339.

Chiao, J. W., and C. Y. Wang (1984), *Cancer Res.* **44**, 1031.

Civin, C. I., J. Mirro, and M. L. Banquerigo (1981), *Blood* **57**, 842.

Civin, C. I., C. L. Strauss, C. Brovall, and J. H. Shaper (1982), *Blood* **60** (Suppl. 1), 95a.

Civin, C. I., L. C. Strauss, M. Fackler, C. Brovall, and J. H. Shaper (1983), *Blood* **62** (Suppl. 1), 149a.

Civin, C. I., L. C. Strauss, C. Brovall, M. J. Fackler, J. F. Schwartz, J. H. J. Shaper, G. P. G. Miller, and J. Puck (1984), *J. Immunol.* **133**, 157.

Clement, L. T., J. E. Lehmeyer, and G. L. Gartland (1983), *Blood* **61**, 326.

Collier, B. S., S. I. Peerschke, L. E. Scudder, and C. A. Sullivan (1983), *J. Clin. Invest.* **72**, 325.

Collins, S. J., F. W. Ruscetti, R. E. Gallagher, and R. C. Gallo (1978), *Proc. Natl. Acad. Sci. USA* **75**, 2458.

Collins, S. J., F. W. Ruscetti, R. E. Gallagher, and R. C. Gallo (1979), *J. Exp. Med.* **149**, 969.

Collins, S. J., A. Bodner, R. Ting, and R. C. Gallo (1980), *Int. J. Cancer* **25**, 213.

Cuttita, F., S. Rosen, A. F. Gazdar, and J. D. Minna (1981), *Proc. Natl. Acad. Sci. USA* **78**, 4591.

Damiani, G., E. Zocchi, M. Fabbi, A. Bargellesi, and F. Patrone (1983), *Exp. Hematol.* **11**, 169.

Davignon, D., E. Martz, T. Reynolds, K. Kürzinger, and T. A. Springer (1981), *Proc. Natl. Acad. Sci. USA* **78**, 4535.

Dimitriu-Bona, A., G. R. Burmester, S. J. Waters, and R. J. Winchester (1983), *J. Immunol.* **130**, 145.

Dimitriu-Bona, A., G. R. Burmester, K. Kelley, and R. J. Winchester (1984), in *Leucocyte Typing: Human Leucocyte Differentiation Antigens Detected by Monoclonal Antibodies* (Bernard, A., L. Boumsell, J. Dausset, C. Milstein, and S. F. Schlossman, eds.), Springer-Verlag, Berlin, p. 434.

Edelman, L., Ph. Rouger, Ch. Dionel, H. Garchon, J. F. Bach, J. Reviron, and Ch. Salmon (1981), *Immunology* **44**, 549.

Edwards, P. A. W. (1980), *Biochem. Soc. Trans.* **8**, 334.

Eisenbarth, G. S., B. F. Haynes, J. A. Schroer, and A. S. Fauci (1980), *J. Immunol.* **124**, 1237.

Ferrero, D., H. E. Broxmeyer, G. L. Pagliardi, S. Venuta, B. Lange, S. Pessano, and G. Rovera (1983a), *Proc. Natl. Acad. Sci. USA* **80**, 4114.

Ferrero, D., S. Pessano, G. L. Pagliardi, and G. Rovera (1983b), *Blood* **61**, 171.

Fialkow, P. J. (1982), *J. Cell. Physiol.* (Suppl. 1), 37.

Fialkow, P. J., R. J. Jacobson, and T. Papayannopoulou (1977), *Am. J. Med.* **63**, 125.

Fialkow, P. J., A. M. Denman, R. J. Jackson, and M. N. Lowenthal (1978), *J. Clin. Invest.* **62**, 815.

Fialkow, P. J., J. W. Singer, J. W. Adamson, R. L. Berkow, J. M. Friedman, R. J. Jacobson, and J. W. Moohr (1979), *New Engl. J. Med.* **301**, 1.

Fialkow, P. J., J. W. Singer, J. W. Adamson, K. Vaidya, K. W. Dow, J. Ochs, and J. W. Moohr (1981), *Blood* **57**, 1068.

Fitchen, J. H., K. A. Foon, and M. J. Cline (1981), *New Engl. J. Med.* **305**, 17.

Foon, K. A., F. Naiem, C. Yale, and R. P. Gale (1979), *Leukemia Res.* **3**, 171.

Fournet, B., J. Montreuil, G. Stecker, L. Dorland, J. Haverkamp, J. F. G. Vliegenthart, J. P. Binette, and K. Schmid (1978), *Biochem.* **17**, 5206.

Fukuchi, Y. S.-I. Hakomori, E. Nudelman, and N. Cochran (1984), *J. Biol. Chem.* (in press).

Gale, R. P. (1979), *New Engl. J. Med.* **300**, 1189.

Girardet, C., S. Ladisch, D. Heumann, J. P. Mach, and S. Carrel (1983), *Int. J. Cancer* **32**, 177.

Golomb, H. M., G. Alimena, J. D. Rowley, J. W. Vardiaman, J. R. Testa, and C. Sovik (1982), *Blood* **60**, 404.

Gooi, H. C., S. J. Thorpe, H. F. Hounsell, H. Rumpold, D. Kraft, O. Forster, and T. Feizi (1983), *Eur. J. Immunol.* **13**, 306.

Graziano, R. F., E. D. Ball, and W. M. Fanger (1983), *Blood* **61**, 1215.

Greaves, M. F. (1981), *Cancer Res.* **41**, 4752.

Greaves, M. F., G. Hariri, R. A. Newman, D. R. Sutherland, M. A. Ritter, and J. Ritz (1983a), *Blood* **61**, 628.

Greaves, M. F., C. Sieff, and P. A. W. Edwards (1983b), *Blood* **61**, 645.

Griffin, J. D. and S. F. Schlossman (1984), in *Leucocyte Typing: Human Leucocyte Differentiation Antigens Detected by Monoclonal Antibodies* (Bernard, A., L. Boumsell, J. Dausset, C. Milstein, and S. F. Schlossman, eds.), Springer-Verlag, Berlin, p. 404.

Griffin, J. D., J. Ritz, L. M. Nadler, and S. F. Schlossman (1981), *J. Clin. Invest.* **68**, 932.

Griffin, J. D., R. P. Beveridge, and S. F. Schlossman (1982), *Blood* **60**, 30.

Griffin, J. D., R. F. Todd, J. Ritz, L. M. Nadler, G. P. Camellos, D. Rosenthal, M. Gallivan, R. Beveridge, H. Weinstein, D. Karp, and S. F. Schlossman (1983a), *Blood* **61**, 85.

Griffin, J. D., R. J. Mayer, H. J. Weinstein, D. S. Rosenthal, F. S. Coral, R. P. Beveridge, and S. F. Schlossman (1983b), *Blood* **62**, 557.

Griffin, J. D., P. Larcom, and S. F. Schlossman (1983c), *Blood* **62**, 1300.

Griffin, J. D., D. Linch, K. Sabbath, P. Larcom, and S. F. Schlossman (1984), *Leukemia Res.* (in press).

Hakomori, S., E. Nudelman, S. Levery, D. Solter, and B. B. Knowles (1981), *Biochem. Biophys. Res. Commun.* **100**, 1578.

Hakomori, S.-I. and R. Kannagi (1983), *J. Natl. Cancer Inst.* **71**, 231.

Hanjan, S. N. S., J. F. Kearney, and M. D. Cooper (1982), *Clin. Immunol. Immunopathol.* **23**, 172.

Hansen, J. A., P. J. Martin, and R. C. Nowinski (1980), *Immunogenetics* **10**, 247.

Hansen, J. A., P. J. Martin, P. G. Beatty, E. A. Clark, and J. A. Ledbetter (1984), in *Leucocyte Typing: Human Leucocyte Differentiation Antigens Detected by Monoclonal Antibodies* (Bernard, A., L. Boumsell, J. Dausset, C. Milstein, and S. F. Schlossman, eds.), Springer-Verlag, Berlin, p. 195.

Hansson, G. C., K.-A. Karlsson, G. Larson, J. M. McKibbin, M. Blaszczyk, M. Herlyn, Z. Steplewski, and H. Koprowski (1983), *J. Biol. Chem.* **258**, 4091.

Harris, J. and E. J. Freireich (1970), *Blood* **35**, 56.

Haynes, B. F., M. E. Memler, D. L. Mann, G. S. Eisenbarth, J. Shelhamer, H. S. Mostowski, C. A. Thomas, J. L. Strominger, and A. S. Fauci (1981), *J. Immunol.* **126**, 1409.

Herrmann, F., B. Komischke, E. Odenwald, and W. D. Ludwig (1983), *Blut* **47**, 157.

Hildreth, J. E. K., F. M. Gotch, P. D. K. Hildreth, and A. J. McMichael (1983), *Eur. J. Immunol.* **13**, 202.

Hogg, N., M. Slusarenko, J. Cohen, and J. Reiser (1981), *Cell* **24**, 875.

Huang, L. C., M. Brockhaus, J. L. Magnani, F. Cuttita, S. Rosen, J. D. Minna, and V. Ginsburg (1983a), *Arch. Biochem. Biophys.* **220**, 318.

Huang, L. C., C. I. Civin, J. L. Magnani, J. H. Shaper, and V. Ginsburg (1983b), *Blood* **61**, 1020.

Kamada, N., K. Okada, and T. Ito (1968), *Lancet* **1**, 364.

Kamoun, M., P. J. Martin, M. E. Kadin, L. G. Lum, and J. A. Hansen (1983), *Clin. Immunol. Immunopathol.* **29**, 181.

Kaneko, Y., J. D. Rowley, H. S. Maurer, D. Variakojis, and J. W. Moohr (1982), *Blood* **60**, 389.

Kemshead, J. T., D. Bicknell, and M. F. Greaves (1981), *Ped. Res.* **15**, 1282.

Kersey, J., A. Goldman, C. Abramson, M. Nesbit, G. Perry, K. Gajl-Peczalska, and T. LeBien (1982), *Lancet* **2**, 1419.

Knapp, W., O. Majdic, H. Rumpold, P. Bettelheim, D. Kraft, K. Liszka, O. Forster, and D. Lutz (1981), in *Leukemia Markers* (Knapp, W., Ed.), Academic Press, London, p. 207.

Knowles, B. B., J. Rappaport, and D. Solter (1982), *Devel. Biol.* **93**, 54.

Kobata, A. and V. Ginsburg (1969), *J. Biol. Chem.* **244**, 5496.

Koeffler, H. P. (1983), *Blood* **62**, 709.

Koeffler, H. P. and D. W. Golde (1980), *Blood* **56**, 344.

Koeffler, H. P., M. Bar-Eli, and M. Territo (1980), *J. Clin. Invest.* **66**, 1101.

Kohler, G. and C. Milstein (1975), *Nature* **256**, 495.

Krensky, A. M., F. Sanchez-Madrid, E. Robbins, J. Nagy, T. A. Springer, and S. J. Burakoff (1983), *J. Immunol.* **131**, 611.

Kung, P. C., G. Goldstein, E. L. Reinherz, and S. F. Schlossman (1979), *Science* **206**, 347.

Kurzinger, K., M. -K. Ho, and T. A. Springer (1982), *Nature* **296**, 668.

LeBien, T. A. and J. H. Kersey (1980), *J. Immunol.* **125**, 2208.

LeBien, T. A., R. W. McKenna, and C. S. Abramson (1981), *Cancer Res.* **41**, 4776.

Lebman, D., M. Trucco, L. Bottero, B. Lange, S. Pessano, and G. Rovera (1982), *Blood* **59**, 671.

Ledbetter, J. A., R. L. Evans, M. Lipinski, C. Cunningham-Rundles, R. A. Good, and L. A. Herzenberg (1980), *J. Exp. Med.* **153**, 310.

Letvin, N. L., R. F. Todd, L. S. Palley, S. F. Schlossman, and J. D. Griffin (1983), *Blood* **61**, 408.

Levine, M. N., J. W. Fray, N. H. Jane, R. S. Metzgar, and B. F. Haynes (1981), *Blood* **58**, 1047.

Levy, R., J. Dilley, R. I. Fos, and R. Warnke (1979), *Proc. Natl. Acad. Sci. USA* **76**, 6552.

Linch, D. C., J. M. Lipton, and D. G. Nathan (1983), *Blood* **62** (Suppl. 1), 151a.

Linker-Israeli, M., R. J. Billing, K. A. Foon, and P. I, Terasaki (1981), *J. Immunol.* **127**, 2473.

Lohmeyer, J., P. Rieber, H. Feucht, J. Johnson, M. Hadam, and G. Reithmuller (1981), *Eur. J. Immunol.* **11**, 997.

Majdic, O., K. Liszka, D. Lutz, and W. Knapp (1981), *Blood* **58**, 1127.

Majdic, O., P. Bettelheim, K. Liszka, and D. Lutz (1982), *Wien. Klin. Wochenschr.* **94**, 387.

Malcolm, A. J., R. C. Shipman, and J. G. Levy (1982), *J. Immunol.* **128**, 2599.

Malcolm, A. J., P. M. Logan, R. C. Shipman, R. Kurth, and J. G. Levy (1983), *Blood* **61**, 858.

Mannoni, P., A. Janowska-Wieczorek, A. R. Turner, L. McGann, and J. M. Turc (1982), *Human Immunol.* **5**, 309.

Mannoni, P., A. Janowska, P. Fromant, B. Weiblen, A. R. Turner, and J. M. Turc (1984), in *Leucocyte Typing: Human Leucocyte Differentiation Antigens Detected by Monoclonal Antibodies* (Bernard, A., L. Boumsell, J. Dausset, C. Milstein, and S. F. Schlossman, eds.), Springer-Verlag, Berlin, p. 410.

Marie, J. P., C. A. Izaguirre, C. I. Civin, J. Mirro, and E. A. McCulloch (1981), *Blood* **58**, 670.

Martin, L. S., J. S. McDougal, S. W. Browning, and D. S. Gordon (1984), in *Leucocyte Typing: Human Leucocyte Differentiation Antigens Detected by Monoclonal Antibodies* (Bernard, A., L. Boumsell, J. Dausset, C. Milstein, and S. F. Schlossman, eds.), Springer-Verlag, Berlin, p. 438.

McCulloch E. A. (1983), *Blood* **62**, 1.

McCulloch, E. A., C. A. Izaguirre, L. J. A. Chang, and L. J. Smith (1982), *J. Cell. Physiol.* (Suppl. 1), 183.

McEver, R. P., N. L. Baenzinger, and P. W. Majerus (1980), *J. Clin. Invest.* **66**, 1311.

McGregor, J. L., J. Brochier, F. Wild, G. Follea, M.-C. Trzeciak, E. James, M. Dechavanne, L. McGregor, and K. J. Clemetson (1983), *Eur. J. Biochem.* **131,** 427.

McKolanis, J. R., M. J. Borowitz, F. L. Tuck, and R. S. Metzgar (1984), in *Leucocyte Typing: Human Leucocyte Differentiaiton Antigens Detected by Monoclonal Antibodies* (Bernard, A., L. Boumsell, J. Dausset, C. Milstein, and D. F. Schlossman, eds.), Springer-Verlag, Berlin, p. 387.

McMichael, A. J., J. R. Pilch, G. Galfre, D. Y. Mason, J. W. Fabre, and C. Milstein (1979), *Eur. J. Immunol.* **9,** 205.

McMichael, A. J., N. A. Rust, R. Pilch, R. Sochynsky, J. Morton, D. Y. Mason, C. Ruan, G. Tobelem, and J. Caen (1981), *Br. J. Haematol.* **49,** 501.

McMichael, A. J., F. M. Gotch, and J. E. K. Hildreth (1982), *Eur. J. Immunol.* **12,** 1002.

Mertelsmann, R., H. T. Thaler, L. To, T. S. Gee, S. McKenzie, P. Schauer, A. Friedman, Z. Arlin, C. Cirincione, and B. Clarkson (1980), *Blood* **56,** 773.

Metzgar, R. S., T. Mohanakumar, and D. S. Miller (1972), *Science* **178,** 986.

Metzgar, R. S., T. Mohanakumar, R. W. Green, D. S. Miller, and D. P. Bolognesi (1974), *J. Natl. Cancer Inst.* **52,** 1445.

Metzgar, R. S., M. J. Borowitz, J. R. McKolanis, F. L. Tuck, and H. Tingye (1984), in *Leucocyte Typing: Human Leucocyte Differentiation Antigens Detected by Monoclonal Antibodies* (Bernard, A., L. Boumsell, J. Dausset C. Milstein, and S. F. Schlossman, eds.), Springer-Verlag, Berlin, p. 656.

Minden, M. D., J. E. Till, and E. A. McCulloch (1978), *Blood* **52,** 592.

Minowada, J., E. Tatsumi, K. Sagawa, M. S. Lok, T. Sugimoto, K. Minato, L. Zgoda, L. Prestine, L. Kover, and D. Gould (1984), in *Leucocyte Typing: Human Leucocyte Differentiation Antigens Detected by Monoclonal Antibodies* (Bernard, A., L. Boumsell, J. Dausset, C. Milstein, and S. F. Schlossman, Eds.), Springer-Verlag, Berlin, p. 519.

Mirro, J., S. Melvin, D. Metzger, A. Look, and S. Murphy (1984), in *Leucocyte Typing: Human Leucocyte Differentiation Antigens Detected by Monoclonal Antibodies* (Bernard A., L. Boumsell, J. Dausset C. Milstein, and S. F. Schlossman, Eds.), Springer-Verlag, Berlin, p. 442.

Mohanakumar, T., R. S. Metzgar, and D. S. Miller (1974), *J. Natl. Cancer Inst.* **52,** 1435.

Mohanakumar, T., D. S. Miller, and R. S. Metzgar (1976), *Blood* **48,** 339.

Mulder, A., J. P. W. van der Veen, M. J. E. Bos, A. E. G. Kr. von dem Borne (1981), in *Leukemia Markers* (Knapp, W., ed.), Academic Press, London, p. 301.

Nadler, L. M., P. Stashenko, R. Hardy, A. van Agthoven, C. Terhorst, and S. F. Schlossman (1981), *J. Immunol.* **126,** 1941.

Nadler, L. M., K. C. Anderson, G. Marti, M. Bates, E. K. Park, J. F. Daley, and S. F. Schlossman (1983), *J. Immunol.* **131,** 244.

Nadler, L. M., K. C. Anderson, M. Bates, E. Park, B. Slaughenhoupt, and S. F. Schlossman (1984), in *Leucocyte Typing: Human Leucocyte Differentiation Antigens Detected by Monoclonal Antibodies* (Bernard, A., L. Boumsell, J. Dausset, C. Milstein, and S. F. Schlossman, Eds.), Springer-Verlag, Berlin, p. 354.

Namikawa, R., S. I. Ogata, R. Ueda, I. Tsuge, K. Nishida, S. Minami, K. Koike, T. Suchi, K. Ota, S. Iijima, and T. Takahashi (1983), *Leukemia Res.* **7**, 375.

Nauseef, W. M., R. K. Root, S. L. Newman, and H. L. Malech (1983), *Blood* **62**, 635.

Newburger, P. E., M. E. Chovaniec, J. S. Greenberger, and H. J. Cohen (1979), *J. Cell. Biol.* **82**, 315.

Papayannopoulou, Th., M. Brice, T. Yokochi, P. S. Rabinovitch, D. Lindsley, and G. Stamatoyannopoulos (1984), *Blood* **63**, 326.

Pigoraro, L., J. Abrahm, R. Cooper, A. Lewis, B. Lange, P. Meo, and G. Rovera (1980), *Blood* **55**, 859.

Perussia, B., D. Lebman, S. H. Ip, G. Rovera, and G. Trinchieri (1981), *Blood* **58**, 836.

Perussia, B., G. Trinchieri, D. Lebman, J. Jankiewicz, B. Lange, and G. Rovera (1982), *Blood* **59**, 382.

Pesando, J. M., J. Ritz, H. Lazarus, S. B. Costello, S. Sallan, and S. F. Schlossman (1979), *Blood* **54**, 1240.

Pesando, J. M., J. Ritz, H. Levine, C. Terhorst, H. Lazarus, and S. F. Schlossman (1980), *J. Immunol.* **124**, 2794.

Pesando, J. M., K. J. Tamaselli, H. Lazarus, and S. F. Schlossman (1983), *J. Immunol.* **131**, 2038.

Pluznik, D. H., and L. Sachs (1966), *J. Cell. Physiol.* **66**, 319.

Raff, H. V., L. J. Picker, and J. D. Stobo (1980), *J. Exp. Med.* **152**, 581.

Reid, M. M. and S. J. Proctor (1982), *Lancet* **2**, 153.

Reinherz, E. L., and S. F. Schlossman (1980), *Cell* **19**, 821.

Reinherz, E. L., P. C. Kung, G. Goldstein, and S. F. Schlossman (1979), *Proc. Natl. Acad. Sci. USA* **76**, 4061.

Reinherz, E. L., P. C. Kung, G. Goldstein, R. H. Levey, and S. F. Schlossman (1980), *Immunology* **77**, 1588.

Ritz, J., J. M. Pesando, S. E. Sallan, L. A. Clavell, J. Notis-McConarty, P. Rosenthal, and S. F. Schlossman (1981), *Blood* **58**, 141.

Robinson, J., C. Sieff, D. Delia, P. A. W. Edwards, and M. Greaves (1981), *Nature* **289**, 68.

Robinson, W. A., J. E. Kurnick, and B. L. Pike (1971), *Blood* **38**, 500.

Robison, W. P., S. L. Melvin, H. N. Sather, G. D. Hammond, and P. F. Coccia (1980), *Am. J. Pediatr. Hematol. Oncol.* **2**, 5.

Rosenberg, S. A., F. S. Ligler, V. Ugolini, and P. E. Lipsky (1981), *J. Immunol.* **126**, 1473.

Rosenthal, P., I. J. Rimm, T. Umiel, J. D. Griffin, R. Osathanadh, and S. F. Schlossman (1983), *J. Immunol.* **131**, 232.

Rovera, G., N. Olashaw, and P. Meo (1980), *Nature* **284**, 69.

Rowley, J. D. (1973), *Ann. Genet.* **16**, 109.

Rowley, J. D. (1977), in *Population Cytogenetics, Proceedings of the Birth Defects Institute Symposium of the New York State Health Department* (Porter, I. H. and E. B. Hood, eds.), Academic Press, New York, p. 189.

Rowley, J. D. (1983), *Cancer Investigation* **1**, 267.

Rowley, J. D., G. Alimena, O. M. Garson, A. Hagemeijer, F. Mitelman, and E. L. Prigogina (1982), *Blood* **59**, 1013.

Ruan, C., G. Tobelem, A. J. McMichael, L. Dronet, Y. Legrand, L. Degos, N. Kieffer, H. Lee, and J. P. Caen (1981), *Br. J. Haematol.* **49**, 511.

Sacks, S. H., and E. S. Lennox (1981), *Vox-Sang.* **40**, 99.

Sallan, S. E., J. Ritz, J. Pesando, R. Gelber, C. O'Brien, S. Hitchcock, F. Coral, and S. F. Schlossman (1980), *Blood* **55**, 395.

Sanchez-Madrid, F., A. M. Krensky, and C. F. Ware (1982) *Proc. Natl. Acad. Sci. USA* **79**, 7489.

Schlossman, S. F., L. Chess, R. E. Humphreys, and J. L. Strominger (1976), *Proc. Natl. Acad. Sci. USA (1976)* **73**, 1288.

Senn, J. S., E. A. McCulloch, and J. E. Till (1967), *Lancet* **2**, 597.

Sieff, C., D. Bicknell, G. Caine, J. Robinson, G. Lam, and M. F. Greaves (1982), *Blood* **60**, 703.

Singer, J. W., I. D. Bernstein, R. Andrews, B. H. Bjornson, A. Keating, and P. J. Fialkow (1984), *Clin. Res.* **32**, 499.

Skubitz, K. M., S. Pessano, L. Bottero, D. Ferrero, G. Rovera, J. T. August (1983a), *J. Immunol.* **131**, 1882.

Skubitz, K. M., Y.-S. Zhen, and J. T. August (1983b), *Blood* **61**, 19.

Smith, L. J., J. E. Curtis, H. A. Messner, J. S. Senn, H. Furthmayr, and E. A. McCulloch (1983), *Blood* **61**, 1138.

Solter, D., and B. B. Knowles (1978), *Proc. Natl. Acad. Sci. USA* **75**, 5565.

Springer, T. A., G. Galfre, D. S. Secher, and C. Milstein (1978), *Eur. J. Immunol.* **8**, 539.

Springer, T. A., D. Davignon, M. K. Ho, K. Kurzinger, E. Martz, and F. Sanchez-Madrid (1982), *Immunol. Rev.* **68**, 111.

Stashenko, P., L. M. Nadler, R. Hardy, and S. F. Schlossman (1980), *J. Immunol.* **125**, 1678.

Stockbauer, P., V. Malaskova, J. Soucek, and V. Chudomel (1983), *Neoplasma* **30**, 257.

Stockinger, H., O. Majdic, K. Liszka, W. Aberer, P. Bettelheim, D. Lutz, and W. Knapp (1984), *J. Natl. Cancer Inst.* (in press).

Strauss, L. C., R. K. Stuart, and C. I. Civin (1983), *Blood* **61**, 1222.

Sutherland, R., D. Delia, C. Schneider, R. Newman, J. Kemshead, and M. Greaves (1981), *Proc. Natl. Acad. Sci. USA* **78**, 4515.

Symington, F. W., I. D. Bernstein, and S.-I. Hakamori (1984), *J. Biol. Chem.* **259**, 6008.

Talle, M. A., P. E. Rao, E. Westberg, N. Allegar, M. Makaowski, R. S. Mittler, and G. Goldstein (1983), *Cell. Immunol.* **18**, 83.

Tatsumi, E., K. Sagawa, J. Mirro, C. I. Civin, H. D. Preisler, E. S. Henderson, and J. Minowada (1981), *Proc. Am. Assoc. Cancer Res.* **22**, 181.

Tetteroo, P. A. T., P. M. Lansdorp, A. H. M. Geurts van Kessel, A. Hagemeijer, and A. E. G. Kr. von dem Borne (1984), in *Leucocyte Typing: Human Leucocyte Differentiation Antigens Detected by Monoclonal Antibodies* (Bernard, A., L. Boumsell, J. Dausset, C. Milstein, and S. F. Schlossman, Eds.), Springer-Verlag, Berlin, p. 419.

Thiagarajan, P., B. Perussia, L. De Marco, K. Wells, and G. Trinchieri (1983), *Am. J. Hematol.* **14**, 255.

Thorley-Dawson, D. A., R. T. Schooley, A. K. Bhan, and L. M. Nadler (1982), *Cell* **30**, 415.

Todd, R. F., and S. F. Schlossman (1982), *Blood* **59**, 775.

Todd, R. F., L. M. Nadler, and S. F. Schlossman (1981), *J. Immunol.* **126**, 1435.

Todd, R. F., A. K. Bhan, S. E. Kabawat, and S. F. Schlossman (1984), in *Leucocyte Typing: Human Leucocyte Differentiation Antigens Detected by Monoclonal Antibodies* (Bernard, A., L. Boumsell, J. Dausset, C. Milstein, and S. F. Schlossman, eds.), Springer-Verlag, Berlin, p. 424.

Ugolini, V., G. Nunez, R. Graham-Smith, P. Stastny, and J. D. Capra (1980), *Proc. Natl. Acad. Sci. USA* **77**, 6764.

Urdal, D. L., T. A. Brentnall, I. D. Bernstein, and S.-I. Hakomori (1983), *Blood* **62**, 190.

Vainchenker, W., J. F. Deschamps, J. M. Bastin, J. Guichard, M. Titeux, J. Breton-Gorius, and A. J. McMichael (1982), *Blood* **59**, 514.

van der Reijden, H. J., D. L. van Rhenen, P. M. Lansdorp, M. B. van't Veer, M. M. A. C. Langenhuijsen, C. P. Engelfriet, and A. E. G. Kr. von dem Borne (1983), *Blood* **61**, 443.

van Rhenen, D. J., J. C. Verhulst, P. C. Huijgen, and M. M. A. C. Langenhuijsen (1980), *Br. J. Haematol.* **46**, 581.

Van Voorhis, W. C., R. M. Steinman, L. S. Hair, J. Luban, M. D. Witmer, S. Koide, and Z. A. Cohn (1983), *J. Exp. Med.* **158**, 126.

Vaughan, W. P., L. C. Strauss, P. J. Burke, K. M. Skubitz, J. F. Schwartz, J. E. Karp, and C. I. Civin (1983), *Proc. Am. Soc. Clin. Oncol.* **23**, 183.

Voak, D., S. Sacks, T. Alderson, F. Takei, E. Lennox, J. Jarvis, and C. Milstein (1980), *Vox-Sang.* **39**, 134.

Weinstein, H. J., R. J. Mayer, D. S. Rosenthal, B. M. Camitta, F. S. Coral, D. G. Nathan, and E. Frei (1980), *New Engl. J. Med.* **303**, 473.

Whittaker, A., J. Witney, D. E. B. Powell, T. E. Parry, and M. Khurshid (1979), *Br. J. Haematol.* **41**, 177.

Wright, S. D., P. E. Rao, W. C. Van Voorhis, L. S. Craigmyle, K. Iida, M. A. Talle, E. F. Westberg, G. Goldstein, and S. C. Silverstein (1983), *Proc. Natl. Acad. Sci. USA* **80**, 5699.

Yamada, K., N. Okabe, H. Saito, R. Suzuki, and K. Kumagai (1983), *Am. J. Hematol.* **15**, 181.

Yamashita, K., Y. Tachibana, T. Nakayama, M. Kitamura, Y. Endo, and A. Kobata (1980), *J. Biol. Chem.* **255**, 5635.

Yunis, J. J., C. D. Bloomfield, and K. Ensrud (1981), *New Engl. J. Med.* **305**, 135.

Yurewicz, E. C., F. Matsumura, and K. S. Moghissi (1982), *J. Biol. Chem.* **257**, 2314.

Zarling, J. M., and P. C. Kung (1980), *Nature* **288**, 394.

Zola, H., P. McNamara, M. Thomas, I. J. Stuart, and J. Bradley (1981), *Br. J. Haematol.* **48**, 481.

Chapter 9

Monoclonal Antibodies as Probes for the Molecular Structure and Biological Function of Melanoma-Associated Antigens

RALPH A. REISFELD

Department of Immunology, Scripps Clinic and Research Foundation, La Jolla, California

1. Introduction

A considerable amount of data that accumulated during the last two decades suggested that antigenic changes on the cell surface often accompany neoplastic transformation. This information has led to attempts by a large number of investigators to identify and characterize antigens associated with human tumor cells to gain a more basic understanding of malignant transformation and to develop new immunologic approaches to the diagnosis, prognosis, and therapy of cancer.

Human malignant melanoma was selected as a model system for study by a relatively large number of immunologists, particularly since, in terms of its interaction with the host's immune system, this disease appeared to be one most influenced by immunological factors (Lewis, 1972; Clark et al., 1977; and Hersey and McCarthy, 1982). The melanoma tumor systems also proved particularly advantageous for study since human malignant melanoma cells are relatively easy to establish in long-term culture, and a number of melanoma antigens are shed into spent culture in amounts that aid their isolation and characterization (Bystryn, 1976; McCabe et al., 1979). In addition, cultured human melanoma cells also provide a relatively stable source of target cells that can be repeatedly tested to classify and define melanoma-associated antigens by serological and immunochemical means (McCabe et al., 1978, 1980).

A number of serological analyses of human melanoma cells revealed different and distinct antigens (Reisfeld, 1982). Thus, different classes of antigens have been distinguished, i.e., individually specific surface antigens (Lewis et al., 1969) and tumor-associated group-specific cytoplasmic antigens (Lewis and Sheikh, 1975). In addition, three classes of antigens and antibodies have been serologically identified, namely tumor-specific antigens on autologous tumors, tumor-associated antigens on some but not all melanomas and astrocytomas, and antigens not restricted to melanoma, but widely distributed among a variety of fresh and cultured tumor cells (Carey et al., 1976; Shiku et al, 1976; Shiku et al., 1977).

During the last ten years, serological assays gradually emerged as technically the most simple and precise means for the measurement of humoral and cellular immune responses in vitro and for the detection of human melanoma-associated antigens. Initially, such assays still had definite limitations, largely because of the lack of truly monospecific antisera. This stricture could only be partly overcome by extensive absorption of multispecific, polyclonal antisera, as reviewed by Old and Stockert (1977).

However, during the last five years, the entire field of human tumor research was most decisively changed and advanced by the generation of specific antibody-secreting hybridomas as pioneered by Kohler and Milstein (1975). The cloning of such antibody-secreting hybridomas established from sensitized mouse splenocyte and mouse myeloma cells has made available a relatively large number of monoclonal antibodies of defined specificities for serological and immunochemical assays. More than any other, this development made it possible to critically evaluate the utility of these reagents for the diagnosis and treatment of cancer.

In the melanoma field in particular, a relatively large number of different monoclonal antibodies to a variety of human melanoma cell-surface antigens stimulated a considerable amount of exciting research directed toward gaining a better understanding of tumor cell biology, and also toward making a critical evaluation of the efficacy of the reagents for the diagnosis and therapy of human malignant melanoma. These efforts were highlighted by two melanoma workshops (Johnson and Riethmuller, 1982; Carrel et al., 1982; Hellstrom et al., 1982; Herlyn et al., 1982; Ross et al., 1982; Harper et al., 1982; Saxton et al., 1982; Stuhlmiller et al., 1982; Lloyd et al., 1982; Kantor et al., 1982). Some of the monoclonal antibodies presented at these workshops are now being applied as excellent molecular probes for the dissection of the melanoma tumor cell surface, to gain knowledge of intracellular transport and

biosynthesis of these antigens and for the initiation of research to delineate the molecular mechanisms involved in neoplastic transformation and
tumor metastasis. The proceedings and data presented at the two melanoma workshops organized by the National Cancer Institute have been
summarized (Reisfeld, 1982) and recently critically reviewed (Reisfeld et
al., 1984).

From a more practical point of view, monoclonal antibodies directed
to melanoma cell surface antigens have made it possible to use nude
mouse model systems for critical evaluation of the usefulness of these reagents for the treatment of malignant melanoma. The availability of these
monoclonal antibodies directed toward specific and relatively narrow
antigenic epitopes also makes it now possible to critically evaluate a potentially useful approach for the treatment of melanoma, namely, the use
of immune effector cells capable of mediating an antitumor killing response by being suitably "directed" by monoclonal antibodies to their
tumor target sites. The concept of the "immunological orchestra" being
used in this manner is most attractive in view of the large amount of information available on the potential role of immunity in the host's defense
against cancer.

It is certainly not the objective of this brief article to critically review
the rather extensive literature in the field of malignant melanoma. Instead, the intent is to simply focus the reader on a few selected reports
that are indicative of the value that monoclonal antibodies may have as
molecular probes for basic tumor biology and biochemistry that ultimately may pave the way for new and effective approaches to aid the diagnosis and therapy of human malignant melanoma.

2. Immunological Characterization of Monoclonal Antibodies

A family of antigens preferentially expressed by human melanoma cells
and tissues designated p97 has been thoroughly investigated in the laboratories of Karl and Ingegard Hellstrom and their collaborators during the
last four years. In initial studies, Woodbury et al. (1980) described the
production and characterization of a particular monoclonal antibody 4.1
of IgG_1 isotype that, when labeled with ^{125}I, bound to a significant extent
with 90% of melanomas tested. This same antibody also reacted in binding assays with 55% of a variety of other tumor cells analyzed. However,
this antibody failed to react with a number of B lymphoblastoid lines or
cultivated fibroblasts. The target antigen for this antibody is expresed on
both cultured cells and biopsy specimens and proved to be a protein with
M_r 97,000, hence the designation p97. These investigators pointed out
that the widespread occurrence of p97 clearly indicates that it is not

melanoma-specific. Although a number of indirect immunoprecipitation studies indicated that p97 is a tumor marker of considerable interest, they also raised the question whether the indirect immunoprecipitation method is sufficiently discriminating to detect even small levels of p97 in normal and neoplastic tissues (Woodbury et al., 1981). In an effort to answer this question, a much improved direct antibody binding assay was developed (Brown et al., 1981d). In this attempt, the ^{125}I-labeled Protein A assay for antibody binding to surface antigens of viable cells was used with eight antibody-secreting hybridomas of IgG_2 isotype that were selected to insure effective binding to Protein A. A key feature of this approach was to isolate and purify the monoclonal antibody by affinity chromatography on Protein A columns and then to label it with [125]I. The eight antibodies detected seven proteins of M_r 23,000, 33,000, 40,000, 80,000, 97,000, 200,000, and 270,000. Five of these proteins, i.e., p23, p33, p40, p200, and p270 were also present on the surface of autologous skin fibroblasts, but two of them, p80 and p97, were absent from fibroblasts and thus were considered potential markers of differentiation or neoplasia. Results from indirect immunoprecipitation analyses agreed with data obtained by the radiobinding assay and indicated that the immunoprecipitation technique was suitable for rapid and informative screening to identify hybridoma-secreting antibodies reactive with protein antigens of cultured human tumor cells (Brown et al., 1981c, 1981d).

Another report described the production of two hybridomas, 5.1 and 6.1, that secrete monoclonal antibodies of IgG_1 and IgM isotype and recognize two cell membrane proteins of M_r 210,000 (p210) and 155,000 (p155), respectively (Loop et al., 1981). Direct binding assays indicated that p210 was expressed by 30% of cultured melanoma cells and 25% of cell lines from other neoplasms. Antigen p155 was detected on 50% of melanoma tumor biopsies tested as well as on some glioblastomas and kidney cell lines. Results of radioimmunoprecipitation analyses indicated that normal adult or fetal tissues and other tumors lacked p155; however, direct radiobinding tests showed that p155 bound to two proteins, one with M_r 60,000 and the other with M_r 250,000. Interestingly enough, antibody 5.1, directed to the M_r 210,000 component, resulted from the fusion of splenocytes of mice immunized with just one melanoma cell line, i.e., M1890; however, antibody 6.1, which recognizes p155, is the product of a hybridoma resulting from the immunization of a mouse with a pool of seven melanoma cell lines. When carefully analyzed, neither of the two monoclonal antibodies seem to be particularly specific for melanoma. Again, as shown with other monoclonal antibodies to melanoma-associated antigens (Mitchell et al., 1981) p155 appears to react with different molecular structures, all bearing at least one identical antigenic determinant (Loop et al., 1981).

In another study, a monoclonal antibody (9.2.27) to a melanoma-associated antigen was produced (Morgan et al., 1981) that was later identified as a glycoprotein chondroitin sulfate–proteoglycan complex (Bumol and Reisfeld, 1982a). One of the key features of the production of 9.2.27 was that the immunogen derived from a $4M$ urea extract of M14 melanoma cells was partially purified by affinity chromatography on lentil lectin Sepharose and by removal of fibronectin, a competing immunogen on gelatin Sepharose. Another important feature of the approach used by these investigators was the use of a radioimmunometric antibody binding assay using chemically defined spent medium of melanoma cells as a solid-phase target to screen for suitable antibody-secreting hybridomas. As pointed out by these investigators (Morgan et al., 1981) the melanoma-associated antigen used was an immunogenic vehicle devoid of competing antigens such as HLA-A,B,C, HLA-DR, and fibronectin. This resulted in the production of 59 antibody-secreting hybridomas (3.7% of 1590 positive wells) that did bind preferentially to melanoma targets. The antigen defined by antibody 9.2.27 appeared as two components by indirect immunoprecipitation and SDS-PAGE, one of very high molecular weight and the other with an approximate M_r of 240,000 (240K). The latter component is highly sensitive to treatment with trypsin, and although it appears to be part of the extracellular matrix, the 240K component is distinctly different from fibronectin by numerous biochemical criteria (Reisfeld et al., 1982a,b).

It is of some interest, as pointed out by Morgan et al. (1981) that a previous report from their laboratory already identified an antigen with very similar characteristics by using a polyclonal xenoantiserum (Galloway et al., 1981). This antigen was subsequently identified as a glycoprotein by intrinsic labeling with several carbohydrate precursors (Morgan et al., 1981). In a subsequent report from this same laboratory, it was pointed out that the antigen recognized by monoclonal antibody 9.2.27 previously considered to be a M_r 240,000 component, associated with a higher molecular weight moiety, actually consists of a prominent component of M_r 250,000 (250K) and a second larger component of $M_r > 780,000$ (Reisfeld et al., 1982a,b).

Dippold et al. (1980) made an extensive analysis of cell surface antigens on human melanoma cells that can be defined by a series of monoclonal antibodies. These investigators selected 18 mouse monoclonal antibodies from an immunization of (BALB/c × C57 BL/6) F_1 female mice with SK-MEL 28 cells and the subsequent fusion of the spleen cells of these animals with the mouse myeloma cell line MOPC-21NS/1. These antibodies were used to define six distinct antigenic systems by serological assays and absorption tests with a panel of 41 cell lines derived from normal and malignant human tissues. The authors stress the need for evaluating the presence or absence of a given antigen on tumor cells by antibody absorption tests that they found more sensitive than direct serological assays. Two of the antigenic systems defined by monoclonal antibodies are glycoproteins of M_r 95,000 (gp 95) and M_r 150,000 (gp 150) as judged by intrinsic radiolabeling with amino acid and carbohydrate precursors.

Another report described the cellular distribution of melanoma-associated antigens recognized by monoclonal antibodies (225.28S and 465.12) on cultured melanoma cell lines and skin biopsies by indirect immunofluorescence (Wilson et al., 1981). Antibody 225.28S is reported to react mainly with a plasma membrane antigen of melanoma cells and nevi consisting of two components of M_r 280,000 and 440,000, whereas antibody 465.12 was found to be reactive with tumor tissues of various histological origins and is considered cytoplasmic in nature, consisting of four, nondisulfide bridge-linked glycopeptides of M_r 94,000, 75,000, 70,000, and 25,000. In an additional manuscript from this same group of investigators, the tissue distribution and molecular profile of the antigen defined by 465.12S was again demonstrated and corroborated (Natali et al., 1982).

A further study described the development and characterization of a monoclonal antibody (F11) that defines an antigen found in the spent medium of human melanoma cells grown continuously in serum-free medium (Chee et al., 1982). This antibody defines an antigen of M_r 100,000 (100K) by indirect immunoprecipitation and SDS-PAGE and reacts by the ABC immunoperoxidase technique with frozen sections of melanomas and carcinomas, whereas it is nonreactive with lymphoblastoid cells and benign nevi. Microscopic examination revealed the presence of the antigen in the cytoplasm, on the plasma membrane of melanoma and some carcinoma cells, and in the lumen of glandular strucutres of breast and colon carcinomas. These investigators caution that although the 100K antigen was not detected on normal tissues, its presence there cannot be ruled out, especially if it is represented in such small quantities that the immunoperoxidase and immunofluorescence techniques will be insufficiently sensitive for detection.

3. Immunochemical and Molecular Profiles of Human Melanoma-Associated Antigens

3.1. Glycoproteins

A comprehensive structural characterization of p97 demonstrated by sequential immunoprecipitation and SDS-PAGE that four different monoclonal antibodies recognized the same p97 molecule (Brown et al, 1981b). Two of these antibodies (4.1 and 8.2) were of IgG_1 isotype, whereas the other two (96.5 and 118.1) were of IgG_{2a} isotype. Antibodies 4.1 and 8.2 recognized the same antigen epitope p97a, whereas antibodies 118.1 and 8.2 defined epitopes p97b and p97c, respectively. It was of interest that these studies also indicated that six additional monoclonal antibodies (M_{17}, L_1, L_{10}, R_{10}, I_{12}, and K_5) reported earlier by others (Dippold et al, 1980) to be specific for a melanoma cell surface protein of M_r 95,000 (gp 95) also bound to the p97 antigen by sequential immunoprecipitation, indicating the p97 and gp 95 are indeed identical. These six monoclonal antibodies also are directed to different epitopes on p97, i.e., M_{17} to p97a, L_1, L_{10}, and R_{19} to epitope 97c. Two new p97 epitopes were discovered as antibodies I_{12} and K_5 defined p97d and p97e, respectively. Brown et al. (1981c) point out the utility of immunoprecipitation and SDS-PAGE as an alternative screening method for hybridomas secreting antibodies directed to different epitopes of the same antigen molecule. Also, since only relatively few distinct proteins, ranging usually from only 5 to 10, are recognized in any one fusion, it is advantageous to vary the immunizing melanoma line and also use different mouse strains to obtain different protein patterns. It is somewhat surprising that there is such a relatively high frequency of hybridomas secreting antibodies to p97. Yet, it is not known whether p97 is particularly immunogenic or is simply present in larger amounts than other antigens on the cell lines used for immunization (K-2 and SK-MEL 28). As far as the quantitation of expression of p97 on SK-MEL 28 melanoma cells is concerend, there are at least 400,000 molecules of p97 per cell based on antibody binding data, i.e., roughly equal to HLA-A,B,C determinants identified by binding of anti-HLA monoclonal antibody W6/32 to these same cells.

Regarding the expression of epitopes p97a, p97b, and p97c on different cell types, it could be demonstrated that a melanoma, a lung carcinoma, as well as a B and T lymphoid cell line all bound each antibody defining these epitopes, but in vastly differing amounts, i.e., the melanoma line bound 300,000–380,000 molecules of each antibody per cell; the lung carcinoma line bound 4000–6200 molecules per cell, whereas the B and T cell lines bound only 250–1400 molecules per cell (Brown et al., 1981a). Concerning the chemical characterization of p97, it was found to be glycosylated and sialylated and consisting of a single polypeptide chain, most likely with some intrachain disulfide bridges. Partial digestion of detergent solubilized p97 with either papain or trypsin produced seemingly identical fragments of M_r 40,000 that were glycosylated and contain the p97a,b,c epitopes, but lack the p97d,e epitopes (Brown et al., 1981b).

Another report delineated the molecular profiles of three distinct human melanoma surface antigens detected by monoclonal anti-melanoma antibodies (Mitchell et al., 1980). One of these antigens identified by antibody 691-13-17 was found to be the human Ia (HLA-DR) antigen with characteristic α and β subunits. This antibody detects the human Ia antigens on all cell types known to express them, including melanoma cells. The authors were able to confirm this by suitable immunodepletion analyses with known anti-HLA-DR antisera. Interestingly enough, antibody 691-13-17 reacts with all HLA-DR phenotypes, but does not detect HLA-DR antigens on normal cutaneous melanocytes of benign lesions. This observation leaves to be explained whether there is any relationship between HLA-DR expression and the transition of melanocytes to a malignant state. Another monoclonal antibody (691-6-37) reacts with a cell surface-located, tissue-specific alloantigen of M_r 80,000 that is not melanoma-specific. This antigen seems to be weakly expressed on many different cell lines, as demonstrated by surface iodination and instrinsic labeling with glucosamine and fucose. Another antibody 691 I5 Nu-4-B recognizes a complex of four associated polypeptide chains of M_r 116,000, 95,000, 29,000, and 26,000, designated α, β, and γ chains, respectively. In the native state, the two smaller chains are covalently linked to the M_r 116,000 unit by disulfide bonds. The M_r 95,000 chain is only attached by noncovalent interactions and cleavage of the two major polypeptides by 2-nitro-5-thiocyanobenzoic acid and subsequent peptide mapping reveals distinct patterns of cleavage suggesting that these two proteins have different primary amino acid structures (Mitchell et al., 1981). What seems particularly intriguing is that one monoclonal antibody directed by definition to a single antigenic determinant facilitates the isolation of a family of four distinct molecules, all of which apparently contain the same antigenic determinant. In this regard, it is of some interest to recall that antibody 691 I5 Nu-4-B is secreted from a hybridoma 691 I5 Nu which, after fusion of the human melanoma line SW691 and the mouse fibroblast cell line IT-22, was shown to contain only human chromosomes 14, 17, and 21, although it retained the tumorigenic potential for the melanoma parent (Koprowski et al., 1978).

The human melanoma associated antigen p97 was reported to be functionally related to transferrin and it was proposed that the two proteins evolved from a common ancestral gene (Brown et al., 1982). This conclusion was based on the amino-terminal amino acid sequence homology between these two molecules, i.e., seven from a total of twelve residues determined were found to be identical. This includes two of the least common amino acids, i.e. tryptophan and cystine. In addition, Brown et al. (1982) contend that their conclusions are further supported by the finding that anitserum to denatured p97 cross-reacted with denatured transferrin and lactotransferrin and also by data indicating that p97 binds iron. Although p97 and transferrin receptors have a similar molecular weight, this same report also showed conclusively that these two molecules are not identical. Thus, following SDS-PAGE under nonreducing conditions, transferrin receptor forms a dimer of M_r 200,000 whereas p97 migrates slightly faster than the reduced protein. In addition, the tissue distribution of the two molecules differs considerably and monoclonal antibody OKT9 that is specific for transferrin receptor does not immunoprecipitate p97 from radioiodinated melanoma cells. The immunological difference of these two molecules was also demonstrated by sequential immunoprecipitation experiments. Finally, p97 also failed to bind to a transferrin–sepharose column. However, although p97 and transferrin receptor are structurally distinct, it was suggested that they may share some of their proposed biological functions, e.g., mediation of cellular uptake of transferrin-bound iron. This suggestion was, however, tempered by the fact that it was not possible to prove this experimentally. In view of the trace amounts of p97 in normal adult tissue, it appears more likely that this function is carried out by transferrin receptor rather than by the p97 molecule (Brown et al., 1982). It seems obvious that distribution of p97, which is more or less restricted to melanoma cells, nevi, and fetal intestine, argues for a more specialized functional role of this molecule that may be restricted to these tissues. However, this contention remains as yet to be substantiated by experimental data.

Finally, still another study describes an antigen expressed on both melanoma and carcinoma cells detected by another monoclonal antibody 376.96S (Imai et al., 1981, 1982). This antigen consists of a single glycoprotein chain of M_r 94,000. Antibody 376.96S is of IgG_{2a} subclass and was found to detect an antigen different from gp 95 described by Dippold et al. (1980) and also distinct from yet another melanoma-associated antigen of similar molecular weight that was reported by Mitchell et al. (1980).

A monoclonal antibody (155.8) produced against purified membranes of human melanoma cells was reported to react with a chondroitin sulfate proteoglycan (CSP) preferentially expressed on such cells. Binding inhibition studies indicated that Mab 155.8 reacts with an epitope different from that recognized by Mab 9.2.27 on the same proteoglycan molecule (Harper et al., 1984). Mab 155.8 binds melanoma cells to a more limited extent than Mab 9.2.27, suggesting that either the antibody recognizes determinant(s) found in smaller numbers on the cell surface or that there is a difference in the affinity constants of the two antibodies. The difference in reactivities of these two monoclonal antibodies with chondroitin sulfate proteoglycan is underlined by results from immunodepletion analysis, which showed that 155.8 determinants are present on only a subgroup of those molecules bearing the 9.2.27 epitope.

The proteoglycan nature of the molecules defined by Mab 155.8 was clearly evident from data of ^3H-leucine incorporation into the high molecular weight component ($M_r > 780,000$) and analysis of $^{35}SO_4{}^{2-}$-labeled material by cellulose acetate electrophoresis following β-elimination of O-linked glycosaminoglycans by alkaline/borohydride treatment. Data from this analysis along with chondroitinase ABC sensitivity confirmed that the sulfated glycosaminoglycans associated with antigen(s) identified by Mab 155.8 indeed contain chondroitin sulfate type A and/or C. Similar to 9.2.27, Mab 155.8 also recognizes determinants on the 250K core glycoprotein and the intact CSP. The disappearance of the CSP and concomitant intensification of the 250K component following chondroitinase digestion of immunoprecipitated proteoglycans proves that the 250K glycoprotein is included in the CSP and is, in fact, its core protein. Harper et al. (1984) have provided clear and direct evidence that Mabs 9.2.27 and 155.8 recognize the proteoglycan in the absence of 250K, thus clearly ruling out the possibility that the proteoglycan does not contain antigenic determinants but is only complexed with the 250K molecule and is merely a "passenger" in immunoprecipitates. Specifically, after resolving antigens extracted from human melanoma cells by $CsCl_2$ density centrifugation in the presence of detergent and high salt, it became possible to immunoprecipitate high density proteoglycans alone as well as the free 250K component from lower density fractions of the gradient.

The topographical distribution of Mab 155.8-defined proteoglycans on the surface of paraformaldehyde-fixed human melanoma cells, when examined by indirect immunofluorescence, shows filamentous structures that sometimes connect cells with the underlying substratum. These molecules were not found distributed as substrate-attached material left behind when cells were removed. This raises interesting questions as to the involvement of CSP in melanoma cell adhesion and spreading on various substrata. In this regard, there is already some evidence that Mabs 9.2.27 and 155.8 inhibit adhesion and, to a greater extent, cytoplasmic spreading of human melanoma cells on plastic and collagen–fibronectin complex substrata (Harper et al., 1984).

The finding of a Mab 155.8-defined CSP on freshly explanted melanoma tissues by indirect immunoperoxidase techniques, underlines its functional relevance. In fact, the distribution of the proteoglycans defined by Mabs 9.2.27 and 155.8 throughout normal fetal and adult tissues as well as other tumor types, suggests that determinants recognized by these antibodies are not found in normal tissues known to be rich in CSP, i.e., cartilage. Consequently, from a strictly functional point of view, CSPs on melanoma cells may play more than simply a structural role proposed for such molecules in normal cartilage and other connective tissues (Harper et al., 1984).

3.2. Glycolipids

Portoukalian et al. (1976) were first to report a large amount of GM_3, GM_2, and GD_3 gangliosides in human melanoma cells. Indeed, these investigators claimed that melanoma patients' sera contained antibody showing a specific immune precipitation with melanoma ganglioside GD_3 (Portoukalian et al., 1978; Portoukalian et al., 1979). Also, the GD_3 level in plasma of patients with melanoma was reported to be greatly elevated and to decrease after surgical treatment of melanoma (Portoukalian et al., 1978). Dippold et al. (1980) were among the first to study monoclonal antibodies that recognized glycolipids. Thus, antigens defined within the R_{24} system by four monoclonal antibodies appeared to be glycolipids, i.e., they were found to be heat-stable and antibody binding could be inhibited with glycolipid fractions of reactive cells. It was shown that monoclonal antibody R_{24}, of IgG_3 isotype, was indeed directed to the disialoganglioside GD_3 that was isolated from melanoma cells. This finding was confirmed by compositional and partial structural analysis and by comparison with authentic GD_3 ganglioside by thin layer chromatography (TLC). The R_{24} antibody reacted specifically with authentic GD_3 and a newly developed glycolipid-mediated immune adherence assay (GMIA) established that melanoma cells and tissues contained GD_3 and GM_3 as major gangliosides, whereas a series of other cells and tissues including other tumor lines, contained these molecules in smaller amounts. One exception in this regard is MOLT-4, a T cell line which shows a relatively large amount of GD_3, as does retina and human brain. In fact, melanoma cells are relatively rich in GD_3, with contents ranging from 31 to 57% of their total ganglioside fraction. This compares favorably with retina (30–40%) and adult human brain (8–10%) (Pukel et al., 1982).

Although the presence of GD_3 is rather ubiquitous and certainly not restricted to melanoma cells, R_{24} was strongly reactive with melanomas and some astrocytomas in serological assays and shows some lower level activity only with normal brain and melanocytes. The characteristic accumulation of GD_3 and GM_3 in melanoma cells is considered to be caused (1) by low levels of N-acetylgalactosaminyl transferase in the Golgi apparatus, where this well-known biosynthetic precursor of gangliosides would likely be concentrated, or (2) by elevated levels of certain sialyltransferases promoting an overabundance of GD_3 and GM_3. The other three antigenic systems, i.e., O_5, M_{19}, and R_8, are not as well characterized, although it appears that O_5 is a glycolipid antigen (Pukel et al., 1982). In fact, none of the antigens defined by their monoclonal antibodies were found to be melanoma-specific since even R_{24}, which is preferentially expressed on melanomas, is also found on astrocytomas, as well as in normal brain and on melanocytes (Dippold et al., 1980).

A monoclonal antibody designated 4.2 was found to react with a surface antigen expressed on most human melanomas (Nudelman et al., 1982). This antigen turned out to be a ganglioside with the carbohydrate structure (Neu Acα2 $\rightarrow$ 8 Neu Acα2 $\rightarrow$ 3 Galβ1 $\rightarrow$ 4 Glcβ1 $\rightarrow$ 1 Cer) that was established by enzymatic degradation and methylation analysis by mass spectrometry. Structurally, this antigen is identical with brain

GD_3 ganglioside, although this melanoma-associated antigen has a ceramide characterized by a predominance of longer chain fatty acids. This is in contrast to brain GD_3, which has mainly C18$\mathfrak{X}$10 fatty acid. Interestingly enough, antibody 4.2 failed to react with gangliosides GT1a and GQ1b, which have a terminal sugar sequence identical to GD_3, i.e., (Neu Acα2 → 8 Neu Acα2 → 3 Gal). Thus, as pointed out by Nudelman et al. (1982), its specificity must therefore be restricted to the Neu Acα2 → 8 Neu Acα2 → 3 Galβ1 → 4 Glc → Cer sequence, including the innermost sugar, Glc residue. Antibody 4.2 was found to react with ~80% of human melanoma cell lines tested; however, this monoclonal antibody does react, although somewhat more weakly, with a variety of nonmelanoma tumor cell lines. One drawback to this antibody is the fact that it fails to be reactive in the overlay technique (Magnani et al., 1980), thus somewhat limiting its usefulness in immunochemical analysis. However, it is clear that antibody 4.2 does react with a GD_3 molecule that differs from ordinary GD_3 found in brain in its ceramide composition, a difference that is postulated by Nudelman et al. (1982) possibly to define the antigenic expression of GD_3 in melanoma. In fact, these authors hypothesize several possibilities why GD_3 acts as an antigen at the surface of melanoma cells. First, an unusually high GD_3 concentration at the melanoma cell surface may provide the necessary threshhold value necessary for recognition by antibody 4.2. Second, GD_3 in normal cell membranes could be cryptic, whereas that in melanoma membranes is highly exposed. A precedent cited by Nudelman et al. (1982) is that of GM_3 in baby hamster kidney cells or globoside in NIL cells that became exposed at the cell surface following transformation by polyoma virus (Hakamori et al., 1968; Gahmberg and Hakamori, 1975). Finally, it is hypothesized that the longer fatty acid chains of the ceramide of melanoma GD_3 are instrumental in arranging its membrane expression in such a way as to make it more antigenic than GD_3 in normal tissues. It is apparent that additional studies are required to distinguish between these various possibilities.

In contrast to the above findings is a report by Pukel et al. (1982), who described a monoclonal antibody (R24) that in earlier work by Dippold et al. (1980) was already reported to react selectively with human melanoma. Antibody R_{24} not only reacts very well in the overlay assay, but clearly recognizes authentic brain GD_3, exhibiting an identical mobility on thin layer chromatography (TLC). This is in contrast to the GD_3 recognized by antibody 4.2 described by Nudelman et al. (1982), which clearly reacts with a GD_3 molecule that differs from authentic brain GD_3 in its ceramide composition and by its mobility on TLC.

Irie et al. (1982) established two long-term human B-lymphoblastoid cell lines (L55 and L72) transformed by Epstein-Barr virus that produced IgMκ antibodies to the human tumor antigen OFA-I. The source of B lymphocytes for establishing these cell lines were peripheral lymphocytes obtained from melanoma patients. When antibody specificity was determined by an immune adherence assay using a variety of human cancer and noncancer tissues as targets, L55 antibody, designated anti-OFA-I-1, was found to react with a variety of tumor types whereas the L72 antibody (anti-OFA-I-2) reacted only with tumor cells of neuroectodermal origin, i.e., melanoma, glioma, and neuroblastoma. In a more recent publication from this same group of investigators, it was reported that OFA-I-1 is chemically distinct from OFA-I-2 since the latter was clearly shown to be the ganglioside GD_2 [Gal NAcβ1 → 4 (Neu Acα2 → 8 Neuα2 → 3) Galβ1 → 4 Glc-ceramide]. This was determined both by specific binding of the L72 antibody to authentic GD_2 and by differential effects of sialidase treatment on melanoma target cells, i.e., binding of L72 to such cells was inhibited, whereas sialidase treatment had no effect on the binding of the L55 antibody. These authors did not yet describe the chemical nature of the OFA-I-1 antigen.

Most recently, monoclonal antibody D1.1 was reported to be specifically reactive with human melanoma tumors and a majority of melanoma cell lines tested (Cheresh et al., 1984). This particular antibody, prepared against the rat B49 cell lines, was repored by Levine et al. (1984) to recognize a ganglioside on developing rat neuroectoderm. Interestingly enough, these investigators found this particular antibody to be highly specific for human melanoma. In fact, the antigen recognized by D1.1 is not found on a variety of fresh frozen fetal tissues and does not react by immunoperoxidase assays with any normal tissues tested, including brain. This antibody also fails to react with a wide variety of fresh frozen tumor tissue sections tested by immunoperoxidase tests. D1.1 also does not react in ELISA binding assays with a large variety of human tumor cell lines and lymphoblastoid lines. However, the antibody does react very well with a variety of human melanoma cell lines and fresh frozen melanoma tumor tissues. These findings set this particular antibody apart from the mouse and human monoclonal antibodies described above, i.e., Mab 4.2, R24, and OFA-I-2 (L72). Cheresh et al. (1984a) could determine by one- and two-dimensional TLC that D1.1 reacts with a ganglioside. Moreover, intermediate ammonia treatment of this ganglioside showed that it contains one or more base-labile O-acyl esters. Mild base hydrolysis of the ganglioside substrate under conditions known to remove O-acyl esters resulted in complete loss of reactivity with antibody D1.1, indicating that the alkali-labile moiety is a critical component of the epitope recognized by this monoclonal antibody. Analysis of the sialic acids of the total gangliosides from [6-^{3}H] glucosamine-labeled melanoma cells showed that ~10% of these molecules are O-acylated. A similar analysis of purified gangliosides indicated that 30% of the sialic acids migrated with authentic 9-O-acetyl-N-acetylneuraminic acid. This observation led to a follow-up study which demonstrated that the antigen specifically detected by antibody D1.1 was indeed a GD_3 diasialoganglioside which was O-acetylated (Cheresh et al., 1984b). The importance of the O-acetyl sialic acid moiety as an antigen epitope specifically recognized by antibody D1.1 was further defined since chemical acetylation of purified GD_3 with N-acetyl-imidazole made this molecule reactive with antibody D1.1 that otherwise does not react with non-acetylated GD_3, as clearly indicated by de-O-acetylation of GD_3 by treatment with ammonia. These data strongly suggest that the ganglioside recognized by antibody D1.1 differs from GD_3 only by a single O-acetyl ester on a sialic acid residue. The data also suggest that GD_3 may serve as a substrate for a specific O-acetyl-transferase responsible for aberrant O-acetylation in human malignant melanoma cells (Cheresh et al., 1984b).

4. Biosynthesis and Structure of Melanoma-Associated Antigens

In a followup study designed to chemically and immunochemically define the antigen recognized by monoclonal antibody 9.2.27, it was found to be a unique glycoprotein–proteoglycan complex preferentially expressed by human melanoma cells (Bumol and Reisfeld, 1982a, 1982b, 1984.) A combination of biosynthetic and enzymatic studies of the antigenic determinant recognized by monoclonal antibody 9.2.27 made it possible to identify this rather unique antigen on human melanoma cells. Specifically, the 9.2.27 antibody recognizes an N-linked, sialylated, glycoprotein of M_r 250,000 (250K) that is associated with a high molecular weight (HMWC) component expressing all the characteristics of a chondroitin sulfate proteoglycan (CSP). The 9.2.27 antibody was also found to recognize both the free pool of core protein and the chondroitin sulfate proteoglycan monomer. The 9.2.27 antibody, while reacting in general preferentially with melanoma cell lines and freshly explanted surgical melanoma specimens also binds to a neuroblastoma cell line. Finally, data obtained by tryptic peptide map analysis and chondroitinase lyase AC and ABC digestion suggest that the 250K molecule is contained within the chondroitin sulfate proteoglycan and possibly represents a "core" protein onto which chondroitin sulfate proteoglycan side chains are added (Bumol et al., 1982a).

In additional studies, the cationic ionophore monensin was found to effectively block the appearance of CSP monomers and ploymers in immunoprecipitates obtained with monoclonal antibody 9.2.27 from detergent extracts of intrinsically radiolabeled melanoma cells that were previously exposed for 18 h to $10^{-7}M$ monensin (Bumol et al., 1984). These findings correlate with those reported previously (Tajiri et al.,

1980), indicating that monensin can effect the biosynthesis of proteoglycans in chondrocytes. Pulse-chase analyses of the endoglycosidase
H-treated antigen complex also suggested that the appearance of CSP is
kinetically linked to biosynthetic functions of the Golgi apparatus, the site
proposed for biosynthesis of proteoglycans involving glycosyltransferases. Bumol et al. (1984) propose that the unique specificity of the
9.2.27 monoclonal antibody for a M_r 250,000, N-linked, sialylated core
glycoprotein associated with a common chondroitin sulfate proteoglycan
suggests that the human melanoma cell may actually express modified or
even unique gene products capable of serving as acceptors or core glycoproteins for common proteoglycan oligosaccharide side chains. These investigators also propose that this type of alteration may account for the
changes in proteoglycans of the membranes and extracellular matrix of
some tumors cells that had been previously reported (Glimelius et al.,
1978).

Another melanoma-associated antigenic molecule was recognized
by yet another monoclonal antibody (F11) by the use of immunochemical
and biosynthetic analyses (Bumol et al., 1982b). As determined by indirect immunoprecipitation and SDS-PAGE, this antibody recognizes a
glycoprotein of M_r 100,000 (100K) in the spent media of melanoma cells
M14, grown in synthetic, serum-free medium; however, a parallel analysis of detergent extracts of these same melanoma cells reveals a more
complex profile of three glycoprotein molecules of M_r 75,000, 77,000,
and 100,000. Pulse-chase studies employed to understand the
biosynthetic relationship among the three molecules indicates the the F11
antibody initially recognizes the molecules of M_r 75/77K early in the
chase in the absence of any detectable 100K antigen. As the 75/77K components increase in intensity until the first appearance of the 100K molecules after 180–240 min into the chase, it is likely that they are
biosynthetic precursors of the larger molecule. The data presented do not
strongly support an alternative explanation, i.e., that F11 simply recognizes a common antigenic site on three distinct glycoproteins. Bumol et
al. (1982b) propose that common antigenic sites can exist on different
molecules within the same cell, which may differ structurally as
biosynthetic intermediates. They base this contention on their data showing sensitivity to degradation of the 77K moles to endoglycosidase H,
thus demonstrating that the N-asparagine-linked oligosaccharides of this
glycoprotein antigen are not processed by the Golgi apparatus. Since this
organelle is considered to be the site of terminal glycosylation of
N-asparagine-linked ligosaccharide biosynthesis, considerable glycosylation could still occur in the Golgi apparatus to form the 100K molecules starting from a lower molecular weight 75/77K core antigen, with
the 100K antigen being destined for secretion into the extracellular milieu
of melanoma cells. The sole addition of sialic acid residues cannot account for all the biosynthetic modifications observed, especially since

treatment of the 100K molecule with neuraminidase reveals a desialylated molecule of M_r 89,000 (Bumol et al., 1982b).

Biosynthetic studies with 72-h fresh surgical melanoma explant cultures indicate that the 77 and 100K components recognized by F11 are also synthesized by these primary tumor cultures, suggesting a strong in vitro/in vivo correlation with antigens recognized by monoclonal antibody F11. Finally, Bumol et al. (1982b) also observed a serologically cross-reactive antigen with F11 that is secreted from neuroblastoma cell lines; however, this antigen has a molecular weight of 90,000. Obviously, two apparently different antigenic structures have a common antigenic determinant. However, this observation again demonstrates what is rapidly becoming a "truism" in tumor immunology, namely that serological identity established by monoclonal antibodies does not necessarily imply complete structural homology of tumor-associated antigens.

5. Function of Melanoma Antigens Defined by Monoclonal Antibodies

5.1. In Vitro Studies

Proteoglycans have been implicated in growth control, cell-substratum interaction, and other functional properties of potential relevance to tumor metastasis (Culp et al., 1979). In an attempt to gather additional evidence in this area, Mab 9.2.27 was used as a specific probe to delineate the possible role of proteoglycans in cell–cell interactions and growth control of human melanoma cells (Harper and Reisfeld, 1983). In this regard, Mab 9.2.27 inhibited anchorage-independent growth of human melanoma cells in soft agar, an event that had been shown to correlate with in vivo tumorigenicity (Shin et al., 1975; Harper and Reisfeld, 1983). Data obtained from the double agar clonogenic assay indicated that the growth inhibitory effect by Mab 9.2.27 in this in vitro system was indeed specific (Harper and Reisfeld, 1983). Thus, monoclonal anti-HLA-A,B,C antibodies that bind to human melanoma cells had no significant effect on their plating efficiency and Mab 9.2.27 also did not affect the plating efficiencies of two 9.2.27 antigen-negative cell lines.

The precise mechanism underlying this phenomenon is not entirely clear at this time. Harper and Reisfeld (1983) postulate that it relates to the physicochemical nature and location of the proteoglycan antigen recognized by Mab 9.2.27 on the surface of human melanoma cells. In this regard, it was shown that human tumor cells maintained on the extracellular matrix exhibited higher growth rates and had lower serum requirements than human tumor cells grown on plastic (Gospodarowicz et al., 1978; Vladavsky et al., 1980). It is believed that the major components of the extracellular matrix, i.e. collagens, laminin, fibronectin, and proteoglycans, work in concert to produce this effect (Gospodarowicz et al., 1978). Although human melanoma cells were shown to lack an organized extracellular matrix (Bumol et al., 1984) immunoperoxidase analysis of freshly explanted melanoma tumor tissue showed that melanoma cells in vivo synthesize and deposit chondroitin sulfate proteoglycans pericellularly among other matrix components (Harper et al., 1982). Thus, when melanoma cells are grown in soft agar containing Mab 9.2.27, cell–cell interactions may actually be disrupted by interference of this antibody with the normal pericellular disposition and organization of the proteoglycans; consequently, Mab 9.2.27 may be involved in interactions important for the growth of melanoma cells in an anchorage-independent fashion.

There are apparently no metabolic constraints on melanoma cells that are attached and spread on a solid substratum since it was observed that binding of Mab 9.2.27 to melanoma cells grown in liquid culture does not affect either DNA or protein synthesis even after 3 d. When taken together, the data of Harper and Reisfeld (1983) strongly suggest that chondroitin sulfate proteoglycans may be among those molecules on the surface of human melanoma cells that are involved in cell–cell interactions important to anchorage-independent growth regulation. Studies of human tumor metastasis, such as these using specific monoclonal antibody probes, may provide a better understanding of the molecules involved in tumor growth and may eventually lead to a more effective treatment and ultimately even prevention of human tumor metastasis.

In attempts to study the functional role of CSPs in human tumor systems, Mab 9.2.27 was found to block early events of melanoma cell spreading on endothelial basement membranes while only slightly inhibiting cell adhesion. These data suggest that CSPs may play a part in stabilizing cell–substratum interactions in this in vitro model for metastatic invasion. Thus, CSPs commonly found in the extracellular matrices of normal cells may have different functional roles in tumor cells lacking a formal structural matrix while maintaining an active biosynthesis of these molecules. This apparently is the case for the melanoma system described by Bumol et al. (1984) that actively synthesizes CSPs but lacks any organized fibronectin matrix.

Certain leukocytes possessing Fc receptors are well known to lyse cells coated with specific antibody (Moller, 1965; Perlmann et al., 1972; Lovchik and Hong 1977). Such an antibody-dependent cell-mediated cytolysis (ADCC) is well illustrated by the lysis of antibody-coated tumor cells by lymphocytes (Greenburg et al., 1975; Handwerger and Koren, 1976) and this classical ADCC reaction has been extensively studied by measuring the lysis of antibody-coated target cells by non-immune effector cells that were not previously exposed to antibody. Interactions of the Fc portion of the antibody molecule with Fc receptors on effector cells are prerequisite for this in vitro reaction; however, this type of reaction is easily inhibited by even low levels of aggregated IgG that competes with target-bound antibody for Fc receptors on effector cells (McLennan, 1972; Larson et al., 1973). It is thus quite obvious that "ADCC like reactions" in vivo would certainly be much impaired by circulating immune complexes that are frequently so very prevalent in the circulation of many cancer patients. One way to avoid inhibition of ADCC by immune complexes is to attach specific antibody to effector cells. This in vitro reaction, i.e., "antibody-directed ADCC," proved more effective and less sensitive to inhibition by immune complexes and aggregates of non-immune IgG than the classical ADCC reaction (Jones and Segal, 1980; Simone, 1982).

In another study, it was observed that monoclonal antibody to human melanoma mediated in vitro ADCC against melanoma cells, without any occurrence of the often-cited "antigenic drift" on tumor cells. This phenomenon did either not occur or failed to influence these reactions since they occurred equally well with recently established cell lines as with those maintained in long-term culture (Steplewski et al., 1979). These investigators raised the possibility that reactivity in ADCC may be partly attributable to Class II histocompatibility antigens expressed on melanoma target cells; however, this possibility appears unlikely since one monoclonal antibody produced by immunizing mice with somatic cell hybrids between human melanoma and mouse fibroblasts failed to react with Class II histocompatibility antigens and may thus specifically recognize a melanoma tumor-associated antigen in the ADCC.

Additional observations were made regarding the possible functional activity of monoclonal antibody-defined melanoma antigen (Yeh et al., 1981). These investigators found that a monoclonal antibody (3.2) of IgG$_{2a}$ isotype which defines an antigen designated 3.1, could mediate a strong ADCC reaction with human melanoma cells expressing this antigen when human peripheral lymphocytes were used as a source of effector (K) cells. Another monoclonal antibody of IgG$_1$ isotype that recognizes another epitope on the same antigenic structure can evoke only weak ADCC. With regard to this finding, it could also be demonstrated that in this experimental system, the presence of the 3.1 antigen was crucial for ADCC to take place (Hellstrom et al., 1981). These observations confirm earlier observations by Herlyn et al. (1979), but also extend them in one important aspect, i.e., human peripheral lymphocytes can funciton equally well as mouse splenocytes as a source of effector (K) cells in the presence of murine monoclonal antibody. These findings also underline the fact that different immunoglobulin classes differ in their ability to evoke ADCC, even if the antibodies are directed to different epitopes on the same antigenic structure.

In another experiment, Schulz et al. (1983) observed that murine effector cells armed with a IgG$_{2a}$ monoclonal antibody highly specific for melanoma (9.2.27) could specifically kill these cells in vitro by a "directed ADCC" reaction. In this case, polyethylene glycol 20,000 (8%) was used to nonspecifically enhance binding of the antibody IgG to effector cells. Thus, effector cells were "armed" as first described by Jones and Segal (1980); however, Schulz et al. (1983) used fetal calf serum rather than phthalate oils as separation medium since the phthalate oils were found more difficult to remove and often cause toxicity in mice when the system was tested in vivo. Data from ^{51}Cr release assays indicated that the directed ADCC was at least twice as effective as the classical ADCC reaction in inducing specific tumor cell killing. In fact, only the directed ADCC reaction clearly exceeded background as it showed a statistically significant reactivity ($p < 0.001$) compared to that of natural killer (NK) cells (Schulz et al., 1983).

The role of macrophages and monocytes as effector cells involved in tumor killing has not yet been critically evaluated in the human melanoma system. However, in a recent report, macrophages and monocytes were clearly implicated as effector cells in the killing of colorectal cancer cells (Steplewski et al., 1983). Fc receptors present in both of these cell types were found to strongly cross-react only with immunoglobulins of $IgG2_a$ isotype. Moreover, macrophages in the presence of murine monoclonal antibody of IgG_{2a} isotype specifically mediated the killing of colorectal tumor cells in vitro. Taken together, all these data from the experiments conducted in several laboratories, strongly support the hypothesis that murine IgG_{2a} monoclonal antibodies directed against human tumor-associated antigens may prove effective in aiding the therapy of human neoplasms.

5.2. In Vivo Studies

Initial experiments performed by Koprowski et al. (1978) demonstrated that monoclonal antibodies to melanoma were able to suppress the growth of human melanoma tumors in athymic (nu/nu) mice. These mice, which received 2×10^6 hybridoma cells secreting monoclonal antibody, 2 d prior to receiving a challenge of 10^7 melanoma cells, were prohibited from establishing tumors that grew rapidly in control animals who expired after 36 d. In another experiment, Bumol et al. (1983) also could suppress melanoma tumor growth in athymic (nu/nu) mice that received multiple doses (40 µg/each) of Mab 9.2.27 2–3 d after the injection of tumor cells. Although it was possible to suppress tumor growth 60% in these experiments, it should be emphasized that residual melanoma cells formed tumors again that ultimately killed the nude mice. Taken together, these data demonstrate that under ideal conditions, administration of monoclonal antibody *per se* may prevent a tumor from establishing itself, but that this regimen will not be useful to effectively inhibit the growth of well-established tumors.

It was against this background of events and the encouraging results obtained in vitro with murine effector cell-antibody conjugates in the directed ADCC that experiments were initiated to test this entire concept in vivo (Schulz et al., 1983). Some encouraging observations were made initially when nude mice implanted subcutaneously with human melanoma cells (7.5×10^6), received 1 d later, several intravenous injections of 2×10^6 effector cells, i.e., mononuclear cells from normal BALB/c mice, "armed" with 40 µg of Mab 9.2.27 IgG. It was only in this group of animals that the tumors remained very small and necrotic and were "biologically dead" once the injection of conjugates was stopped after 12 d. Another group of animals that received an equal number of injections of 40 µg 9.2.27 IgG *per se* showed ⁻60% suppression of tumor growth, similar to that observed under these conditions by Bumol et al. (1983) in previous experiments. Again, as in these previous experiments, the effect was transient. This was also true when effector cells either alone or treated with 8% polyethylene glycol were administered to several groups of animals. In other words, at day 32, when the experiments were terminated, tumors were growing rapidly in all treatment groups, with the notable exception of those animals that received the effector cells "armed" with Mab 9.2.27 (Schulz et al., 1983).

It should be pointed out, however, that the results from these experiments did not establish that effector cells "armed" with a specific antitumor monoclonal antibody can effectively inhibit the growth of established tumors. This concept was tested very recently by Schulz et al. (1984), and it was discovered that a single intravenous injection of 2×10^7 effector cells plus 400 µg Mab 9.2.27 IgG could completely eliminate relatively large (mean volume = 90 mm³) melanoma tumors that were well established in the nude mice for 14 d prior to any injection of effector cell–antibody conjugates (Schulz et al., 1984).

6. Conclusions

The purpose of this selective review was to document the decisive impact made by monoclonal antibodies on structural and functional studies dealing with human melanoma-associated antigens. Indeed, these highly specific reagents have served as excellent molecular probes and contributed considerably to recent progress made not only in melanoma antigens, but in the entire field of tumor biology. This brief review has also attempted to point out some of the limitations of monoclonal antibodies, especially when dealing with highly complex populations of tumor cells. It is hoped that the reader realizes that at this time the application of monoclonal antibodies to the diagnosis and therapy of human cancer is still very much at the beginning. It is obvious that new and imaginative ways will have to be explored to produce and apply monoclonal antibodies in such a way that they will effectively contribute towards the elimination of cancer.

Acknowledgments

The author's research has been supported in part by NIH grant CA 28420. The author also would like to acknowledge that his colleagues, Drs. J. R. Harper, G. Schulz, and D. A. Cheresh kindly made some of their data available that are either currently in press or submitted for publication. The author wishes to thank Ms. Bonnie Pratt Filiault for her excellent assistance in the typing of this manuscript.

References

Brown, J. P., R. G. Woodbury, C. E. Hart, I. Hellstrom, and K. E. Hellstrom (1981a), *Proc. Natl. Acad. Sci., USA* **78,** 539.

Brown, J. P., K. Nishiyama, I. Hellstrom, and K. E. Hellstrom (1981b), *J. Immunol.* **127,** 539.

Brown, J. P., P. W. Wright, C. E. Hart, R. G. Woodbury, K. E. Hellstrom, and I. Hellstrom (1981c), *J. Biol. Chem.* **255,** 4980.

Brown, J. P., K. E. Hellstrom, and I. Hellstrom (1981d), *Clinical Chem.* **27,** 1592.

Brown, J. P., R. M. Hewick, I. Hellstrom, K. E. Hellstrom, R. F. Doolittle, and J. W. Dreyer (1982), *Nature* **296,** 171.

Bumol, T. F. and R. A. Reisfeld (1982a), *Proc. Natl. Acad. Sci., USA* **79,** 1245.

Bumol, T. F., D. O. Chee, and R. A. Reisfeld (1982b), *Hybridoma* **1,** 283.

Bumol, T. F., Q. C. Wang, R. A. Reisfeld, and N. O. Kaplan (1983), *Proc. Natl. Acad. Sci., USA* **80,** 529.

Bumol, T. F., L. E. Walker, and R. A. Reisfeld (1984), *J. Biol. Chem.*, in press.

Bystryn, J. C. (1976), *J. Immunol.* **116,** 302.

Cahan, L. D., R. F. Irie, R. Singh, A. Cassidenti, and J. C. Paulson (1982), *Proc. Natl. Acad. Sci., USA* **79,** 7629.

Carey, T. E., T. Takahashi, L. E. Resnick, H. F. Oettgen, and L. J. Old (1976), *Proc. Natl. Acad. Sci., USA* **73,** 3278.

Carrel, S., M. Schreyer, A. Schmidt-Kessen, and J. P. Mach (1982), *Hybridoma* **1,** 387.

Chee, D. O., R. H. Yonemoto, P. L. Leong, G. F. Richards, V. R. Smith, J. L. Klotz, R. N. Goto, R. L. Gascon, and M. M. Drushella (1982), *Cancer Res.* **42,** 3142.

Cheresh, D. A., A. P. Varki, N. M. Varki, W. B. Stallcup, J. Levine, and R. A. Reisfeld (1984a), *J. Biol. Chem.*, **259,** 7453.

Cheresh, D. A., L. E. Wolff, A. P. Varki, and R. A. Reisfeld (1984b), *Science*, in press.

Cifone, M. A. and I. J. Fidler (1980), *Proc. Natl. Acad. Sci., USA* **77,** 1039.

Clark, W. H., R. R. Reimer, M. Greene, A. M. Ainsworth, and M. J. Mastrangelo (1977), *Adv. Cancer Res.* **24**, 267.

Culp, L. A., B. A. Murray, and B. J. Rollins (1979), *J. Supramol. Struct.* **11**, 401.

Dippold, W. G., K. O. Lloyd, T. L. Li, H. Ikeda, H. F. Oettgen, and L. F. Old (1980), *Proc. Natl. Acad. Sci., USA* **77**, 6114.

Gahmberg, C. G. and S. Hakamori (1975), *J. Biol. Chem.* **250**, 2438.

Galloway, D. R., R. P. McCabe, M. A. Pellegrino, S. Ferrone, and R. A. Reisfeld (1981), *J. Immunol.* **126**, 62.

Glimelius, B., B. Norling, B. Westernmark, and A. Wasteson (1978), *Biochem. J.* **172**, 443.

Gospodarowicz D., D. Greenburg, and C. R. Birdwell (1978), *Cancer Res.* **38**, 4155.

Greenberg, A. H., L. Shen, and G. Medly (1975), *Immunol.* **21**, 79.

Hakamori, S., C. Teather, and H. Andrews (1968), *Biochem. Biophys. Res. Commun.* **33**, 563.

Handwerger, B. J. and H. S. Koren (1976), *Clin. Immunol.* **5**, 272.

Harper, J. R., T. F. Bumol, and R. A. Reisfeld (1982), *Hybridoma* **1**, 423.

Harper, J. R. and R. A. Reisfeld (1983), *J. Natl. Cancer Inst.* **71**, 259.

Harper, J. R., T. F. Bumol, and R. A. Reisfeld (1984), *J. Immunol.*, in press.

Hellstrom, I., K. E. Hellstrom, and M. Y. Yeh (1981), *Int. J. Cancer* **27**, 281.

Hellstrom, I., J. P. Brown, and K. E. Hellstrom (1982), *Hybridoma* **1**, 399.

Herlyn, D., M. Herlyn, Z. Steplewski, and H. Koprowski (1979), *Eur. J. Immunol.* **9**, 657.

Herlyn, M., Z. Steplewski, B. F. Atkinson, C. S. Ernst, and H. Koprowski (1982), *Hybridoma* **1**, 403.

Hersey, P. and W. H. McCarthy (1982), In *Melanoma: Antigens and Antibodies,* (R. A. Reisfeld and S. Ferrone, eds.), Plenum Press, New York, pp 211–233.

Imai, K., A. K. Ng, and S. Ferrone (1981), *J. Natl. Cancer Inst.* **66**, 489.

Imai, K., B. S. Wilson, A. Bigotti, P. G. Natali, and S. Ferrone (1982), *J. Natl. Cancer Inst.,* **68**, 761.

Irie, R. F., L. L. Sze, and R. E. Saxton (1982), *Proc. Natl. Acad. Sci., USA* **79**, 5666.

Johnson, J. P. and G. Riethmuller (1982), *Hybridoma* **1**, 381.

Jones, J. F. and D. M. Segal (1980), *J. Immunol.* **125**, 926.

Kantor, R. S., A. K. Ng, P. Giacomini, and S. Ferrone (1982), *Hybridoma* **1**, 473.

Kohler, G. and C. Milstein (1975), *Nature* **256**, 495.

Koprowski, H., Z. Steplewski, D. Herlyn, and M. Herlyn (1978), *Proc. Natl. Acad. Sci., USA* **75**, 3405.

Larson, A., P. Perlmann, and J. B. Natvig (1973), *Immunol.* **25**, 675.

Levine, J., L. Beasley, and W. B. Stallcup (1984), *J. Neurochem.*, in press.

Lewis, M. G., R. C. Ilonopisov, R. C. Naiem, T. M. Phillips, and P. Alexander (1969), *Brit. Med. J.* **3**, 547.

Lewis, M. G. (1972), *Ser. Haematol.* **5**, 44.

Lewis, M. G. and K. M. A. Sheikh (1975), *Behring Inst. Mit.* **56**, 78.

Lloyd, K. O., A. Albino, and A. Houghton (1982), *Hybridoma* **1**, 461.

Loop, S. M., K. Nishiyama, I. Hellstrom, R. G. Woodbury, J. P. Brown, and
    K. E. Hellstrom (1981), *Int. J. Cancer* **27**, 775.
McLennan, I. C. M. (1972), *Clin. Exp. Immunol.*, **10**, 275.
Magnani, J. F., D. F. Smith, and V. Ginsburg (1980), *Anal. Biochem.* **109**, 399.
McCabe, R. P., S. Ferrone, M. A. Pellegrino, D. H. Kern, E. C. Holmes, and
    R. A. Reisfeld (1978), *J. Natl. Cancer Inst.* **60**, 773.
McCabe, R. P., D. R. Galloway, S. Ferrone, and R. A. Reisfeld (1979), In *Current Trends in Tumor Immunology*, (S. Ferrone, R. Herberman, L. Gorine,
    R. A. Reisfeld, eds.) Garland STPM Press, New York, pp 269–286.
McCabe, R. P., F. Indiveri, D. R. Galloway, S. Ferrone, and R. A. Reisfeld
    (1980), *J. Natl. Cancer Inst.* **65**, 703.
Nikulski, S. M. and M. Chirigos (1979), *J. Immunopharmacol.* **1**, 311.
Mitchell, K. F., J. P. Fuhrer, Z. Steplewski, and H. Koprowski (1980), *Proc.
    Natl. Acad. Sci., USA* **77**, 7287.
Mitchell, K. F., J. P. Fuhrer, Z. Steplewski, and H. Koprowski (1981), *Molec.
    Immunol.* **18**, 207.
Moller, E. (1965), *Science* **147**, 873.
Morgan, A. C., D. R. Galloway, and R. A. Reisfeld (1981), *Hybridoma* **1**, 27.
Natali, P. G., B. S. Wilson, K. Imai, K. Bigotti, and S. Ferrone (1982), *Cancer
    Res.* **42**, 583.
Nudelman, E., S. Hakamori, R. Kannagi, S. Levery, M. Y. Yeh, K. E.
    Hellstrom, and I. Hellstrom (1982), *J. Biol. Chem.* **257**, 12752.
Old, L. J. and E. Stockert (1977), *Ann. Rev. Genet.* **11**, 127.
Perlmann, P., and H. Perlmann (1972), *Cell Immunol.* **1**, 300.
Portoukalian, J., G. Zwingelstein, J. F. Dore, and J. J. Bourgnoin (1976),
    Biochemie (Paris) **58**, 1285.
Portoukalian, J., G. Zwingelstein, N. Abdul-Malak, and J. F. Dore (1978),
    Biochim. Biophys. Res. Commun. **85**, 916.
Portoukalian, J., G. Swingelstein, and J. F. Dore (1979), *Eur. J. Biochem.* **94**,
    19.
Pukel, C. S., K. O. Lloyd, L. R. Travassos, W. G. Dippold, H. F. Oettgen, and
    L. Old (1982), *J. Exp. Med.* **155**, 1113.
Reisfeld, R. A. (1982), *Nature* **298**, 325.
Reisfeld, R. A., D. R. Galloway, and A. C. Morgan (1982a). In *Melanoma Antigens and Antibodies*, (R. A. Reisfeld and S. Ferrone, eds.) Plenum Press,
    New York, pp. 317–337.
Reisfeld, R. A., A. C. Morgan, and T. F. Bumol (1982b). In *Hybridoma in
    Cancer Diagnosis and Treatment*, (M. S. Mitchell and H. F. Oettgen, eds.)
    Raven Press, New York, pp 183–186.
Reisfeld, R. A., J. R. Harper, and T. F. Bumol (1984). In *Critical Reviews in
    Immunology*, (M. Z. Atassi, ed.) CRC Press, Inc., Boca Raton, FL, vol. 5,
    pp. 27–53.
Ross, A. H., K. F. Mitchell, Z. Steplewski, and H. Koprowski (1982),
    Hybridoma **1**, 413.
Saxton, R. E., B. O. Mann, D. L. Morton, and M. W. Burk (1982), *Hybridoma*
    1, 433.
Schulz, G., T. F. Bumol, and R. A. Reisfeld (1983), *Proc Natl. Acad. Sci.,
    USA* **80**, 5407.

Schulz, G., G. Dennert, and R. A. Reisfeld (1984), to be submitted.

Shiku, A., T. Takahashi, H. F. Oettgen, and L. J. Old (1976), *J. Exp. Med.* **114,** 873.

Shiku, A., T. Takahashi, L. Resnick, H. F. Oettgen, and L. F. Old (1977), *J. Exp. Med.* **115,** 788.

Shin, S. V. Freedman, R. Risser, and R. Pollak (1975), *Proc. Natl. Acad. Sci., USA* **72,** 4435.

Simone, C. B. (1982), *Nature,* **297,** 294.

Steplewski, Z., M. Herlyn, D. Herlyn, W. H. Clark and H. Koprowski (1979), *Eur. J. Immunol.* **89,** 94.

Steplewski, Z., M. D. Lubeck, and H. Koprowski (1983), *Science* **221,** 865.

Stuhlmiller, G. M., M. J. Borowitz, B. P. Croker, and H. E. Seigler (1982), *Hybridoma* **1,** 447.

Tajiri, K., N. Uchida, and M. L. Tanzer (1980), *J. Biol. Chem.* **255,** 6036.

Vladavsky, I., G. M. Lui, and D. Gospodarowicz (1980), *Cell* **19,** 607.

Wilson, B. S., K. Imai, P. G. Natali, and S. Ferrone (1981), *Int. J. Cancer* **28,** 293.

Woodbury, R. G., J. P. Brown, M. Y. Yeh, I. Hellstrom and K. E. Hellstrom (1980), *Proc. Natl. Acad. Sci., USA* **77,** 2183.

Woodbury, R. G., J. P. Brown, S. M. Loop, K. E. Hellstrom, and I. Hellstrom (1981), *Int. J. Cancer* **27,** 145.

Yeh, M. Y., I. Hellstrom, and K. E. Hellstrom (1981), *J. Immunol.* **126,** 1312.

Chapter 10

Lung Cancer Markers as Detected by Monoclonal Antibodies

JAMES L. MULSHINE, FRANK CUTTITTA,
AND JOHN D. MINNA

National Cancer Institute—Navy Medical Oncology Branch, Clinical Oncology Program, Division of Cancer Therapy, National Institutes of Health, Bethesda, Maryland

1. Introduction

Over 120,000 new cases of lung cancer occur annually in the United States and the incidence is increasing (Silverberg, 1982). Ninety percent of those individuals with lung cancer die from their disease, making lung cancer the single most lethal malignancy, accounting for 25% of all cancer fatalities (Silverberg, 1982). Other than surgical resection of early lesions, the effectiveness of most other forms of therapy has been marginal (Aisner and Hansen, 1981; Minna et al., 1982). In considering lung cancer, one must deal with at least four major histologies, sharing variable degrees of relatedness (Matthews, 1981; Gazdar, 1984). Clinically, the distinction is often made between small cell lung cancer (SCLC) and the remaining histologies collectively referred to as the nonsmall-cell lung cancers (NSCLC) due to the distinct natural history and response to therapy of the two different groups (Cohen, 1978; Gazdar, 1983). The NSCLC histologies include squamous cell, adenocarcinoma, and large cell and share the properties of poor response to chemotherapy, but frequently complete response to surgical resection at an early stage. In contrast, SCLC tends to metastasize early precluding surgical resection, but has a high initial response rate to combination chemotherapy. Therefore, major treatment decisions hinge upon the distinction between SCLC and

NSCLC (Minna et al., 1982), so considerable interest has been focused on developing reagents which would distinguish pathologically between the two forms (Gazdar, 1983). Innovative approaches to these problems are needed. One such approach would be to utilize monoclonal antibodies in the diagnosis and therapy of this disorder. The work of Miller, Levy, and coworkers (1982) using a monoclonal antiidiotypic antibody for therapy in a patient with follicular lymphoma demonstrates that these reagents can be effective in the setting of advance cancer recalcitrant to standard therapy. Monoclonal antibodies offer the advantage of a replenishable, homogeneous source of a monospecific reagent that may be utilized for many clinical and laboratory applications. Investigators have already made progress in describing a role for these agents in the therapy of various nonpulmonary malignancies (Levy, 1983; Ritz and Schlossman, 1982; Oldham, 1983). The search for relevant tumor markers for lung cancer, however, has been problematic. Previous work with lung cancer markers involved the use of heteroantisera. This work has been fully summarized in the previous edition of this text (McIntire, 1982). The use of such antisera had little direct application in the clinical management of patients with NSCLC. Our hope is that the applications of monoclonal antibodies will bridge the void between laboratory and clinical applications.

Design considerations are critical factors as the the nature of immunization and screening assays govern the likelihood of "seeing" a hybridoma clone with the desired predetermined characteristics. From our initial published experience (Cuttitta et al., 1981), we have evolved more tailored selection conditions to enhance production of monoclonals possessing predetermined characteristics. In this manuscript we shall review the techniques for production and utilization of monoclonal antibodies directed against human lung cancer based on the experience of our laboratory.

2. Methods

The methods of immunization and screening have been previously published (Cuttitta et al., 1981; Minna et al., 1981), so we will summarize them briefly. Immunizations were done with whole live cells initially innoculated intraperitoneally into previously pristine primed rodents. For subsequent immunizations, boosts were done intraperitoneally or subcutaneously followed with a final intavenous boost administered three days before cell fusion. Rats or mice were used in all experiments without discernable differences in results. Hybridizations were accomplished using standard fusion techniques with a mouse myeloma cell line as the fusion partner (Kohler and Milstein, 1975; Galfre, 1977). The resulting hybridoma cells were plated out into 96 well microtiter plates and grown in mouse spleen-conditioned media. At 7–10 d, wells showing growth were tested for specific antibody production using an indirect radio-immunoassay (RIA). The RIA were performed using 96 well target plates containing solid phase glutaraldehyde fixed tumor cells plated at a density of 1×10^5 cells per well. The hybridoma supernatants were incubated for 30 min at room temperature, washed with phosphate-buffered saline (PBS) and then incubated with an appropriate species-specific secondary antibody. The plates were again washed with PBS and incubated with ^{131}I-labeled staphlococcal protein A for 30 min. Plates were then washed again with PBS and then analyzed for counts. Results were expressed as binding ratios (total counts − background counts/background counts).

Our screening strategy evolved as our experience with the characterization of antibodies developed. Initially, we selected antibodies that recognize SCLC but not autologous B lymphocytes, reasoning that antigens expressed exclusively on the neoplastic cells were more likely to be central to the malignant process (Cuttitta et al., 1981). With antibodies generated against NSCLC, as shown in Fig. 1, we added an additional condition that they not react with either SCLC cells, or autologous B cells (Mulshine et al., 1983c). Hybridomas secreting such antibodies were successively "minicloned" (Nowinski et al., 1979) at least three times and then single-cell cloned using limiting dilution techniques. Antibodies that maintain specificity after these procedures were propagated in mouse ascites to assure availability of large quantities of antibodies. One significant exception was the immunization and characterization of the monoclonal generated against amphibian neuropeptide bombesin. This immunizaton was accomplished using Lys-3-bombesin conjugated to bovine serum albumin. The immunization schedule was identical to that used for the other monoclonal antibodies. The screening technique also differed in that solid-phase peptides were used as targets in the initial radioimmunoassays. The goal was to select for antibodies that bound to bombesin, but not to other peptides such as substance P, physalaemin, or neurotensin. Hybridomas which met these criteria were cloned and propagated as outlined previously.

3. Characterization Studies

Monoclonal antibodies maintaining specific antibody production through the preliminary screens were tested for binding by radioimmunoassay (RIA) with all available lung cancer cell lines, as well as representative cell lines of other tumors. This was done to establish the spectrum of binding activity of various antibodies. Further analysis entailed using immunohistochemical assays, for which we used the avidin–biotin com-

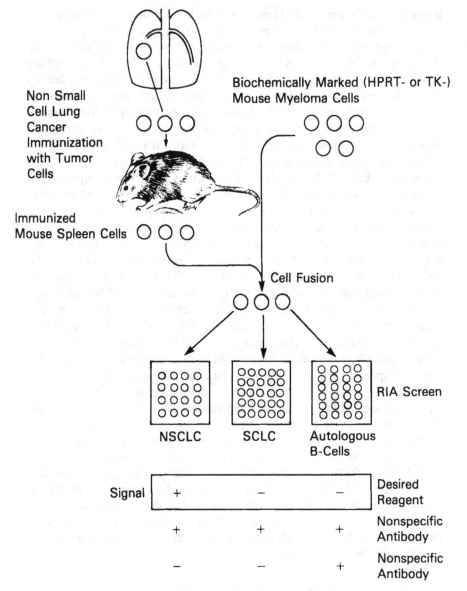

Fig. 1. Immunization and screening strategy for generation of an anti-nonsmall-cell lung cancer monoclonal antibody.

plex technique (Hsu et al., 1981). In all these assays we used saturating quantities of primary antibodies (10 µg/mL) incubated at room temperature for at least 1 h in a humidity chamber. We routinely employed nickel chloride-modified diaminobenzidene as the substrate for the peroxidase as it gives superior contrast in comparison to conventional diaminobenzidene methods, especially when used with a methyl green counterstain (Hsu and Soban, 1982). Another advantage of this technique is that the precipitate does not fade with time as the conventional diaminobenzidene precipitates. To determine the nature of antigen expression *in situ*, we initially screened formalin-fixed nude mouse xenografts of tumor cell lines (Gazdar et al., 1981), and then specimens direct from patients. The density of antigen expression on tumor tissue recognized by two anti-lung cancer monoclonal antibodies is demonstrated in Figs. 2A and 2B. Immunohistochemical assays were routinely performed to determine the expression of tumor-associated antigens on normal tissues as well. Our routine normal tissue screen included a panel with at least one well-preserved example of nine major human organs. A summary of representative data generated in this kind of analysis is shown on Table 1. Such antibodies frequently bind to antigens expressed discreetly on cell subsets within normal organs (Fig. 3). The selectivity of the binding to normal tissue structures is striking. Most of the anti-SCLC monoclonal generated by Rosen et al. (1984) reacted with elements of normal lung. An example of such reactivity is shown in Fig. 3A. The selectivity of antigen expression recognized by these antibodies is demonstrated with an anti-SCLC monoclonal binding to myoepithelial cells of human prostate (Fig. 3B). In a few cases, the binding was very focal in nature, not always correlating well with the known microanatomy. An example of this is shown in Fig. 3C with another anti-SCLC monoclonal antibody binding to some non-islet cell acinar structures in the pancreas. Such focal reactivity with distinct subsets of cells could be important in analyzing microanatomy from a new perspective. This immunoanatomy, defined by well-characterized monoclonal antibodies, may facilitate the understanding of developmental processes, as well as structure function relationships previously undecipherable.

Certain antibodies appear to have a restricted expression by screening formalin-fixed paraffin-embedded material (Table 1); however, we would have to perform more extensive analysis before suggesting that any monoclonal antibodies evaluated to date in our laboratory recognize an antigen uniquely expressed on malignant tissue. Based on our current understanding of tumor biology, we have speculated that such unique tumor-specific antigens are exceedingly rare. We have concentrated on selecting monoclonal antibodies that bind antigens with either a very limited distribution or a very well-defined distribution on normal tissues. In this fashion, one can restrict the utilization of such reagents to situations in which cross-reactivity would not be a problem.

4. Monoclonal Antibodies to Small-Cell Lung Cancer

The first monoclonal reported by our laboratory was 534F8, which was generated against SCLC (Cuttitta et al., 1981). This antibody bound to a

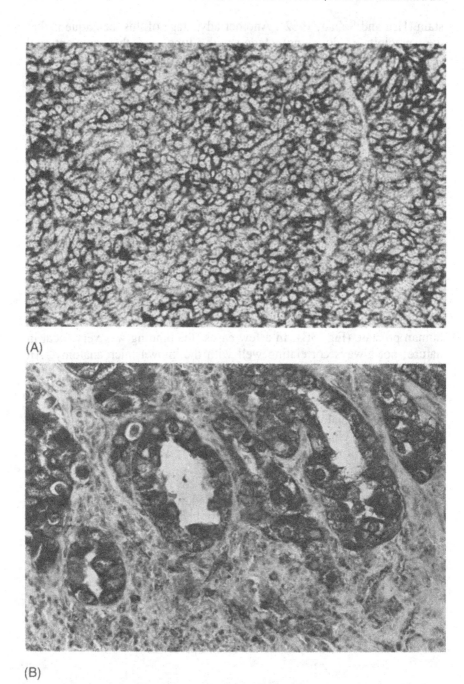

(A)

(B)

Fig. 2. Monoclonal antibodies generated against lung cancers used in an immunohistochemical assay system (Hsu and Soban, 1982). (A) Anti-small-cell antibody strongly binding to a small cell tumor. Antigen expression is demonstrated by areas of black. (B) Anti-nonsmall-cell lung cancer (adenocarcinoma) with tumor cells in gland-like structures showing positive reaction.

surface antigen that was expressed on most SCLC tumor and approximately half of NSCLC tumors. The antigen was also expressed on certain normal tissues including bronchial epithelium (Table 1) (Coombs et al.,1984). In collaboration with the laboratory of Victor Ginsburg of the NIH we were able to establish that the antigen recognized by the antibody was the carbohydrate lacto-*N*-fucopentaose III (LNFP III) (Huang et al., 1983a; Ginsburg et al., 1984). This antigen was originally characterized as a human milk fat sugar (Kobata and Ginsburg, 1969), but has been found to be expressed in a variety of systems including mouse embryonal carcinoma, murine embryos (SSEA-1), (Hakomori et al, 1983; Gooi et al., 1981), and human myeloid cells (Huang et al., 1983b). This oligosaccharide is also very immunodominant in a variety of malignancies including lung cancer, colon cancer, breast cancer, promyelocytic leukemia (Huang et al., 1983b; Magnani and Ginsburg, 1983; Hakomori and

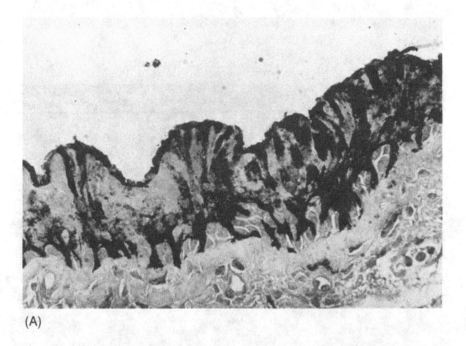

(A)

Fig. 3. Anti-SCLC monoclonals demonstrating pattern of antigen expression on normal adult tissues in immunohistochemical assays. (A) Reactivity of a monoclonal with bronchial epithelium. The ciliated cells are the most heavily stained cells of the bronchus. (B) Reactivity with prostate reveals very focal reactivity seen exclusively with the myoepithelial elements of the prostatic glands and the vas deferens. (C) Focal reactivity with acinar-like elements in the pancreas is demonstrated. Exact morphological structure expressing this antigen is not clear.

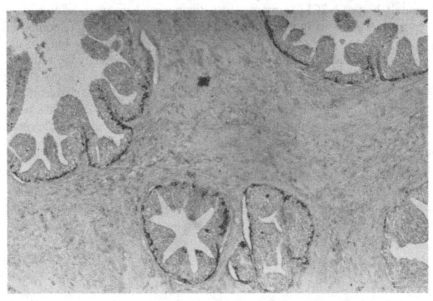

(B)

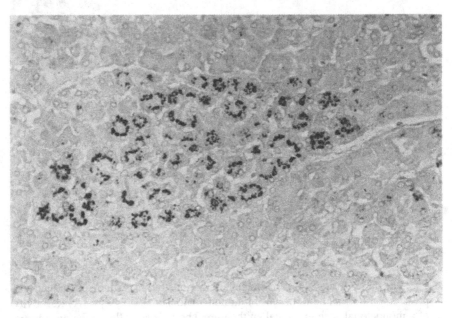

(C)

Table 1
Normal Tissue Distribution of Antigens as Recognized by Anti-Lung Cancer Monoclonal Antibodies in Immunohistochemical Assays[a]

Monoclonal antibody	Antigen	Lung[b]		Liver		Pancreas	
		Mucosa	Chondrocytes	Kupffer	Epithelium	Islet	Parenchyma
534F8[c]	LNFP3	+		+		+	
600D11[d]	LNFP3	+		+	+	+	+
624A6	LNFP3	+	+	+		+	+
624A12	LNFP3	+	+			+	
625B5	LNFP3	+					
602G2	LNFP3	+					
703D4[c]	p31	−				+	
704A1	p31	−					

[a]All assays done under identical conditions, on serial sections of formalin-fixed paraffin-embedded material.
[b]Sites evaluated include: bronchial mucosa, bronchial chondrocytes, Kupffer cells, hepatic epithelium, islet cells, and pancreatic parenchyma.
[c]Cuttitta et al., 1981.
[d]Rosen et al., 1984.
[e]Mulshine et al., 1983.

Kannagi, 1983). Competition studies with anti-Leu M1, an antibody that binds to the malignant cells of Hodgkin's disease (Hanjan et al., 1982), suggest that Leu M1 is also directed against the LNFP III antigen (Hsu at al., 1984). LNFP III is expressed principally as a glycolipid in SCLC. However this antigen is expressed as a glycoprotein Hodgkin's disease (150,000 kdaltons) (Hsu et al., 1984). Of interest, we have been able to generate several different antibodies with specificity for LNFP III as determined on thin layer chromotography, and hapten inhibition studies (Huang et al., 1983a; Rosen et al., 1984). All of these antibodies have been found to be IgM class despite extensive hyperimmunization. In several of the assay systems, each performed under constant conditions, the individual antibodies directed against LNFP III gave disparate results (Table 2). These differences could be due to several reasons. The affinities of the individual antibodies for the antigen may be different. The antigen LNFP III may have multiple epitopes or accessibility to the antigen may vary as a function of its location in relationship to adjacent carbohydrates (Hakomori and Kannagi, 1983; Ginsburg et al., 1984). We have recently determined that the level of expression of this and other glycolipids may be useful in distinguishing among subsets of lung cancers and this possibility is being actively explored (Mulshine et al., 1984).

4.1. Analysis of Antigen Expression in Small-Cell Lung Cancer

Fargion and coworkers (1984) used a panel of seven independent monoclonal antibodies generated against SCLC (Rosen et al., 1984) in a

Table 2
Assays with Anti-Small-Cell Monoclonal with Specificity for
Lacto-N-Fucopentaose III

Monoclonal antibody	Radioimmunoassay, binding ratio		Immunohistochemistry, number positive/total number		
	SCLC glycolipid extract[a]	Pooled meconium[b]	SCLC cell lines[c]	SCLC cell lines	SCLC patient specimens
600D11	20	2	8/12	3/8	7/7
624A6	70	12	8/12	6/8	5/7
624A12	100	24	11/12	6/8	5/7
625B5	67	11	10/12	4/8	4/7
602G2	18	4	11/12	1/8	1/7

[a]Glycolipid extracts of SCLC lung cancer cells were prepared as previously described (Huang et al., 1983) and then analyzed in a solid-phase system.

[b]Pooled meconium is a rich source of glycolipid and a useful preliminary screening material (solid phase) when assessing for the presence of glycolipid.

[c]Positive binding ration >2.

formal analysis of antigen expression. These assays including immuno-histochemistry, radiobinding, and cell analysis led to several observations about antigen expression. Considerable heterogeneity of antigen expression exists between tumors of similar histologies. In radiobinding assays, binding ratios varied as much as two logs among various specimens of the same tumor type. These observations were consistent using fresh tumor tissue as well as cell lines of human lung cancers, and not attributable to differences in cell kinetics. In an analysis of multiple tumor cell lines established from independent sites from individual patients, this same pattern existed. These differences were also independent of cell cycle. Preliminary analysis of tumor cell lines for the mode of transmission of antigen expression revealed that this heterogeneous pattern of antigen expression was preserved within all clones, suggesting that heterogeneity of antigen expression is an intrinsic property of tumor cells. A possible implication of this research is that either therapeutic or diagnostic applications of monoclonal antibodies may require development of panels of antigens to insure recognition and/or destruction of all neoplastic cells in a particular host.

5. Monoclonal Antibodies to Nonsmall-Cell Lung Cancer

Two anti-NSCLC monoclonal antibodies (7O3D4 and 7O4A1) were generated using a large-cell lung cancer cell line (NCI-H157). Both antibodies were IgG2A$_k$ isotype. The large cell histology was selected since it appears morphologically to be the least differentiated of the NSCLC types, so that it may possess antigens common to all forms of NSCLC. Preliminary work with the two antibodies used in immunohistochemical assays (Fig. 2B) suggests that these monoclonal antibodies may be of help in distinguishing NSCLC from SCLC in a clinical setting (Mulshine et al., 1983a). In use with a series of 41 formalin-fixed clinical tumor specimens these two antibodies recognized over 90% (23/25) of the NSCLC while binding to only 19% (3/16) of SCLC (Mulshine et al., 1983a). Only one of the "false positive" SCLC tumors had classic histologic appearance. The other two SCLC tumors had atypical features. We use single-dimension polyacrlyamide gel electrophoresis (PAGE) analysis of metabolically labeled cellular lysates of tumor cells from cell lines to analyze the antigen recognized by the monoclonal antibodies. The two anti-NSCLC antibodies bound to a determinant with an apparent molecular mass of 31 kdaltons (p31). Although the proteins identified by the PAGE appeared to be identical, further analysis with direct radiobinding competition studies suggests that the two antibodies bound to different epitopes. In generating the anti-NSCLC monoclonals we were interested in selecting antibodies with specificities for antigens that were expressed selectively on NSCLC but not expressed on SCLC, and as previously discussed, we attempted to make our screening criteria more focused (Fig. 1). In contrast to our experience with anti-SCLC monoclonals, which react with both the SCLC and NSCLC forms of lung cancer the anti-NSCLC antibodies are more selective for the NSCLC form (Mulshine et al., 1983b). The latter also have a more restricted normal tissue reactivity that may be an unexpected benefit of our more stringent screening conditions. To corroborate these preliminary findings of specificity with the anti-NSCLC antibodies, we are now prospectively correlating antigen expression with diagnosis and clinical course in a series of carefully staged lung cancer patients. In this fashion we should develop a precise knowledge of their clinical utility.

6. Monoclonal Antibodies to Defined Proteins of Lung Cancer

Our group has collaborated with investigators from Johns Hopkins in using two dimensional PAGE techniques to determine novel antigens that are expressed selectively on lung cancer. Baylin et al. (1982) used this technique with radioiodinated lung cancer membrane preparations to describe a distinct surface phenotype for the two major forms of lung cancer. SCLC cells express 12 distinctive low molecular mass proteins (40–70 kdaltons), whereas NSCLC cells express nine different distintive low molecular mass proteins, as well as five high molecular mass proteins (>100,000 kdaltons). Bernal et al. (1983) using similar techniques, analyzed the expression of cytoskeletal proteins of the two forms of lung cancer. Certain cytoskeletal elements also distinguished the two major forms of lung cancer. We are currently attempting to exploit these findings to generate useful new monoclonal antibodies. Protein bands that appeared to be restricted either to SCLC or NSCLC are used as immunogens to generate hybridomas. The hybridomas are then screened for specific activity using the appropriate PAGE-purified antigens as target in radiobinding assays. If successful, this offers a novel strategy for generating tumor type-specific antibodies.

In our laboratory, Doyle and collaborators (1983) have demonstrated a difference in the expression of the major histocompatability antigens between the two main forms of lung cancer. Using monoclonal antibodies against the HLA framework protein and B_2-microglobulin, low or absent expression of these antigens was found on eight different SCLC cell lines, whereas nine NSCLC cell lines had marked expression of these surface antigens. Preliminary molecular analysis reveal that the defect is at the translational level. Further work is being conducted to study the dynamics of this process, especially to determine if modulation of expression can be achieved. Lack of expression of HLA elements may frustrate immune surveillance, allowing propagation of the malignant process.

7. Imaging Lung Cancer with Monoclonal Antibodies

Preliminary in vivo work includes use of the rat anti-SCLC monoclonal antibody (Rosen et al., 1984) in a radioimaging trial using nude mouse bearing lung cancer xenografts (Zimmer et al., 1983). The antibody (600D11) used in this study is an IgM, with definite binding to an antigen (LNFP III) expressed on normal tissues (Table 1). Nonetheless, using ^{131}I as the nuclide, over 10% of the total injected dose concentrated in tumor tissue by 48 h with significant tumor to normal organ gradient permitting excellent imaging. Further work in model systems such as this may help determine the dynamics of antibody and antigen biodistribution in vivo to establish the critical characteristics of monoclonal antibodies that will allow for sucessful use in imaging studies.

8. Monoclonal Antibodies with Therapeutic Applications

A major goal of immunobiologists is to use monoclonal antibodies therapeutically to help control or destroy tumors. Monoclonal antibodies given alone may have a therapeutic impact. This effect may be enhanced by putting toxins, chemotherapy agents, radionuclides or effector cells on the antibody. We have initiated preliminary studies to sort out the value of these various possibilities.

8.1. In Small-Cell Lung Cancer Variants

In our laboratory, the first therapeutic application of monoclonal antibodies in an in vivo system involved a rat monoclonal antibody generated by Fargion, et al. (1984). The antibody 1IG11 is of rat IgM class, which was derived against a small-cell variant (SCLC-v), NCI-N417. The SCLC-v subset of SCLC is an emerging distinct biological (Carney et al., 1983b; Little et al., 1983; Gazdar, 1984) and clinical entity (Radice et al.,1982). Cell lines of SCLC-v have shorter doubling time and higher cloning effiencies than classic SCLC. This may be associated with a very aggressive clinical behavior. A SCLC-v cell line was chosen as the immunogen to try to identify a marker for this biological subset. The monoclonal antibody 1IG11 bound strongly (K_A of $0.9 \times 10^9 M^{-1}$ with 1.5×10^6 binding sites/cell) to an antigen expressed on SCLC-v as well as many other forms of malignancy and on certain normal structures as well. The normal structures expressing this antigen included bronchial epithelium, normal skin, and renal tubules. The immunohistochemical assay of antigen density on lung cancer tissue markedly exceeded that on normal pulmonary tissue. From cellular kinetic analysis, we know that the expression of this antigen is cell-cycle independent. Of interest, this antibody when coincubated for 2 h in the absence of complement with human lung cancer cell lines expressing the antigen, inhibits their clonal growth in soft agarose up to 80% without direct cytotoxicity. This effect is also documented in a mass culture system analyzed for DNA synthesis by thymidine incorporation. Preliminary work with intravenous 1IG11 injected twice weekly into nude mice demonstrated inhibition of successful engraftment of as many as 10^7 tumor cells injected subcutaneously. Preliminary analysis using radio-binding competition assays of many other known hormones and growth factors including transferrin fails to alter this effect suggesting that this inhibition may be mediated through a previously undefined receptor. Experiments are now under way to see if this monoclonal antibody has any effect on established heterotransplants of lung cancer cell lines.

8.2. In Small-Cell Lung Cancer

Another approach to therapeutic interventions utilizing monoclonal antibodies entails a mouse monoclonal antibody with specificity for the binding site of the neuropeptide, bombesin (Cuttitta et al., 1984). This monoclonal antibody was generated to bombesin after the description of this neuropeptide as a marker for small-cell lung cancer (Moody et al., 1981). Bombesin or bombesin-like immunoreactivity has been found in at least 90% of SCLC, but rarely in NSCLC. Subsequent work with this peptide demonstrates that it has autotrophic effect on the growth of small-cell lung cancer cells as demonstrated in a serum-free defined media system (Carney et al., 1983a). Specific receptors for this peptide have been recently characterized (K_d 1.0 nM) (Moody et al., 1983) and are found at low density (2000 sites/cell) on many SCLC cell lines. This monoclonal antibody, 2A11, is an IgG I class and has high affinity for bombesin (K_A 3.5 × $10^9 M^{-1}$). This antibody also binds to closely related peptides including gastrin-releasing peptide, but not to a variety of other neuropeptides including physaelamine and substance P. Although it binds to small-cell lung cancer tumors it has very limited reactivity with normal human tissues. The antigen is expressed on pulmonary endocrine cells that are relatively common in fetal lung (Fig. 4) but very scarce in normal adult lungs. These factors suggested a role for 2A11 as a potential therapeutic tool. In vitro analysis using a soft agarose stem-cell assay confirmed that the autotrophic effect of bombesin could be inhibited with equivalent concentrations of the monoclonal antibody 2A11. In preliminary nude mouse experiments conducted by Cuttitta et al. (1984) cell lines were injected (10^7 live tumor cells) and allowed to grow to approxi-

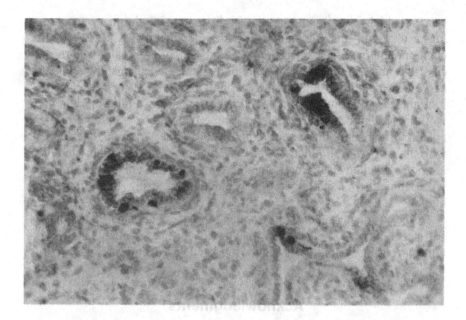

Fig. 4. Human 20-wk fetal lung demonstrating a positive reaction in immunohistochemical assay of the antibombesin monoclonal with neuroendocrine cells. Two large aggregates of positively stained cells in the upper right are neuroepithelial bodies.

mately 0.5 cm in diameter. From that point on, the monoclonal antibody 2A11 was administered intraperitoneally on a twice weekly schedule. Established small-cell lung cancer heterotransplants completely regressed and remained without any evidence of growth for at least one month after the initiation of antibody therapy (Minna, 1984).

The current positive results suggest a fundamentally new approach to tumor therapy. Identification of essential growth factors and then utilization of monoclonal antibodies to deny the tumor such growth factors is a new strategy with potential for broad application. Further experiments are being conducted with the monoclonal antibody, but application to human therapy will be evaluated.

9. Summary

Monoclonal antibodies generated against small-lung cancer have provided reagents for exploring the chemistry of membrane glycolipids. These reagents have been useful for probing the nature of antigen expression, which may allow for more rational application of immunotherapy strategies. The antibodies generated against NSCLC may prove useful in distinguishing the non-small-cell forms from the small-cell forms of lung cancer, which is an important clinical distinction. Preliminary encouraging results with imaging studies in nude mice bearing SCLC xenografts using monoclonal IgM anti-SCLC antibodies may eventually lead to successful human applications. The antibody generated against the clinically aggressive small cell lung cancer variants has been successful in inhibiting the clonal growth of tumor cells in soft agarose. Preliminary in vivo work in nude mice suggests that this property could be exploited for therapeutic application. In a more completely defined system, interference with the autocrine stimulation of SCLC by bombesin using a monoclonal antibody resulted in dramatic tumor regression in nude mice, and provides impetus for initiation of a clinical trial using this strategy in humans.

The ultimate value of the applications of monoclonal antibodies is still speculative. Diseases such as lung cancer are excellent model systems to explore biological, diagnostic, and therapeutic aspects of this question.

Acknowledgments

We would like to thank Drs. A. F. Gazdar and D. C. Ihde for their helpful comments on the manuscript and Dr. Gazdar for preparation of photomicrographs.

The opinions or assertions contained herein are the private views of the authors and are not to be construed as official or as reflecting the views of the Department of the Navy or the Department of Defense.

References

Aisner, J., and H. H. Hansen (1981), *Cancer Treat. Rep.* **65,** 979.

Baylin, S. B., A. F. Gazdar, J. D. Minna, S. D. Bernal, and J. H. Shaper (1982), *Proc. Natl. Acad. Sci.*, **79,** 4650.

Bernal, S. D., S. B. Baylin, J. H. Shaper, A. F. Gazdar, and L. B. Chen (1983), *Cancer Res.* **43,** 1798.

Carney, D. N., H. Oie, T. Moody, A. Gazdar, F. Cuttitta, and J. D. Minna (1983a), *Proc. Amer. Fed. for Clin. Res.* **31,** 404.

Carney, D. N., A. F. Gazdar, and J. D. Minna (1982), *Pathobiol. Annual* **12,** 115.

Carney, D. N., J. B. Mitchell, and T. Kinsella (1983b), *Cancer Res.* **43,** 2806.

Cohen, M. H., and M. J. Matthews (1978), *Semin. Oncol.* **5,** 234.

Coombs, S. G., R. J. Marder, J. D. Minna, J. L. Mulshine, M. R. Polovina, and S. T. Rosen (1984), in press, *J. Histochem. Cytochem.*

Cuttitta, F., D. N. Carney, J. Mulshine, and J. D. Minna (1984), in press, *Proc. Amer. Assoc. Cancer Res.*

Cuttitta, F., S. Rosen, A. F. Gazdar, and J. D. Minna (1981), *Proc. Natl. Acad. Sci. USA.* **78,** 4591.

Cuttitta, F., T. W. Moody, D. N. Carney, J. Fedorko, J. Mulshine, P. Bunn, and J. Minna (1983), *Proc. Amer. Fed. Clin. Res.* **31,** 404.

Doyle, A., and F. Cuttitta (1983), *Proc. Amer. Soc. Clin. Oncol.* **2,** 12.

Fargion, S., D. N. Carney, F. Cuttitta, P. A. Bunn, J. Fedorko, J. Mushine, A. F. Gazdar, and J. D. Minna (1983), *Proc. Amer. Soc. Clin. Oncol.* **2,** 55.

Fargion, S., F. Cuttitta, J. Mulshine, D. N. Carney, P. A. Bunn, and J. D. Minna (1983), *Proc. Amer. Asso. Cancer Res.* **24,** 221.

Galfre, G., S. C. Hoew, C. Milstein, G. W. Butcher, and J. C. Howard (1977), *Nature* (London) **266,** 550.

Gazdar, A. F. (1984), in *Endocrine Lung in Health and Disease* (Becker, K. and Gazdar, A. F., eds.) W. B. Saunders Co., Philadelphia.

Gazdar, A. F., D. N. Carney, H. L. Simms, and A. Simmons (1981), *Int. J. Cancer* **28,** 777.

Gazdar, A. F., D. N. Carney, and J. D. Minna (1983), *Sem. Oncol.* **10,** 3.

Ginsburg, V., P. Fredman, and J. L. Magnani (1984), in *Genes and Antigens in Cancer Cells: The Monoclonal Antibody Approach*, Karger Verlag, Basel.

Gooi, H. C., T. Feizi, A. Kapadla, B. B. Knowles, D. Solter, and M. J. Evans, (1981), *Nature* (London) **292,** 156.

Hakomori, S., and R. Kannagi (1983), *J. Natl. Canc. Inst.* **71,** 231.

Hanjan, S. N., J. F. Kearney, and M. D. Cooper (1982), *Clin. Immunol. Immunopathol.* **23,** 172.

Hsu, S., L. Raine, and H. Fanger (1981), *J. Histochem. Cytochem.* **30,** 1079.

Hsu, S., and E. Soban (1982), *J. Histochem. Cytochem.* 29, 577.

Hsu, S., L. C. Huang, J. Mulshine, F. Cuttitta, and E. Jaffe, (1983), unpublished data.

Huang, L. C., M. Brockhaus, J. L. Magnani, F. Cuttitta, S. Rosen, J. D. Minna, and V. Ginsburg (1983a), *Arch. Biochem. and Biophys.* **220,** 318.

Huang, L. C., C. I. Civin, J. L. Magnani, J. H. Shaper, and V. Ginsburg (1983b), *Blood* **61,** 1020.

Kobata, A., and V. Ginsburg (1969), *J. Biol. Chem.* **244,** 5496.

Kohler, G., and C. Milstein (1975), *Nature* (London) **256,** 495.

Levy, R., R. A. Miller (1983), *Annual Rev. Med.* **34,** 107.

Little, C. D., M. M. Nau, D. N. Carney, A. F. Gazdar, and J. D. Minna (1983), *Nature* (London) **306,** 194.

Magnani, J. L., and V. Ginsburg (1983), in *Monoclonal Antibodies in Cancer* (Langman, R. and Dulbecco, R., eds.), Academic Press, New York.

Matthews, M. J., and A. F. Gazdar (1981), in *Lung Cancer*, (Livinston, R. B., ed.) Martinus Nijhoff, Boston, p. 283.

McIntire, K. R. (1982), in *Human Cancer Markers*, (S. Sell and B. Wahren, eds.), Humana Press, Clifton, p. 359.

Miller, R. A., D. G. Maloney, R. Warnke, and R. Levy (1982), *N. Engl. J. Med.* **306,** 517.

Minna, J. D., *Proc. Amer. Assoc. Cancer Res.* **25,** 393.

Minna, J. D., F. Cuttitta, S. Rosen, P. A. Bunn, D. N. Carney, A. F. Gazdar, and S. Krasnow (1981), *In Vitro* **17,** 1058.

Minna, J. D., G. A. Higgins, E. J. Glatstein (1982), in *Principles and Practice of Oncology*, (DeVita, V., T. Hellman, S. Rosenberg, eds.), J. B. Lippincott, Philadelphia, p. 396.

Moody, T. W., C. B. Pert, A. F. Gazdar, D. N. Carney, and J. D. Minna (1981), *Science* **214,** 1246.

Moody, T. W., V. Bertness, and D. N. Carney (1983), *Peptides* **4,** 683.

Mulshine J. L., F. Cuttitta, M. Bibro, J. Fedorko, S. Fargion, C. Little, D. N. Carney, A. F. Gazdar, and J. D. Minna (1983c), *J. Immunol.* **131,** 497.

Mulshine, J., F. Cuttitta, C. Little, S. Fargion, J. Fedorko, M. Bibro, D. Carney, M. Matthews, A. Gazdar, and J. Minna (1983a), *Proc. Amer. Soc. Clin. Oncol.* **2,** 15.

Mulshine, J. L., S. Rosen, F. Cuttitta, S. Fargion, M. Bibro, M. Matthews, J. Minna, and A. F. Gazdar (1983b), *Proc Amer. Assoc. Canc. Res.* **24,** 221.

Mulshine J. L., F. Cuttitta, S. Rosen, D. N. Carney, J. Minna, and A. Gazdar (in press), *Proc. Amer. Soc. Clin. Oncol.*

Nowinski, R. C., M. E. Lostrom, M. R. Tam, M. R. Stone, and W. N. Burnette (1979), *Virology* **93,** 111.

Oldham, R. K., (1983), *J. Clin. Oncol.* **1,** 582.

Radice, P. A., M. J. Matthews, D. C. Ihde, A. F. Gazdar, D. N. Carney, P. A. Bunn, M. A. Cohen, B. E. Fossieck, R. W. Makuch, and J. D. Minna (1982), *Cancer* **50,** 2894.

Ritz, J., and S. F. Schlossman (1982), *Blood* **59,** 1.

Rosen, S., J. L. Mulshine, F. Cuttitta, J. Fedorko, D. N. Carney, A. F. Gazdar, and J. D. Minna (1984), *Cancer Res.* **44,** 2052.

Silverberg, E. (1982), *CA-A-Journal for Physicians* **32,** 15.

Zimmer, A. M., S. M. Spies, S. Rosen, E. A. Silverstein, M. Polovina, and J. D. Minna (1983), *Proc. Soc. Nucl. Med.*

Chapter 11

Human Breast Cancer Markers Defined by Monoclonal Antibodies

J. SCHLOM[1], J. GREINER[1], P. HORAN HAND[1],
D. COLCHER[1], G. INGHIRAMI[1], M. WEEKS[1], S. PESTKA[2],
P. B. FISHER[3], P. NOGUCHI[4], AND D. KUFE[5]

Laboratory of Tumor Immunology and Biology, National Cancer Institute, National Institutes of Health, Bethesda, Maryland[1]; Roche Institute of Molecular Biology, Nutley, New Jersey[2]; Institute of Cancer Research, Columbia University, New York, New York[3]; Office of Biologics, National Center for Drugs and Biologics, Food and Drug Administration, Bethesda, Maryland[4]; Dana Farber Cancer Institute, 44 Binney Street, Boston, Massachusetts[5]

1. Introduction

Numerous monoclonal antibodies (Mab) have been described that are reactive with human mammary carcinomas. In general, they can be classified into three groups based on the immunogen used to generate the Mab; these are Mab derived using (a) breast tumor cell lines, (b) milk fat globule membrane, or (c) membrane enriched extracts of breast carcinoma metastases as immunogen. Each of the Mab thus far described (Colcher et al., 1981a; Sloan and Omerod, 1981; Taylor-Papadimitriou et al., 1981; To et al., 1981; Arklie et al., 1982; Epenetos et al., 1982a,b; Foster et al., 1982; Gatter et al., 1982; Nuti et al., 1982; Rasmussen et al., 1982; Colcher et al., 1983a; Hand et al., 1983; Menard et al., 1983; Papsidero et al., 1983; Thompson et al., 1983) including those prepared by several different groups to milk fat globule membrane, appears to be unique with respect to either percent of reactive mammary tumors, percent of reactive cells within tumors, location of reactive antigen within the tumor cell, or degree of reactivity with nonmammary tumors as well as normal tissues.

The rationale of the studies reviewed here was to utilize membrane-enriched extracts of human metastatic mammary tumor cells as immunogens in an attempt to generate and characterize Mab reactive with determinants that would be maintained on metastatic human mammary carcinoma cells. Metastatic tumor cells were used with the hypothesis that primary tumor masses may contain a subpopulation of cells with a predefined metastatic potential; the possibility may therefore exist that antibodies made against determinants present on the vast majority of breast carcinoma cells in primary lesions may not be reactive with cells in metastatic lesions. Similarly, mammary tumor cell lines were avoided as immunogens. The hypothesis set forth here is that cell lines are the products of great selective pressure on cell populations found in vivo; the antigenic phenotype of those cells selected for their ability to grow in culture may therefore be quite different from the antigenic phenotype of those cells in primary or metastatic masses. One of the antibodies (B72.3) described below has just such properties. Multiple assays (Colcher et al., 1981a; Nuti et al., 1981; Nuti et al., 1982; Colcher et al., 1983a; Colcher et al., 1983b; Hand et al., 1983) using tumor cell extracts, tissue sections, and live cells in culture have been employed to reveal the range of reactivities and diversity of the monoclonal antibodies generated.

2. Generation of Monoclonal Antibodies

Mice were immunized with membrane-enriched fractions of human metastatic mammary carcinoma cells from either of two involved livers (designated Met 1 and Met 2) from two different patients. Spleens of immunized mice were fused with nonimmunoglobulin secreting NS-1 murine myeloma cells to generate 4250 primary hybridoma cultures. All hybridoma methodology and assay methods employed have been described previously (Herzenberg et al., 1979; Colcher et al., 1981a). Supernatant fluids from hybridoma cultures were first screened in solid phase radioimmunoassays (RIA) for the presence of immunoglobulin that is reactive with extracts of metastatic mammary tumor cells from involved livers and not reactive with extracts of apparently normal human liver. Following passage and double-cloning by endpoint dilution of cultures secreting immunoglobulins demonstrating preferential reactivity with breast carcinoma cells, the monoclonal antibodies from eleven hybridoma cell lines were chosen for further study. The isotypes of all eleven antibodies were determined; ten were IgG of various subclasses and one was an IgM (Table 1).

Table 1
Reactivity of Monoclonal Antibodies in Solid Phase Radioimmunoassays

| Monoclonal antibody | Isotype | Cell extracts[a] | | | Live cells[b] | | | | |
| | | Met 1 | Met 2 | Liver | Mammary carcinoma | | | Melanoma, sarcoma[c] | Normal[d] |
					BT-20	MCF-7	ZR-75-1		
B6.2	IgG₁	++++	++	Neg	+++	+++	++	Neg	Neg
B14.2	IgG₁	++++	++	Neg	+	+++	+	Neg	Neg
B39.1	IgG₁	++++	++	Neg	+++	+++	++	Neg	Neg
F64.5	IgG₂ₐ	++++	++++	Neg	++	+++	++	Neg	Neg
F25.2	IgG₁	++++	++++	Neg	+++	+++	+	Neg	Neg
B84.1	IgG₁	++	+	Neg	++	++	Neg	Neg	Neg
B50.4	IgG₁	++++	+	Neg	Neg	+	Neg	Neg	Neg
B50.1	IgG₁	++	++	Neg	Neg	Neg	Neg	Neg	Neg
B25.2	IgM	Neg	+++	Neg	Neg	Neg	Neg	Neg	Neg
B72.3	IgG₁	+++	Neg	Neg	Neg	+	+++	Neg	Neg
B38.1	IgG₁	+	+	Neg	+++	+	Neg	Neg	Neg
W6/32	IgG₂ₐ	Neg	Neg	++	++	+	+++	++	++
B139	IgG₁	++	+	++	++	+	Neg	++	++

[a] Solid-phase RIA. Neg, <500; +, 500–2000 cpm; ++, 2001–5000 cpm; +++, >5000 cpm. Met 1 and Met 2 designate breast tumor metastases to the liver from two individual patients.

[b] The live cell immunoassay was performed on human cells. Neg, <300 cpm; +, 300–1000 cpm; ++, 1001–2000 cpm; +++, > 2000 cpm.

[c] Rhabdomyosarcoma (A204), fibrosarcoma (HT-1080), and melanoma (A375, A101D, A875, A3875).

[d] Human cell lines were derived from apparently normal breast (HSo584Bst, HSo578Bst), embryonic skin (Detroit 550, 551), fetal lung (WI-38, MRC-5), fetal testis (HSo181Tes), fetal thymus (HSo208Th), fetal bone marrow (HSo074BM), embryonic kidney (FLOW-4000), fetal spleen (HSo203Sp), and uterus (HSo769Ut).

The eleven monoclonal antibodies could immediately be divided into three major groups based on their differential reactivity to Met 1 versus Met 2 in solid phase RIA (Table 1). The immunogen used in the generation of monoclonal B72.3 was Met 1, while the immunogen used for the generation of monoclonal B25.2 was Met 2. All eleven antibodies were negative when tested against similar extracts from normal human liver, a rhabdomyosarcoma cell line, the HBL-100 cell line derived from cultures of human milk cells, mouse mammary tumor and fibroblast cell lines, disrupted mouse mammary tumor virus and mouse leukemia virus, purified carcinoembryonic antigen (CEA), and ferritin. Two monoclonal antibodies were used as positive controls in all these studies: (a) W6/32, a commercially available antihuman histocompatibility antigen (Barnstable et al., 1978), and (b) B139, which was generated in our laboratory against a human breast tumor metastasis, and which demonstrates reactivity to all human cells tested (Table 1).

To determine whether the monoclonals bound cell surface determinants, each antibody was tested for binding to live cells in culture, i.e., established cell lines of human mammary carcinomas. The nine monoclonals grouped together on the basis of their binding to both metastatic cell extracts could be further separated into three different groups on the basis of their differential binding to cell surface determinants (Table 1). Many of the monoclonals also bound to the surface of selected nonbreast carcinoma cell lines (Kufe et al., 1983). None of the eleven monoclonal antibodies, however, bound to the surface of sarcoma or melanoma cell lines, nor to the surface of over 24 cell lines derived from apparently normal human tissues (Table 1, Colcher et al., 1981a; Kufe et al., 1983). Control monoclonals W6/32 or B139, however, did bind all of these cells (Table 1).

To further define the specificity and range of reactivity of each of the eleven monoclonal antibodies, the immunoperoxidase technique was employed on formalin-fixed tissue sections. All the monoclonals reacted with mammary carcinoma cells of primary mammary carcinomas, both infiltrating ductal and lobular. The percentage of primary mammary tumors that were reactive varied for the different monoclonals and in many of the positive primary and metastatic mammary carcinomas, not all tumor cells stained; both of these points will be discussed in detail below. A high degree of selective reactivity with mammary tumor cells, and not with apparently normal mammary epithelium (except in the area of the tumor), stroma, blood vessels, or lymphocytes of the breast was also observed.

Experiments were then carried out to determine if the eleven monoclonals could detect mammary carcinoma cell populations in regional nodes and at distal sites. Since the monoclonals were all generated using metastatic mammary carcinoma cells as antigens, it was not unexpected that the monoclonals all reacted, but with different degrees, to various metastases. None of the monoclonals reacted with normal lymphocytes or stroma from any involved or uninvolved nodes. The monoclonals were then tested for reactivity to normal and neoplastic nonmammary tissues. Most of the monoclonals showed reactivity with some nonbreast carcinomas such as adenocarcinoma of the colon as well as with selected normal epithelial cells, but showed no staining to sarcomas and lymphomas. Monoclonals B72.3 and B6.2 were chosen for further study since they appeared to be noncoordinately expressed in different breast tumor cells and reacted with approximately 50 and 75%, respectively, of 39 formalin-fixed infiltrating ductal carcinomas tested via the immunoperoxidase technique. The major cross-reactivity to normal tissues of monoclonal B6.2 was to subsets of circulating polymorphonuclear leukocytes. Thus far, monoclonal B72.3 has demonstrated the most selective degree of reactivity for tumor tissues in that no reactivity with adult normal human tissues has been detected. However, fetal tissue has not yet been carefully examined nor has absolutely every tissue type in the body. It would be naive to assume that any antigenic determinant consisting of a few amino acids would be expressed only on carcinoma cells, and at no time during development in the embryo, or at various stages of cell differentiation within the spectrum of adult tissues.

Since monoclonal B72.3 (an IgG_1) displayed the most restricted range of reactivity for human mammary tumor versus normal cells, this antibody was used for further studies to determine the effect of antibody concentration on the staining intensity and the percent of tumor cells stained in immunoperoxidase assays. Since one cannot titrate antigen in the fixed tissue section, an antibody dilution experiment was performed to give an indication of the relative titer of reactive antigen within a given tissue. A 500-fold range of antibody concentration, varying from 0.02 to 10 μg of purified B72.3 immunoglobulin (per 200 μL) per tissue section, was used on each of four mammary carcinomas from different patients. The results (Table 2) demonstrate that: (a) different mammary tumors may vary in the amount of the antigen detected by B72.3, (b) a given mammary tumor may contain tumor cell populations that vary in antigen density, and (c) some mammary tumors may score positive or negative depending on the dose of antibody employed. These studies point out a concept that must be kept in mind if tissue sections are to be used in prospective or retrospective prognostic studies using monoclonal antibodies. As seen in Table 2, using 4 μg of B72.3, Tumor 4 appears to have an antigenic phenotype different from that of the other three. However, when 1 μg of B72.3 is used in the assay, Tumor 3 now is the one that appears to have the unique phenotype. Thus, studies on tissue sections should always include antibody titrations and be evaluated on the basis of dose of antibody employed.

Table 2
Dose of Monoclonal Antibody B72.3 vs Reactivity of Human
Mammary Carcinoma Cells in
Immunoperoxidase Assay

B72.3,[b] μg	Tumor staining intensity[a]		% Reactive tumor cells	
	Tumor 1	Tumor 2	Tumor 3	Tumor 4
10	1+(90) 2+(10)	3+(100)	3+(80)	Neg
4	1+(5)	2+(100)	3+(80)	Neg
2	Neg	1+(80)	3+(70)	Neg
1	Neg	Neg	3+(70)	Neg
0.2	Neg	Neg	2+(50)	Neg
0.02	Neg	Neg	2+(30)	Neg

[a]Staining intensity: 1+ weak, 2+ moderate, 3+ strong.
[b]0.02 μg of B72.3 is equivalent to a 1:100,000 dilution of B72.3 produced in mouse ascites fluid.

To further characterize the range of reactivity of B72.3, the immunoperoxidase technique was used to test a variety of malignant, benign, and normal mammary tissues. Using 4 μg of monoclonal per slide the percent of positive primary breast tumors was 46% (19/41); 62% (13/21) of the metastatic lesions scored positive (Nuti et al., 1982). Several histologic types of primary mammary tumors scored positive: there were infiltrating ductal (Figs. 1A and B), infiltrating lobular, and comedo carcinomas. Many of the *in situ* elements present in the above lesions also stained (Fig. 1C) None of the six medullary carcinomas tested were positive. Approximately two-thirds of the tumors that showed a positive reactivity demonstrated a cell-associated membrane and/or diffuse cytoplasmic staining (Fig. 1B), approximately five percent showed discrete focal staining of the cytoplasm (Fig. 1D), and approximately one-fourth of the reactive tumors showed an apical or marginal staining pattern. Metastatic breast carcinoma lesions that were positive were in axillary lymph nodes, and at the distal sites of skin, liver, lung, pleura (Fig. 1D), and mesentery. Fifteen benign breast lesions were also tested; these included fibrocystic disease, fibroadenomas, and sclerosing adenosis. Two of these 15 specimens showed positive staining: one case of fibrocystic disease where a few cells in some ductals were faintly positive, and a case of intraductal papillomatosis and sclerosing adenosis with the majority of cells staining strongly. Monoclonal B72.3 was also tested against normal breast tissue from noncancer patients and showed no reactivity. A variety of nonbreast tissues were tested and were also negative; these included uterus, liver, spleen, lung, bone marrow, colon, stomach, salivary gland, lymph node, and kidney.

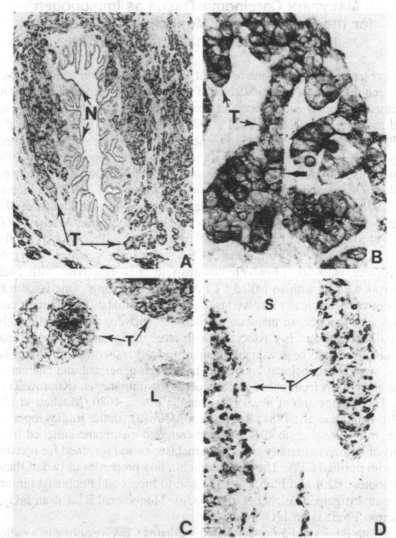

Fig. 1.   Immunoperoxidase staining of fixed tissue sections of primary and metastatic mammary carcinomas of four different patients with monoclonal antibody B72.3: (A) Infiltrating ductal carcinoma: at the center of the field is a negative large normal ductal (N) surrounded by positively staining infiltrating tumor cells (T). 54 ×; (B) Infiltrating ductal carcinoma; note the intense membrane and faint cytoplasmic staining of the tumor cells (T). The broad arrow indicates a negative tumor cell flanked by positive tumor cells. 540 ×; (C) *In situ* element (T) of an infiltrating ductal carcinoma: note the stroma and lymphocytes (L) that are negative. 130 ×; (D) Breast tumor metastasis in the pleura. This is an example of the focal pattern of staining: intense stain is concentrated in the cytoplasm of tumor cells (T). The stroma (S) is negative, 330 ×.

3. Mammary Carcinoma Tissue as Immunogen for the Preparation of Monoclonal Antibodies to Carcinoembryonic Antigen (CEA)

The presence of high plasma levels of CEA (Gold and Freedman, 1964) has been reported to be an indicator of the possible presence of metastatic disease in patients with cancers of the digestive system, breast, lung, as well as other sites (Hansen et al., 1974; Krebs et al., 1978; Gold et al., 1979). Using assays based on antibodies to colonic CEA, elevated plasma levels of CEA (above 2.5 ng/mL) have been reported in 38–79% of patients with mammary carcinomas (Chu and Nemoto, 1973; Hansen et al., 1974; Steward et al., 1974; Menendez-Botet et al., 1976; Lokich et al., 1978; Waalkes et al., 1978; Chatal et al., 1980; Wilkinson et al., 1980). There have been several reports (Pusztaszeri and Mach, 1973; Vrba et al., 1975; Chism et al., 1977; Dent et al., 1980; Rogers et al., 1981b), however, indicating that "CEA" is a heterogeneous family of glycoproteins, some of which demonstrate cross-reactivity with each other as well as with so called "CEA-related" proteins. One issue that has not yet been clearly resolved is the possibility that different tumor cell types may produce, or maintain on their cell surface, a CEA that is only partially related to CEA associated with other malignancies. Monoclonal antibodies should be a valuable reagent toward resolving this point. To date, several monoclonal antibodies have been generated and characterized using CEA from colon carcinomas as the immunogen (Koprowski et al., 1979; Miggiano et al., 1979; Accolla et al., 1980; Mitchell et al., 1980; Kupcik et al., 1981; Rogers et al., 1981a). In the studies reported here, monoclonal antibodies were generated to membrane-enriched fractions of human mammary carcinoma metastases and screened for reactivity with purified CEA. The differential binding properties of two of these antibodies (B1.1 and F5.5.) to CEA and to breast and nonbreast tumors were investigated (Colcher et al., 1983a). Monoclonal B1.1 is an IgG_{2a}, whereas F5.5. is an IgG_1.

Both B1.1 and F5.5 precipitated iodinated CEA, resulting in a radiolabeled peak at approximately 180,000 daltons. No precipitation of purified CEA was obtained using monoclonal antibody B6.2, B72.3, nor with any of the monoclonals described above. Purified immunoglobulin preparations of monoclonals B1.1 and F5.5 were then titered for binding to five CEA purified from five different patients with colon cancer; significant binding was observed with both antibodies to all five CEA. Monoclonals B1.1 and F5.5 were shown to be clearly reactive with different epitopes on the CEA molecule, however, as evidenced by their differential binding to the various CEA preparations. Specifically, monoclonal F5.5 reacted similarly with all five CEA preparations whereas B1.1 exhibited preferential binding to different CEA preparations.

Monoclonals B1.1 and F5.5 were tested for binding to live cells in culture to further define their range of reactivities, and to ascertain if they bound to antigenic determinants present on the cell surface. Both monoclonals bound to the same three of six established human mammary carcinoma cell lines and to the two colon carcinoma cell lines, but not to the lung carcinoma or vulva carcinoma cell lines. No surfacing binding was observed with either antibody to 13 cell lines derived from apparently normal human tissues, but both bound to the surface of peripheral blood polymorphonuclear leukocytes (Colcher et al., 1983a). The two monoclonals could be distinguished, however, by their differential reactivity to the surface of melanoma cell lines. B1.1 bound to three of four melanoma cell lines tested, whereas F5.5 did not bind to any of the four. To further identify the range of reactivities of monoclonals B1.1 and F5.5 with human mammary carcinomas, the immunoperoxidase technique was used on formalin-fixed tumor sections. Monoclonals F5.5 and B1.1 reacted positively with 55 and 66%, respectively, of the mammary carcinomas tested. The positive mammary tumors included infiltrating ductal, *in situ*, and medullary carcinomas. Monoclonals B1.1 and F5.5 also reacted positively with metastatic mammary tumor cells in lymph nodes and at distal sites. It is anticipated that studies can now be undertaken to determine if the presence of, the intensity of, or the cellular localization of these reactions, using either or both of these monoclonals with tissue sections of primary breast lesions, is of any prognostic value. A previous study (Sehested et al., 1981) performed using heterologous anti-CEA polyclonal antisera and small cell carcinomas of the lung, has indicated that CEA reactivity of tissue sections may have prognostic significance.

4. Identification and Purification of Mammary Tumor-Associated Antigens

As a first step in the identification of the best source of antigens reactive with the monoclonal antibodies described, monoclonal antibodies were screened by solid phase RIA for reactivity with a variety of mammary tumor extracts including primary and metastatic tumors and established cells lines. Monoclonals B1.1 and B6.2 reacted similarly with tissue extracts and extracts of cell lines. Antibody B72.3, however, showed very strong reactivity with approximately 50% of extracts of human breast tumors, but reacted poorly with virtually all mammary tumor cell lines. Two breast tumor metastases to the liver were thus chosen as the prime sources for antigen identification and purification on the basis of their broad immunoreactivity with all the monoclonal antibodies.

An extract of a breast tumor metastasis to the liver was detergent-disrupted and separated using molecular sieving on Ultrogel AcA34; the column fractions were assayed for reactivity with monoclonals B1.1, and B6.2, and B72.3 by solid phase RIA; the appropriate immunoreactive fractions were then pooled and labeled with [125]I. SDS-PAGE analyses of the immunoprecipitates generated are seen in Fig. 2. B72.3 immunoprecipitated a complex of four bands with molecular weights of approximately 220,000–400,000 dalton. B1.1 immunoprecipitated a heterogenous component with an average estimated molecular weight of 180,000. B6.2 immunoprecipitated a 90,000 dalton component as did several other monoclonal antibodies. An extract of a breast tumor metastasis to the liver, which demonstrated strong immunoreactivity with B72.3, was therefore used as the starting material for purification of the 220,000–400,000 dalton high molecular weight complex. Following detergent disruption and high speed centrifugation, the supernatant was subjected to molecular sieving using Ultrogel AcA34. Immunoreactive fractions were then passed through a B72.3 antibody affinity column and eluted with 3M KSCN. Radiolabeled aliquots from the various purification steps were analyzed by SDS-PAGE (Fig. 3). Only minimal radioactivity in the high molecular weight range was seen in gel patterns of the AcA34 pool, whereas the B72.3 antibody affinity column eluant demonstrated the four distinct bands of the 220,000–400,000 dalton com-

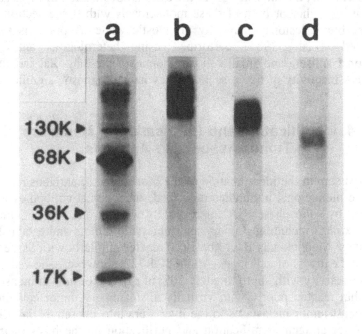

Fig. 2.   Immunoprecipitation of ^{125}I-labeled extract of a human breast tumor metastases. Lane a: markers, immunoprecipitation by monoclonal antibodies B72.3 (lane b), B1.1 (lane c) and B6.2 (lane d).

Extract   AcA-34   Affinity
(100,000xg)   (Pool-B)   (B72.3)

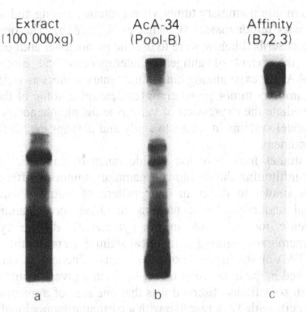

a   b   c

Fig. 3.   Purification of mammary tumor-associated antigen reactive with monoclonal B72.3. SDS-PAGE of ^{125}I-labeled extract from breast tumor metastasis at various purification steps. An equal amount of each ^{125}I-labeled sample was loaded onto the gel. Lane: (a) 100,000g supernatant of crude extract; (b) pool of AcA34 fractions reactive with B72.3; (c) pool of eluant of B72.3 affinity column fractions.

plex. This ^{125}I-labeled B72.3 affinity purified antigen was also shown to be immunoreactive by solid phase RIA. Normal human liver extract was subjected to the identical method of purification; at no step within the purification scheme was any reactivity with B72.3 detected.

5. Antigenic Modulation and Evolution Within Human Mammary Carcinoma Cell Populations

In 1954, Foulds documented the existence of distinct morphologies in different areas of a single mammary tumor. Since then, several investigators have reported the occurrence of heterogeneity in a variety of tumor cell populations (Kerbel, 1979; Hart and Fidler, 1981). Using a variety of methods and reagents including heterologous antisera, heterogeneity has also been observed with respect to the antigenic properties of tumor cell populations (Prehn, 1970; Pimm and Baldwin, 1977; Kerbel, 1979; Miller and Heppner, 1979; Poste et al., 1981). Consistent with this finding, we have observed antigenic heterogeneity, as defined by the expression of tumor-associated antigens (TAA) detected by monoclonal antibodies to mouse mammary tumor virus proteins, among and within murine mammary tumor masses (Colcher et al., 1981b). The objectives of the studies described below were to use the monoclonal antibodies to: (a) determine the extent of antigenic heterogeneity and modulation of specific TAA that exist among human mammary tumors as well as within a given mammary tumor population; (b) determine some of the parameters that mediate the expression of various antigenic phenotypes; and (c) develop model systems in which to study and perhaps eventually control these phenomena.

Our studies have revealed a wide range of antigenic phenotypes present in infiltrating ductal human mammary tumors. Different tumors have been shown to differ in their pattern of staining with a given monoclonal antibody. These patterns included focal staining (representing dense foci of TAA in the cytoplasm), diffuse cytoplasmic staining, membrane staining, and apical staining (representing a concentration of TAA on the luminal borders of cells). Phenotypic variation was also observed in the expression of TAA within a given mammary tumor. One pattern sometimes observed was that one area of a mammary tumor contained cells with TAA reactive with a particular monoclonal antibody, whereas another area of the same tumor contained cells that were unreactive with the identical antibody. A more common type of antigenic heterogeneity was observed among cells in a given area of a tumor mass. This type of antigenic diversity, termed "patchwork," reveals tumor cells expressing a specific TAA directly adjacent to tumor cells negative for the same antigen (Fig. 1B). Patterns of reactivity with a specific monoclonal antibody were also observed to vary within a given tumor mass, i.e., antigen was detected in the cytoplasm of cells in one part of the tumor mass, and on the luminal edge of differentiated structures in a different part of the same mass.

In an attempt to elucidate the phenomenon of antigenic heterogeneity in human mammary tumors, model systems were examined. The MCF-7 human mammary tumor cell line was tested for the presence of TAA using the cytospin/immunoperoxidase method (Nuti et al., 1982; Hand et al., 1983). This cell line was shown to contain various subpopulations of cells as defined by variability in expression of TAA reactive with monoclonal antibody B6.2 or B1.1, i.e., positive MCF-7 cells are seen adjacent to cells that scored negative.

Studies were conducted to determine if the antigenic heterogeneity observed in MCF-7 cells was (1) the result of at least two stable genotypes or phenotypes, or (2) was the reflection of a modulation of cell surface antigen expression of a single phenotype, or (3) the result of both phenomena. In experiments designed to monitor cell surface antigen expression in different phases of cell growth, it was observed that MCF-7 cells at contact inhibition expressed less antigen on their surface, as detected by monoclonal B6.2, than cells in active proliferation. Using fluorescence activated cell sorter analyses, it has been shown that two of the monoclonal antibodies developed (B6.2 and B38.1) are most reactive with the surface of MCF-7 cells during S-phase of the cell cycle (Fig. 4, Kufe et al., 1983). For this reason, all the experiments using cell lines described below were performed with cells in log phase.

Studies were undertaken to determine if any change in antigenic phenotype occurs during extended passage of cells in culture. The BT-20 human breast cancer cell line, obtained at passage 288, was serially passaged and assayed at each passage level during logarithmic growth. As seen in Table 3, a cell surface HLA antigen, detected by anti-HLA monoclonal W6/32, was present at all passage levels, as was the antigen detected by monoclonal antibody B38.1. The antigen detected by

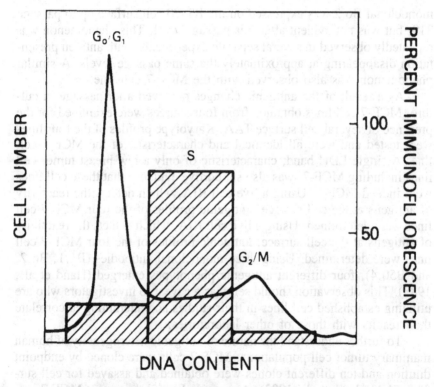

Fig. 4. Analysis of effects of cell cycle on the expression of cell surface tumor-associated antigens. MCF-7 cells were grown to confluency and 24 h after passage were stained with Hoechst dye (5 µg/mL for 1 h at 37°C). Approximately $1–2 \times 10^6$ cells were treated with 0.1 mL of monoclonal antibody B6.2 at a concentration of 0.2 µg/1 mL, and then reacted with 0.1 mL of a 1:40 dilution of goat anti-mouse fluorosceinisothiocyanate. Cells were then analyzed by flow cytometry and indirect immunofluorescence (Kufe et al., 1983).

Table 3
Differential Expression of Tumor Associated Antigens in BT-20
Cells upon Passage[a]

Mab	Passage number					
	316	317	318	319	320	323
W6/32	690[b]	1620	750	620	700	500
B38.1	2560	2280	1380	1640	1550	1320
B6.2	1620	2910	560	710	Neg[c]	Neg
B14.2	1600	1380	Neg	Neg	Neg	Neg

[a]Monoclonal antibodies were tested for binding to the surface of BT-20 mammary tumor cells in a live cell RIA.

[b]Values are expressed as cpm above background.

[c]Neg = <200 cpm.

monoclonal B6.2 was expressed on the BT-20 cell surface up to passage 319, but was not evident after this passage level. This phenomenon was repeatedly observed in several separate experiments, with antigen presentation disappearing at approximately the same passage levels. A similar phenomenon was also observed with the MCF-7 cell line.

As a result of the antigenic changes observed after passage in culture, MCF-7 cell lines obtained from four sources were examined for the presence of several cell surface TAA. Karyotype profiles of the four lines were tested and were all identical and characteristic of the MCF-7 cell line. A single LDH band, characteristic of only a few breast tumor cell lines including MCF-7, was also supportive evidence that these cell lines were indeed MCF-7. Using a live cell RIA, which detects the reactivity of antigens at the cell surface, antigenic profiles of the four MCF-7 cell lines were determined. Using a live cell RIA, which detects the reactivity of antigens at the cell surface, antigenic profiles of the four MCF-7 cell lines were determined. Using three monoclonal antibodies (B1.1, B6.2, and B50.4), four different antigenic phenotypes emerged (Hand et al., 1983). This observation should serve as a caveat to investigators who are utilizing established cell lines in their studies and attempting to correlate their results with those of other laboratories.

To further understand the nature of antigenic heterogeneity of human mammary tumor cell populations, MCF-7 cells were cloned by endpoint dilution and ten different clones were obtained and assayed for cell surface TAA (Hand et al., 1983). As seen in Fig. 5, the parent MCF-7 culture reacts most strongly with monoclonal antibody B1.1 and least with monoclonal B72.3. Clone 6F1 (Fig. 5B) exhibits a similar phenotype to that of the parent (Fig. 5A). At least three additional major phenotypes were observed among the other clones. For example, clone 10B5 is devoid of detectable expression of any of the antigens assayed (Fig. 5C), although it does contain HLA and human antigens detected by

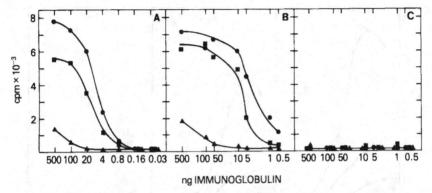

Fig. 5. Reactivity of monoclonal antibodies with the surface of the parent MCF-7 mammary adenocarcinoma cell line and cloned MCF-7 cell populations. Using a live cell radioimmunoassay, increasing amounts of monoclonal antibodies B1.1 (closed circle), B6.2 (closed square), and B72.3 (closed triangle), were tested for binding to the parent MCF-7 cell line (Panel A), MCF-7 clone 6F1 (Panel B), and MCF-7 clone 10B5 (Panel C).

monoclonal antibodies W6/32 and B139, respectively (Hand et al., 1983).

To determine the stability of the cell surface phenotype of the MCF-7 clones, each line was monitored through a four month period and assayed during log phase at approximately every other passage. Although some of the MCF-7 clones maintained a stable antigenic phenotype throughout the observation period, a dramatic change in antigenic phenotype, i.e., antigenic evolution, was observed in some of the clones (Fig. 6).

Antigenic variability of TAA among and within human mammary tumor cell populations presents a potential problem in the development and optimization of immunodiagnostic and therapeutic procedures for breast cancer. Knowledge about the nature of this antigenic heterogeneity may therefore be helpful in the prediction or control of the expression of specific antigenic phenotypes. The studies described here have enabled us to demonstrate the extent of specific antigenic variability in vivo as well as within human mammary tumor cell populations in vitro. The variability observed in cell surface expression of some antigens in different stages of the cell cycle indicates that the "patchwork" antigenic heterogeneity observed in tissue sections may reflect, in part, cells in different phases of growth. The studies involving the MCF-7 cell clones indicate that some stable antigenic phenotypes may exist, but other clones demonstrated an antigenic evolution, i.e., the gradual expression of specific cell surface TAA with extended passage. One can thus hypothesize that the antigenic phenotype of a given tumor mass in situ, as defined by monoclonal antibodies, may differ at the time of detection versus later stages of tumor progression. This concept must be further investigated if

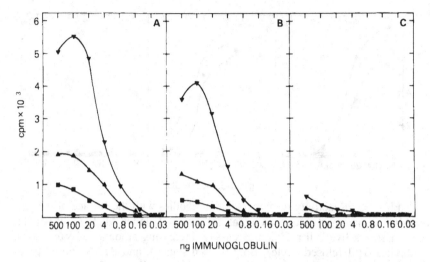

Fig. 6.   Detection of TAA in a MCF-7 cloned population with continued cell passage. Using a live cell RIA to detect cell surface antigen expresson, increasing amounts of monoclonal antibodies B1.1 (Panel A), B6.2 (Panel B), and B72.3 (Panel C) were tested for binding to MCF-7 clone 10B5 at passage 6 (circles); passage 9 (squares); passage 12 (triangles); and passage 15 (inverted triangles).

monoclonal antibodies are to play a useful role in diagnosis, prognosis, and therapy of breast cancer.

6. Differential Reactivity of a Monoclonal Antibody (DF3) with Human Malignant vs Benign Breast Tumors

Mab DF3 was generated using a membrane-enriched fraction from a human metastatic mammary carcinoma (Kufe et al., submitted for publication). The molecular weight of the reactive antigen is approximately 290,000 daltons, and it is found on the surface of mammary carcinoma cells. Whereas Mab DF3 is reactive with the vast majority of several histologic types of malignant and benign human breast tumors, it shows a strong differential reactivity to cytoplasmic antigen in carcinomas versus reactivity to antigen concentrated on apical borders in benign breast lesions (Kufe et al., in press).

Several histologic types of human malignant mammary carcinomas were examined for reactivity with MAb DF3 using the ABC immunoperoxidase method and 5-μm sections of formalin-fixed tissues. Mab DF3 was reactive with 78% of 32 infiltrating ductal carcinomas (IDC), with the proportion of tumor cells staining within each of the 25 IDC ranging from a few to over 90% (Fig. 7). Further, the staining pat-

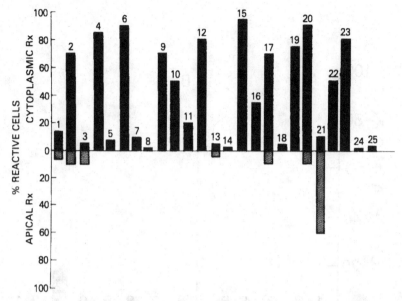

Fig. 7.   Reactivity of Mab DF3 with 5 μm sections of infiltrating ductal carcinomas using the ABC immunoperoxidase method. Each bar represents a different patient. The dark areas represent the percent of tumor cells with a cytoplasmic reaction; the striped areas represent the percent of tumor cells displaying Mab DF3 reactivity on apical borders.

tern for these carcinomas was primarily cytoplasmic (Fig. 7). A similar staining pattern was observed for mammary carcinomas containing both infiltrating ductal and intraductal elements. The percent reactive cells varied for individual tumors, and the infiltrating elements of each tumor displayed a higher degree of cytoplasmic reactivity than the intraductal component. Similar staining patterns were observed with *in situ*, medullary, and infiltrating lobular carcinomas. The three infiltrating lobular carcinomas and one medullary carcinoma showed only cytoplasmic staining. In contrast, the *in situ* carcinomas had varying degrees of cytoplasmic and apical border reactivity.

In contrast to the cytoplasmic reactivity observed with the malignant breast tissues, Mab DF3 reacted principally with the apical borders of all benign breast lesions. A similar pattern of reactivity was observed with a lactating breast tissue. Approximately 10–20% of normal ducts from breast tumor patients also showed a slight apical staining. However, none of five fibroadenomas (Fig. 8A), only one of eight fibrocystic disease specimens (Fig. 8B), and no normal duct cells showed any evidence of cytoplasmic Mab DF3 reactive antigen.

In scoring the reactivity (cytoplasmic and apical) of Mab DF3 with human breast tumors, 87% of 52 malignant lesions, and 100% of 13 benign lesions were positive. If reactivities were scored on the basis of only

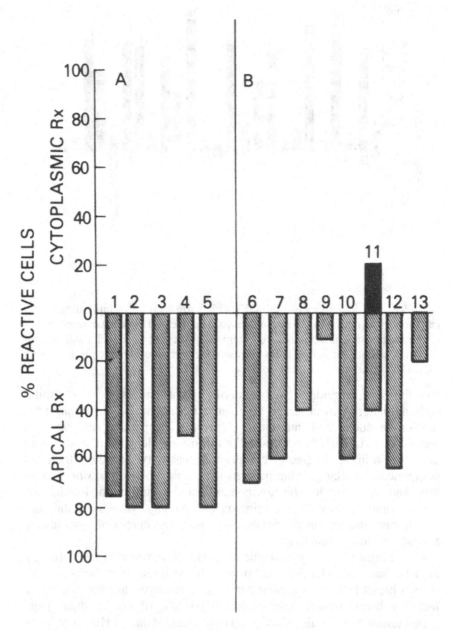

Fig. 8.   Reactivity of Mab DF3 with 5 μm sections of benign mammary tumors using the immunoperoxidose method. panal A represents 5 fibro-adenomas, and Panel B represents eight fibrocystic disease specimens. The dark areas represent the percent of tumor cells with a cytoplasmic reaction; the striped areas represent the percent tumor cells displaying Mab DF3 reactivity on apical borders.

cytoplasmic staining, however, 78% of malignant lesions were positive, whereas only one of thirteen benign lesions displayed this pattern of reactivity.

Primary and metastatic breast carcinomas from three patients were also examined for reactivity with Mab DF3; all 14 metastases to axillary lymph nodes and distal sites were positive. The pattern of reactivity for distal metastatic disease was uniformly cytoplasmic as was observed with the primary breast carcinomas. One exception was one lung metastasis obtained from one patient that also revealed some degree of apical staining. The reactivity of Mab DF3 with breast tumor metastasis is demonstrated in Fig. 9. Figure 9A shows the strongly staining breast carcinoma cells metastatic to ovary. Figure 9B reveals strongly reactive metastatic disease in the bone marrow of the same patient.

Since the immunogen used to prepare Mab DF3 was a membrane-enriched fraction of a human mammary carcinoma metastatic to liver, we compared reactivity of this antibody with the similarly prepared Mabs B6.2, B72.3, and B1.1. Mab B72.3 is reactive with a 220–400 kilodalton glycoprotein complex, whereas Mab B1.1 is reactive with the 180 kilodalton glycoprotein CEA. In contrast, Mab DF3 reacts with a 290 kilodalton antigen detectable in metastatic tumor but not in uninvolved liver. Furthermore, there was no correlation in terms of reactivity of Mab DF3 and B72.3 with 20 primary breast carcinomas. Similarly, there was noncoordinate expression of antigens reactive with Mab DF3, B6.2, and B1.1 in 10 primary breast carcinomas (Kufe et al.)

It was of further interest to determine whether the immunoperoxidase staining of human breast tumors with Mab DF3 is related to cell surface expression of the reactive antigen. The reactivity of Mab DF3 with MCF-7 breast carcinoma cells was demonstrated using indirect immunofluorescence. MCF-7 and the BT-20 mammary carcinoma cells were also assayed for surface antigen using a live-cell radioimmunoassay. Mab DF3 bound to the surface of both cell lines. In contrast, there was no evidence of Mab DF3 binding to the surface of two human colon carcinoma cell lines (Kufe et al., in press).

The above results have shown that the DF3 antigen is present in high levels on apical borders of differentiated secretory mammary epithelial cells and in the cytosol of less differentiated cells. This finding could have prognostic significance. For example, the prognostically more favorable in situ carcinomas demonstrated predominantly apical reactivity with Mab DF3. Tubular breast carcinomas, another pathologic category of favorable outcome, also reacted with Mab DF3 along apical borders. Immunoperoxidase staining of large numbers of primary breast tumors as a correlate of disease-free survival will now be required to resolve the prognostic value of reactivity with this antibody.

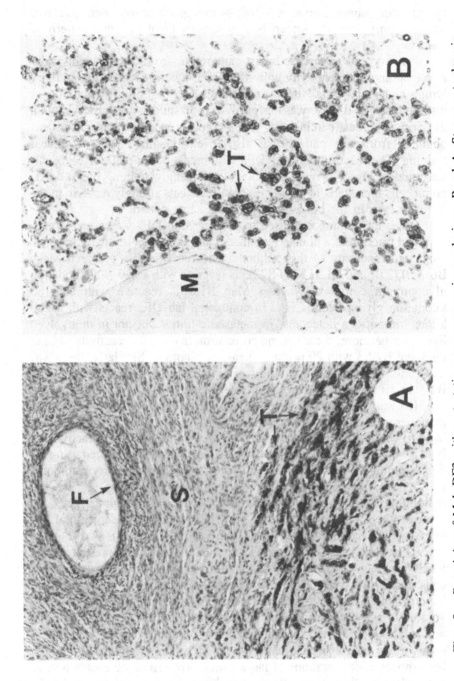

Fig. 9. Reactivity of Mab DF3 with metastatic mammary carcinoma lesions. Panel A: Strong cytoplasmic reactivity with a mammary tumor metastases (T) in the ovary; S is stroma; F is follicular cyst, 130 ×. Panel B is positive metastatic mammary tumor cells (T) in the bone marrow (M), 220 ×.

7. Radiolocalization of Human Mammary Tumor Transplants in Athymic Mice by a Monoclonal Antibody

With the development of the hybridoma technology, homogenous populations of Mabs to TAA can now be utilized in either lymphoscintigraphy, to detect mammary tumor lesions in nodes of the axilla and internal mammary chain, or to detect distal metastases. In the studies described here, Mab B6.2, which may be useful in lymphoscintigraphy procedures, was utilized. B6.2 IgG was purified, and F(ab')$_2$ and Fab' fragments were generated by pepsin digestion. All three forms of the antibody were radiolabeled and assayed to determine their utility in the radioimmunolocalization of transplanted human mammary tumor masses (Colcher et al., 1983b).

The IgG and its fragments were labeled with ^{125}I using the iodogen method to specific activities of 15–50 µCi/µg. The labeled antibody was shown to bind to the surface of live MCF-7 cells and retained the same specificity as the unlabeled antibody. Better than 70% of the antibody remained immunoreactive in sequential saturation solid-phase RIA after labeling.

Athymic mice bearing the Clouser transplantable human mammary tumor were injected with 0.1 µg of ^{125}I-Mab B6.2. The ratio of radioactivity/mg of tissue in the tumor compared to that of various tissues rose over a 4-d period and then fell at 7 d. The tumor to tissue ratios were 10:1 or greater in the liver, spleen, and kidney at day 4 (Colcher et al., 1983b). Ratios of the counts in the tumor to that found in the brain and muscle were greater than 50:1 and as high as 110:1. When the mammary tumor bearing mice were injected with ^{125}I-F(ab')$_2$ fragments of B6.2, higher tumor to tissue ratios were obtained. The tumor to tissue ratios in the liver and spleen were 15–20:1 at 96 h. This was probably a result of the faster clearance of the F(ab')$_2$ fragments, as compared to the IgG. Athymic mice bearing a human melanoma (A375), a tumor that shows no surface reactivity with B6.2 in live cell RIAs, were used as controls and were negative for nonspecific binding of the labeled antibody or antibody fragments to tumor tissue. Similarly, no localization was observed when either normal murine IgG or MOPC-21 IgG$_1$ (the same isotype as B6.2 from a murine myeloma), or their F(ab')$_2$ fragments, were radiolabeled and inoculated into athymic mice bearing human mammary tumor or melanoma transplants. Athymic mice bearing Clouser mammary tumors were also injected with ^{125}I-labeled B6.2 Fab'. The clearance rate of the Fab' fragment was considerably faster than the larger F(ab')$_2$ fragment and the intact IgG. Acceptable tumor to tissue ratios were obtained, but the fast clearance rate resulted in a large amount of the labeled Fab' being found in the kidney and bladder, resulting in low tumor to kidney ratios. These studies therefore indicate that F(ab')₂ fragments are superior to Fab' or intact IgG in the radiolocalization studies in mice with monoclonal antibody B6.2.

Studies were undertaken to determine whether the localization of the ¹²⁵I-labeled antibody and fragments in the tumors was sufficient to detect using a gamma camera (Colcher et al., 1983b). Athymic mice bearing the Clouser mammary tumor or the A375 melanoma were injected iv with approximately 30 μCi of ¹²⁵I-B6.2 IgG. The mice were scanned and then sacrificed at 24 h intervals. The Clouser tumors were easily detected at 24 h (Fig. 10A) using radiolabeled B6.2 IgG, with a small amount of activity detectable in the blood pool. The tumor remained strongly positive over the 4-d period with the background activity decreasing to the point where it was barely detectable at 96 h (Fig. 10B). The 0.5 cm diameter tumors localized in Figs. 10A and 10B appear bigger than their actual size; this may be due to the dispersion of rays through the pinhole collimeter. No tumor localization was observed using radiolabeled B6.2 IgG in mice bearing the control human melanoma transplants (Fig. 10C).

Mice were also injected with ¹²⁵I-B6.2 F(ab')₂ fragments. The mice cleared the fragments faster than the intact IgG and a significant amount of activity was observed in the two kidneys and bladder at 24 h (Fig. 11A), but tumors were clearly positive for localization of the ¹²⁵I-B6.2 F(ab')₂ fragments. The activity was cleared from the kidneys and bladder by 48 h and the tumor to background ratio increased over the 4-d period of scanning, with little background and good tumor localization observed at 96 h (Fig. 11B). No localization of activity was observed with the radiolabeled B6.2 F(ab')₂ fragments in the athymic mice bearing the A375 melanoma (Fig. 11C).

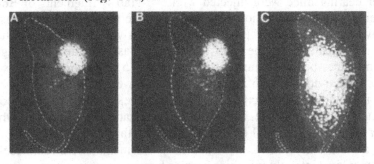

Fig. 10.   Gamma camera scanning of athymic mice bearing transplanted human tumors using ¹²⁵I-labeled B6.2 IgG. Athymic mice bearing a transplantable human mammary tumor (Clouser, Panels A and B) or a human melanoma (A375, Panel C) were inoculated with approximately 30 μCi of ¹²⁵I-B6.2 IgG. The mice were scanned after various time intervals (24 h, Panel A, C; 96 h, panel B) until an equal number of counts were detected in each field.

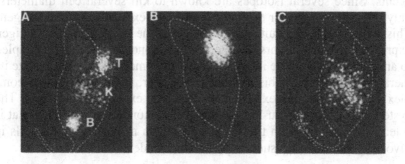

Fig. 11. Gamma camera scanning of athymic mice bearing transplanted human tumors using ^{125}I-labeled B6.2 F(ab')$_2$. Athymic mice bearing a transplantable human mammary tumor (Clouser, Panels A and B) or a human melanoma (A375, Panel C) were inoculated with approximately 30 μCi of ^{125}I-B6.2 F(ab')$_2$. The mice were scanned after various time intervals (24 h, Panel A; 96 h, Panels B and C) until an equal number of counts were detected in each field. (T = tumor, K = kidney, B = bladder).

The ^{125}I labeled antibody and fragments all successfully localized tumors with the F(ab')$_2$ fragment giving the overall highest tumor to tissue ratios. The Fab' or F(ab')$_2$ fragments may be the better forms to use because of the potential problem of Fc receptors on a variety of cells binding the labeled IgG and yielding a higher nonspecific distribution of the antibody. The use of an antibody without the Fc portion should also reduce its immunoreactivity in patients and thus minimize an immune response. The smaller fragments also clear the body faster than intact immunoglobulin and should thus result in a lower whole body radiation-absorbed dose to the host.

Radiolabeled monoclonal antibodies that are reactive with the surface of human mammary carcinoma cells may eventually prove useful in several areas in the management of human breast cancer. The detection of occult metastatic lesions at distal sites via gamma scanning could serve as an adjunct in determining which patients should receive adjuvant therapy, and subsequent scanning may reveal which tumors are responding to therapy. At present, only axillary lymph nodes, removed at mastectomy, are examined for tumor involvement for use in staging; the extent of nodal tumor involvement in the internal mammary chain is not determined. The use of radiolabeled monoclonal antibodies in lymphoscintigraphy of the internal mammary chain may thus eventually increase the reliability of staging of nodal involvement as a prognostic indicator. Along with their potential in the diagnosis and prognosis of breast cancer, monoclonal antibodies coupled with isotopes decaying via high energy transfer with short range radiation may eventually prove useful as radiotherapeutic agents. Since several isotopes are known to kill several cell diameters, only one cell of a cluster of tumor cells needs express the target antigen. This approach may be quite useful in light of the heterogeneity of antigen expression in some tumors. Furthermore, a monoclonal antibody coupled to an isotope need not be internalized by the tumor cell for it to realize its therapeutic potential. This approach, however, is obviously quite complex and would require extensive studies in an experimental system. The system described here, using a radiolabeled monoclonal antibody that is selectively reactive with the surface of human mammary tumor cells in vivo may provide one such experimental model.

8. The Use of Recombinant Interferon to Enhance Detection of Human Carcinoma Antigens by Monoclonal Antibodies

As shown above, a high degree of antigenic heterogeneity exists in many human carcinoma cell populations. Such heterogeneity will undoubtedly compromise the effectiveness of Mab for the detection and/or therapy of human carcinomas. In fact, if Mab are to be used successfully for the *in situ* detection or therapy of human carcinoma lesions the phenomenon of antigenic heterogeneity must be modified so that most, if not all, cells of a tumor mass express a given tumor-associated antigen (TAA). One approach would be to investigate whether well defined substances that (a) alter states of cell differentiation and (b) have potential clinical applicability may also possess the capability of modifying the expression of cell surface TAA. Native interferon (Attallah et al., 1979; Imai et al., 1981; Grant et al., 1982; Fellous et al., 1982) and recombinant human leukocyte interferon (IFN-αA) (Fisher et al., 1983; Pestka, 1983) meet those two criteria. Because of its homogeneity, stability, and extensive degree of characterization, recombinant human leukocyte (clone A) interferon (IFN-αA) (Staehlin et al., 1981a; Staehlin et al., 1981b; Pestka, 1983) was thus evaluated for its ability to enhance the detection of TAA on the surface of human carcinoma cells by Mab (Greiner et al., 1984).

IFN-αA was first titrated on the human mammary carcinoma cell line MCF-7 for its ability to enhance the detection of tumor-associated as well as normal cell surface antigens (Greiner et al., 1984). A solid-phase RIA with live cells and various concentrations of purified monoclonal immunoglobulin was used to detect antigen expression. A 5×10^4 quantity of cells, with or without various amounts of IFN-αA, was seeded in 96 well plates. As seen in Fig. 12, 10, 100, or 1000 U/mL of IFN-αA enhanced the detection of the 90K (Fig. 12C), the 180K CEA (Fig. 12D), and the 220–400K (Fig. 12E) TAA by Mab B6.2, B1.1, and B72.3, respectively, in a dose-dependent manner. Mab directed against two anti-

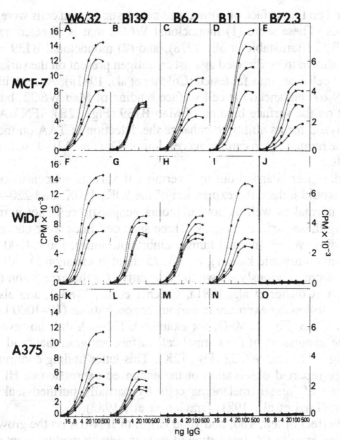

Fig. 12.   The effect of recombinant IFN-αA on the expression of human tumor-associated and normal cell surface antigens. The live cell solid phase RIA used has been described previously (Hand et al., 1983). Panels A–E are MCF-7 human mammary carcinoma cells; Panels F–J are WiDr colon carcinoma cells; panels K–O are A375 melanoma cells (FLOW 4000 human embryonic kidney, and WI-38 human embryonic lung cell gave similar results.). Monoclonal IgG were affinity-purified and used at the amounts indicated. Mab W6/32 (Panels A, F, K) and Mabs B139 (Panels B, G, L), B6.2 (C, H, M), B1.1 (D, I, N), and B72.3 (E, J, O) are described in the text. 5×10^4 cells were incubated at 37°C for 24 h at which time the medium containing the appropriate Mab was added. After 1 h at 37°C, cells were washed 2× and 75,000 cpm (in 50 μL) of ^{125}I-labeled goat anti-mouse IgG was added. After 1 h at 37°C, cells were washed 3× and the cpm bound was determined. IFN-αA was obtained and purified as previously described (Staehlin et al., 1981a). The specific activity of the preparation used was 2×10^8 U/mg protein when tested on MDBK (bovine kidney) cells. Amounts of IFN-αA/mL used were 10 U (squares), 100 U (triangles), 1000 U (diamonds). Control buffer, RPMI 1640, containing 1% BSA is denoted by circles.

gens found on the surface of normal and neoplastic human cells were used as controls. These were (1) monoclonal W6/32 that is directed against HLA-A,B,C (Barnstable et al., 1978), and (2) monoclonal B139 which has been shown to be directed against an antigen present on the surface of all human cell lines thus far tested (Colcher et al., 1981a). As seen in Fig. 12A, IFN-αA enhanced the cell surface binding of Mab W6/32, but had no effect on the surface binding of Mab B139 (Fig. 12B). IFN-αA was then analyzed for its ability to enhance the detection of TAA on the surface of the human colon carcinoma cell line WiDr (Fig. 12F–J) with similar results.

Studies were carried out to determine if various concentrations of IFN-αA would induce the expression of the 90K, 180K, and 220–400K TAA on normal as well as noncarcinoma neoplastic cells not normally expressing these surface antigens. Three such cell lines were chosen for these studies: WI-38 (normal human embryonic lung), Flow 4000 (normal human embryonic kidney), and A375 (human melanoma). All three cell lines were previously shown to be negative for the expression of the three TAA (Colcher et al., 1981a; Colcher et al., 1983a), and also remained so following exposure to various concentrations (10–1000 U/mL) of IFN-αA (see Fig. 12M–O, for example). IFN-αA did, however, increase the expression of the normal cell surface antigens that bind Mabs B139 (Fig. 12L) and W6/32 (Fig. 12K). This latter finding confirms the previously reported observation of the enhanced expression of HLA on the surface of human melanoma cells by partially purified leukocyte interferon (Imai et al., 1981; Braylon et al., 1982).

The effect of ten, 100, and 1000 U/mL of IFN-αA on the growth of MCF-7 was monitored. Incubation of cells in growth medium containing 10 or 100 U/mL IFN-αA for 6 d had no appreciable effect on cell growth; incubation with 1000 U/mL IFN-αA for 6 d reduced the total cell number by approximately 46%. However, no effect on cell number was observed 1, 2, or 4 d following IFN-αA addition at any dose level. Similar results were found using WiDr cells. Since IFN-αA effects on the expression of surface TAA were maximal after 24 h and since all determinations were made at this time interval and similar results were observed using either 100 or 1000 U/mL, the enhanced TAA expression appears to be independent of changes in cell proliferation.

The dose and temporal dependence for the enhancement of TAA expression by IFN-αA were also studied. The binding of B1.1 to the surface of MCF-7 cells exhibited a dose-dependent increase up to approximately 100 U IFN-αA/mL. The addition of higher units (and more cytotoxic) IFN-αA was less effective in enhancing the expression of the TAA. The IFN-αA-mediated enhancement of TAA expression on the surface of MCF-7 and WiDr cells was also temporally dependent. For example, an increased level of binding for Mab B1.1 to the surface of MCF-7 cells could be detected 4 h after the addition of 1000 U IFN-αA to the growth medium. The increase of B1.1 binding continued to rise with time and became maximal 16–24 h following IFN-αA addition.

The enhanced TAA expression on the surface of human breast and colon carcinoma cells mediated by recombinant human leukocyte interferon could be caused by a variety of cellular and/or molecular changes that include (1) the increased expression of TAA on a subpopulation of cells already expressing the TAA, (2) the induction of the expression of a given TAA on a population of cells not previously expressing the antigen, (3) a change in the surface area of the cell, or (4) a combination of any of these phenomena. To explore such possibilities, Mab B1.1 was reacted with WiDr human carcinoma cells in the presence or absence of 1000 U/mL IFN-αA and the cells were analyzed with a cell sorter. The background analysis of WiDr cells in the absence of addition of Mab B1.1, with or without IFN-αA, is shown in Fig. 13A. Figure 13B shows a heterogeneous population of cells, depicted as a spectrum of fluorescence intensities (X-axis), expressing various levels of the cell surface 180K protein. Following a 24 h incubation with 1000 U/mL IFN-αA, a dramatic shift is observed (Fig. 13C) in both the percentage of cells expressing the 180K antigen (vertical Z-axis), and the fluorescence intensity per cell (X-axis). No difference in DNA content of cells (Fig. 13, Y-axis) or the relative size of the individual WiDr cells was observed after interferon treatment. Thus, following the addition of IFN-αA, computer analysis revealed both an increase in mean fluorescence intensity per cell, and more than 98% of tumor cells now binding the Mab B1.1. These findings suggest that the increase of TAA expression induced by recombinant IFN-αA is a result of more antigen that is expressed per cell and a "recruitment" of new cells to express the antigen.

One of the potential clinical applications of Mab is the use of radiolabeled immunoglobulins to detect micrometastases in regional nodes and at distal sites. Mab B6.2 and B72.3 have already been used to detect human carcinoma transplants in athymic mice (Colcher et al., 1983b). One of the major considerations of radiolocalization studies is reducing the amount of radiolabeled Mab required to bind and detect a given tumor mass *in situ*; the use of lower levels of radioactively labeled Mab would increase "signal to noise" ratios and thus make detection of smaller lesions more efficient. A reduction in the amount of Mab required to give an equally efficient signal for surface binding of a Mab may be possible by a prior or concomitant treatment with interferon and have potential clinical application for the *in situ* detection of carcinoma lesions with radiolabeled Mab or in the use of Mab for immunotherapy. The ability of recombinant human leukocyte interferon to somewhat selectively

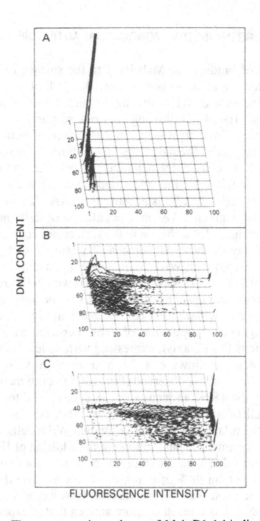

Fig. 13. Flow cytometric analyses of Mab B1.1 binding the surface of WiDr cells following treatment with IFN-αA. Each figure is a three-dimensional isometric display of DNA content (Y-axis), fluorescence intensity, i.e., cell surface 180K CEA expression as reflected by Mab B1.1 binding (X-axis), with the Z-axis representing the number of cells. 10^7 WiDr cells were incubated for 24 h at 37°C with or without 1000 U/mL IFN-αA. The cells were then harvested, washed, and incubated in medium containing 2 µg Mab B1.1/10^6 cells. After incubation the cells were washed and incubated with fluoresceinated sheep anti-mouse antibody. The cells were washed, centrifuged at 500g, and resuspended at a concentration of 10^6 cells/0.3 mL. The cells were then fixed, pelleted, resuspended, and stained for 4 h at room temperature, 10^6 cells/mL in PBS with propidium iodide (PI) and ribonuclease A. The stained cells were analyzed on an Ortho Cytofluorograf System 50H with blue laser excitation of 200 mW at 488 nm. Under these conditions PI bound to nuclear DNA fluoresces red, whereas surface immunofluorescence bound to the 180K antigen fluoresces green. Data from 25,000 cells were stored on an Ortho Model 2150 computer system and used to generate the figures shown here. A, WiDr cells stained for DNA content (with or without IFN), but with no Mab B1.1. B, WiDr cells stained for both nuclear DNA and Mab B1.1 binding. C, WiDr cells treated with 1000 U IFN-αA for 24 h and stained as in B.

enhance the expression of monoclonal-defined TAA in carcinoma cell lines may also prove useful in defining the role of specific TAA in the expression of the transformed phenotype.

References

Accolla, R. S., S. Carrel, and J. P. Mach (1980), *Proc. Natl. Acad. Sci. U.S.A.* **77,** 563.

Arklie, J., J. Taylor-Papadimitriou, W. Bodmer, M. Egan, and R. Millis (1982), *Int. J. Cancer* **28,** 23.

Attallah, A., C. Needy, P. Noguchi, and B. Elisberg (1979), *Int. J. Cancer* **24,** 49.

Barnstable, C. J., W. F. Bodmer, G. Brown, G. Galfre, C. Milstein, A. F. Williams, and A. Ziegler (1978), *Cell* **14,** 9.

Braylon, R., N. Benson, V. Nourse, and H. Kouth (1982), *Cytometry* **2,** 337.

Chatal, J. F., F. Chupin, G. Ricolleau, J. L. Tellier, A. le Mevel, P. Fumoleau, O. Godin, and B. P. le Mevel (1980), *Eur. J. Cancer* **17,** 233.

Chism, S. E., L. W. Noel, J. V. Wells, P. Crewther, S. Hunt, J. J. Marchalonis, and H. H. Fudenberg (1977), *Cancer Res.* **37,** 3100.

Chu, T. M. and T. Nemoto (1973), *J. Natl. Cancer Inst.* **51,** 1119.

Colcher, D., P. Horan Hand, M. Nuti, and J. Schlom, (1981a), *Proc. Natl. Acad. Sci. U.S.A.* **78,** 3199.

Colcher, D., P. Horan Hand, Y. A. Teramoto, D. Wunderlich, and J. Schlom (1981b), *Cancer Res.* **41,** 1451.

Colcher, D., P. Horan Hand, M. Nuti, and J. Schlom (1983a), *Cancer Invest.* **1,** 127.

Colcher, D., M. Zalutsky, W. Kaplan, D. Kufe, F. Austin, and J. Schlom (1983b), *Cancer Res.* **43,** 736.

Dent, P. B., S. Carrel, and J. P. Mach (1980), *J. Natl. Cancer Inst.* **64,** 304.

Epenetos, A. A., K. E. Britton, S. Mather, J. Shepherd, M. Granowska, J. Taylor-Papadimitriou, C. C. Nimmon, H. Durbin, L. R. Hawkins, J. S. Malpas, and W. F. Bodmer (1982a), *Lancet* Nov. 6, 1000.

Epenetos, A. A., G. Canti, J. Taylor-Papadimitriou, M. Curling, and W. Bodmer (1982b), *Lancet* Nov. 6, 1004.

Fellous, M., U. Nir, D. Wallach, G. Merlin, M. Rubinstein, and M. Revel, (1982), *Proc. Natl. Acad. Sci. U.S.A.* **79,** 3082.

Fisher, P. B., A. F. Miranda, L. E. Babiss, S. Pestka, and I. B. Weinstein (1983), *Proc. Natl. Acad. Sci. U.S.A.* **80,** 2961.

Foster, C. S., P. A. W. Edwards, E. A. Dinsdale, and A. M. Neville (1982), *Virchows Arch [Pathol, Anat.]* **394,** 279.

Foulds, L. (1954), *Cancer Res.* **14,** 327.

Gatter, K. C., Z. Abdulaziz, P. Beverly, J. R. F. Corvalan, C. Ford, E. B. Lane, M. Mota, J. R. G. Nash, K. Pulford, H. Stein, J. Taylor-Papadimitriou, C. Woodhouse, and D. Y. Mason (1982), *J. Clin. Pathol.* **35,** 1253.

Gold, P. and S. O. Freedman (1964), *J. of Exp. Med.* **121,** 439.

Gold, P., S. O. Freedman and J. Shuster (1979), in *Immunodiagnosis of Cancer* (R. B. Herberman and K. R. McIntire, eds.), Marcel Dekker, Inc., New York, p. 147.

Grant, S., K. Bhalla, I. B. Weinstein, S. Pestka and P. B. Fisher (1982), *Biochem. Biophys. Res. Commun.* **108,** 1048.

Greiner, J. W., P. Horan Hand, P. Noguchi, P. B. Fisher and J. Schlom (1984), *Cancer Res.* **44,** 3208.

Hand, P., M. Nuti, D. Colcher, and J. Schlom (1983), *Cancer Res.* **43,** 728.

Hansen, H. J., J. J. Snyder, E. Miller, J. P. Vandevoorde, O. N. Miller, L. R. Hines,and J. J. Burns (1974), *Human Pathology* **5,** 139.

Hart I. R. and I. J. Fidler (1981), *Biochem. Biophys. Acta* **651,** 37.

Herzenberg, L., L. A. Herzenberg, and C. Milstein (1979), in *Handbook of Experimental Immunology,* (D. M. Weir, ed.) Blackwell Scientific, London, 25.1.

Imai, K., A.-K. Ng, M. K. Glassy, and S. Ferrone (1981), *J. Immunol* **127,** 505.

Kerbel, R. S. (1979), *Nature* **280,** 358.

Koprowski, H., Z. Steplewski, K. Mitchell, M. Herlyn, D. Herlyn, and P. Fuhrer (1979), *Somatic Cell Genet.* **5,** 957.

Krebs, B. P., C. M. Lalanne and M. Schneider, eds., (1978) *Clinical Application of Carcinoembryonic Antigen Assay,* Excerpta Medica, Oxford.

Kufe, D. W., L. Nadler, L. Sargent, H. Shapiro, P. Horan Hand, F. Austin, D. Colcher, and J. Schlom (1983), *Cancer Res.* **43,** 851.

Kufe, D, G. Inghirami, M. Abe, D. Hayes, H. Justi-Wheeler, and J. Schlom, *Hybridoma,* in press.

Kupcik, H. Z., V. R. Zurawski Jr., J. G. R. Hurrell, N. Zamcheck, and P. H. Black (1981), *Cancer Res.* **41,** 3306.

Lokich, J. J., N. Zamcheck, and M. Lowenstein (1978), *Annals of Internal Med.* **89,** 902.

Menard, S., E. Tagliabue, S. Canevari, G. Fossati, and M. I. Colnaghi (1983), *Cancer Res.* **43,** 1295.

Menendez-Botet, C. J., J. S. Nisselbaum, M. Fleisher, P. P. Rosen, A. Fracchia, G. Robbins, J. A. Urban, and M. K. Schwartz (1976), *Clin. Chem.* **22,** 1366.

Miggiano, V., C. Stahli, P. Haring, J. Schmidt, M. LeDain, B. Glatthaar, and T. Staehlin (1979), *Twenty-Eighth Colloquium,* Pergamon Press, Oxford, p. 501.

Miller, F. R. and G. H. Heppner, (1979), *J. Natl. Cancer Inst.* **63,** 1457.

Mitchell, K. F. (1980), *Cancer Immunol. Immunother.* **10,** 1.

Nuti, M., D. Colcher, P. Horan Hand, F. Austin, and J. Schlom (1981), in *Monoclonal Antibodies and Development in Immunoassay,* (A. Albertini and R. Ekins, eds.), Elsevier/North Holland Biomedical press, North Holland, 87.

Nuti, M., Y. A. Teramoto, R. Mariani-Costantini, P. Horan Hand, D. Colcher, and J. Schlom (1982), *Int. J. Cancer* **29,** 539.

Papsidero, L. D., and G. A. Croghan, M. J. O'Connell, L. A. Valenzuela, T. Nemoto, and T. M. Chu (1983), *Cancer Res.* **43,** 1741.

Pestka, S. (1983), *Arch. Biochem. Biophys.* **221,** 1.

Pimm, M. V. and R. W. Baldwin (1977), *Int. J. Cancer* **20,** 37.

Poste, G., J. Doll, and I. J. Fidler (1981), *Proc. Natl. Acad. Sci. U.S.A.* **78,** 6226.

Prehn, R. T. (1970), *J. Natl. Cancer Inst.* **45,** 1039.

Pusztaszeri, G. and J. P. Mach (1973), *Immunochemistry* **10,** 197.

Rasmussen, B. B., S. Hilkens, J. Hilgers, H. H. Nielsen, S. N. Thorpe, and C. Rose (1982), *Breast Cancer Res.* **2,** 401.

Rogers, G. T., G. A. Rawlins, and K. D. Bagshawe (1981a), *Br. J. Cancer* **43,** 1.

Rogers, G. T., G. A. Rawlins, P. A. Keep, E. H. Cooper, and K. D. Bagshawe (1981b), *Br. J. Cancer* **44,** 371.

Sehested, M., F. R. Hirsch, and K. Hou-Jensen (1981), *Eur. J. Cancer Clin. Oncol.* **17,** 1125.

Sloane, J. P. and M. G. Omerod (1981), *Cancer* **47,** 1786.

Staehlin, T., D. S. Hobbs, H.-F. Kung, C.-Y. Lai, and S. Pestka (1981a), *J. Biol. Chem.* **256,** 9750.

Staehlin, T., D. S. Hobbs, H.-F. Kung and S. Pestka (1981b), in *Interferons, Methods in Enzymology,* Vol. 78 (S. Pestka, ed.), Academic Press, New York, p. 505.

Steward, A. M., D. Nixon, N. Zamcheck, and A. Aisenberg (1974), *Cancer* **33,** 1246.

Taylor-Papadimitriou, J., J. A. Peterson, J. Arklie, J. Burchell, R. L. Ceriani, and W. Bodmer (1981), *Int. J. Cancer* **28,** 17.

Thompson, C. H., S. L. Jones, R. H. Whitehead, and I. F. C. McKenzie (1983), *J. Natl. Cancer. Inst.* **70,** 409.

To, A., D. V. Coleman, D. P. Dearnley, M. G. Omerod, W. Steele, and A. M. Neville (1981), *J. Clin. Pathol.* **34,** 1326.

Vrba, R., E. Alpert, and K. J. Isselbacher (1975), *Proc. Natl. Acad. Sci. U.S.A.* **72,** 4602.

Waalkes, T. P., C. W. Gehrke, D. C. Tormey, K. B. Woo, K. C. Kuo, J. Snyder, and H. Hansen (1978), *Cancer* **41,** 1871.

Wilkinson, E. J., L. L. Hause, E. A. Sasse, R. A. Pattillo, J. R. Milbrath, and J. D. Lewis (1980), *Amer. J. Clin. Pathol.* **73,** 669.

Chapter 12

Antigens of Normal and Malignant Human Exocrine Pancreatic Cells

MICHAEL A. HOLLINGSWORTH AND
RICHARD S. METZGAR

*Department of Microbiology and Immunology, Duke University
Medical Center, Durham, North Carolina*

1. Introduction

Pancreatic cancer is currently the fourth leading cause of cancer-related death in the United States (Cohn, 1976). The diagnosis of pancreatic adenocarcinoma is usually a late event in the disease, which has a 5-yr survival rate of less than 2% (Hirayama et al., 1980). Early signs and symptoms of this disease are often vague or lacking, except for occasional obstructive jaundice or major vascular involvement. Ascites, liver involvement, and other signs of advanced disease are often the presenting physical findings. It is not yet clear whether the low survival rate is due to a late stage of disease presentation, the early development of metastases, or other factors. The few survivors, however, are almost exclusively patients in whom a tumor was detected fortuitously and surgically excised at an early, premetastatic stage. This fact suggests that early diagnosis could substantially improve the prognosis for the disease and has stimulated many attempts at defining systems for early diagnosis including: exploratory surgery and biopsy (Mikal, 1964; Wave, 1975); ultrasonic scanning (Filly and Fiemanis, 1970); selective arteriography with hypotonic duodenography (Suzuki et al., 1974); computerized transaxial tomography

(Sorabella et al., 1974); endoscopic retrograde cholangiopancreatography (Fukumoto et al., 1974); and pancreatic functional tests (Cohn, 1976). Unfortunately, to date such attempts have not been useful as cancer-screening tests.

Several investigators have applied immunological techniques to the study of pancreatic cancer. Results of some of these studies will be described in this chapter. However, some other antigens that have been measured in pancreatic cancer patients, such as carcinoembryonic antigen (CEA) and alphafetoprotein will not be considered, as they are the subject of separate chapters in this volume. Many studies of pancreatic malignancies have attempted to define antigens that are shed into body fluids at concentrations sufficient for meaningful measurement and diagnosis of the disease state. Early studies were directed at defining organ- or tissue-specific antigens of normal pancreas or at discovering tumor-specific antigens that were not expressed on normal tissue. Though some claims of tumor-specific antibodies have been made, these reagents were not screened against a sufficient number of normal and neoplastic tissues to certify the claimed specificity, and were subject to the problems which will be cited below for tumor-associated antigens (TAA).

There are numerous studies on the existence of TAA on pancreatic cancers. Although these antigens are expressed on some normal tissues, certain malignancies are distinguishable by a quantitative increase in antigen expression (on cells or in body fluids). Some TAA were initially thought to be tumor-specific since they were not detected on normal pancreatic tissue, but were present on some malignant cells of that tissue. These early studies were often misleading since the techniques used to detect the antigens were either not very sensitive or not quantifiable. In addition, the methods often were not capable of detecting antigen-positive normal cells at the single cell level. The TAA antibodies were usually polyclonal xenoantisera raised against pancreatic cell lines, tumors, or fetal tissues. Absorption with normal adult cells and/or tissues, to render them tumor-specific, reduced antibody titers and few studies were able to use these antibodies to purify the antigens and detail their molecular properties. With the advent of hybridoma technology and the ability to produce monoclonal antibodies to pancreatic tumors, it was hoped that some of the earlier specificity and antigen characterization problems could be resolved. Although there have been numerous monoclonal antibody studies reported for some human tumors, relatively few have been published on antigens of pancreatic carcinomas. Therefore, this chapter will review data on both polyclonal and monoclonal antibodies to human pancreatic normal and tumor antigens.

2. Human Pancreatic Cell Antigens Defined by Polyclonal Antibodies

2.1. Polyclonal Antibodies Elicited to Normal Adult Pancreas or to Pancreatic Secretions

In 1929, Witebsky (1929) reported that pancreas contained organ-specific antigens. Later attempts to demonstrate that an autoimmune disease could be experimentally produced to this tissue failed and instead, pancreas-specific alloantigens were detected (Witebsky, et al., 1960). Although the initial studies were done in rabbits, subsequent work indicated that pancreas-specific alloantigens could also be detected in monkeys and man (Metzgar, 1964a; Metzgar, 1964b; Metzgar, 1980). The antigens were noted to be exocrine cell products, but the molecular nature of the antigens was never established (Metzgar, 1980). Antibodies to known pancreatic enzymes have also been shown to be good markers of the exocrine pancreas.

Greene et al. (1975) later reported the presence of two pancreas specific antigens in normal human urine. One of these demonstrated esterase enzymatic activity. More recently, Nerenberg et al. (1980) described a human pancreas specific protein that was defined by a rabbit antiserum to crushed gel sections of preparative polyacrylamide gel gradient electrophoresis fractions from saline extracts of the pancreas. The antigen was partially purified and appeared to be a glycoprotein with a molecular mass of 2.25×10^5 daltons (Table 1). It was destroyed by perchloric acid, trypsin, and neuraminidase, but was unaffected by DNase or RNase. The antiserum reacted by radial immunodiffusion assay with pancreatic extracts, but not with extracts from many other organs. The antiserum did not react with purified pancreatic secretory enzymes or insulin. A radioimmunoassay using this antiserum detected elevated concentrations of this antigen in serum of some patients with pancreatitis, but no data was presented on the presence of the antigen in the serum of pancreatic cancer patients.

Chu and his colleagues described a pancreas specific antigen (PaA) which was isolated from saline extracts of normal pancreas (Table 1) (Loor et al., 1981). This antigen was purified by ammonium sulfate precipitation followed by chromatography on DEAE cellulose and Con A Sepharose, gel filtration on Sephadex G-200, and preparative isoelectric focusing. The purified antigen was used to immunize a rabbit, and the resulting antiserum was similar to an antiserum to pancreas that had been absorbed with normal human serum, liver, lung, and colon. The antise-

Table 1

Characteristics of Antigens Defined by Polyclonal Rabbit Antisera to Normal Human Adult and Fetal Pancreas

Antigen	Reference	Immunizing material	Molecular weight	Antigen epitope		Characteristics
				Affected by	Unaffected by	
Undesignated	Nerenberg et al., 1980	PAGE separated normal adult pancrease extract	2.25×10^5	Perchloric acid, trypsin, neuraminidase	DNase, RNase	Glycoprotein; noncross-reacting with secretory enzymes or insulin; present in serum of some patients with pancreatitis
PaA	Loor et al., 1982	Normal adult pancreas extract	4.4×10^4	Trypsin, pepsin, carboxypeptidase B perchloric acid, 70° C for 10 min	Neuraminidase, and β-glucosidase	Found in pancreatic juice; no enzymatic activity; localized in acinar cell cytoplasm; elevated serum concentration in benign and malignant pancreatic disease
OPA	Knapp, 1981	Fetal pancreas homogenate	4×10^4	Trypsin, pepsin, papain	DNase, RNase, neuraminidase	Increased serum levels in patients with pancreatic adenocar-

Antigen	Source	Reference	MW	Sensitive to	Resistant to	Comments
						...cinoma and other diseases; detected in fetal pancreatic tissue; pancreatic carcinomas; reportedly cross-reacts with POA
POA	Fetal pancreas	Gelder et al., 1978	7–9×10^5	Trypsin, pepsin, papain, pronase	DNase, RNase, neuraminidase	Glycoprotein; increased serum levels in some carcinomas and other nonmalignant disorders; detected in tissues from fetal pancreas, fetal small bowel, stomach contents, adult small bowel, stomach, pancreatic adenocarcinoma
POP	Fetal pancreas	Mihas, 1978	NR[a]	Trypsin, chymotrypsin	Neuraminidase	Detected in fetal pancreas, pancreatic adenocarcinoma

[a]Not reported.

rum to PaA reacted in rocket immunoelectrophoresis and crossed immunoelectrophoresis with pancreas, but not with most other tissues. The PaA antigen had a molecular mass of 44,000 daltons, showed α to β migration in immunoelectrophoresis, was sensitive to treatment with trypsin, pepsin, carboxypeptidase B, perchloric acid, and head (70°C for 10 min), but was resistant to neuraminidase and β-glucosidase treatment. PaA was found in pancreatic juice, but did not demonstrate any enzymatic activity. Immunoperoxidase and immunofluorescence staining revealed that the antigen was localized in the cytoplasm of acinar, but not ductal, cells in normal pancreas, and in the cytoplasm of tumor cells from patients with pancreatic adenocarcinoma (presumably of ductal origin). An enzyme-linked immunoassay (ELISA) was developed for PaA and used to determine its concentration in sera of various patients (Loor et al., 1982; Loor et al., 1981). The antigen concentrations in serum from normal individuals was less than 21.5 μg/mL in 96% of the cases. PaA concentrations greater than this value were present in less than 8% of serums taken from patients with lung, colorectal, breast, and prostate cancer. Patients with pancreatic malignancies had elevated PaA serum concentrations in 66% of the cases. Twenty-five percent of patients with pancreatitis and 38% of patients with cholelithiasis also had elevated levels.

An interesting finding was recently reported by Gold et al. (1983). These investigators immunized rabbits with purified human pancreatic duct mucin (PDM). After absorption with human type AB red blood cells, the antisera detected a single band in immunodiffusion against PDM or a crude pancreatic extract. The tissue distribution of the antigen was analyzed by an indirect immunoglucoseoxidase technique. The antigen was found in mucin-producing organs including pancreatic ductal epithelium, salivary glands, stomach, duodenum, jejunum, ileum, cecum, colon, bile duct, trachea, and bronchus, but was not found in pancreatic acinar cells or islet cells, esophagus, liver, gallbladder, lungs, heart, spleen, kidney, ovary, cervix, endometrium, breast, or bladder. In an effort to improve the specificity of the mucin staining, an antiserum was absorbed with mucinous ovarian cystadenocarcinoma fluid. This removed all reactivity except for pancreatic ductal epithelium and goblet cells of the distal colon. Further absorption of the antiserum with purified colonic mucin rendered the antiserum specific for pancreatic ductal epithelium. This reactivity could be removed by absorption with PDM. This antigen was also localized by the immunoglucose-oxidase assay in two pancreatic adenocarcinoma cell lines grown as tumors in nude mice. An immunologically identical PDM was purified from these tumors.

In previous work (Gold et al., 1978), this group reported that similar antibody absorption studies using purified colonic mucin yielded an antiserum specific for colon mucin. These polyclonal antibody studies, as well as some of the monoclonal studies to be described later, suggest that tissue- or organ-specific antigenic determinants may be expressed as part of the complex antigenic structure of mucin molecules, and that antibodies to epitopes on mucin-like antigens may be helpful in the detection and classification of adenocarcinomas.

2.2. Polyclonal Antibodies Elicited to Fetal Pancreas

In 1974, Banwo et al. (1974) raised antisera in rabbits to fresh fetal pancreas homogenate. Their work was based on earlier work with oncofetal antigens such as CEA and alphafetoprotein. An antiserum, after absorption with adult pancreas, defined five precipitin lines in two-dimensional immunoelectrophoresis. One of the bands with an α_2 mobility was detected only in fetal pancreatic tissue and in pancreatic carcinomas. This antigen was also detected in 36 of 37 sera from patients with pancreatic carcinoma, but was unreactive with other patients' sera. Further biochemical characterization of this antigen was not reported.

Gelder et al. (1978) also described a pancreatic oncofetal antigen (POA) that was detected by a rabbit antiserum to fetal pancreas that had been absorbed with normal adult pancreatic tissue (Table 1). Double immunodiffusion tests of fetal and adult tissues indicated that in addition to fetal pancreas, the antigen was expressed on some fetal small bowel cells and stomach contents, and to a lesser extent on some cells of adult small bowel and stomach. The POA was purified by Sepharose 6B chromatography to a single peak with a molecular mass from 700,000–900,000 daltons. The antigen is a glycoprotein with an α–β mobility in immunoelectrophoresis. Its immunoreactivity was destroyed by treatment with trypsin, papain, pronase, and pepsin, but was not affected by DNase or RNase. Neuraminidase treatment reduced, but did not eliminate antibody binding. The antigen would bind to Con A Sepharose, but not to Sepharose alone, and it stained with the periodic acid-Shiff reaction, suggesting a carbohydrate moiety. The analysis of sera from normal subjects for POA by quantitative rocket immunoelectrophoresis revealed antigen concentrations of less than 20 μg/mL. Sera from patients with different types of carcinomas and from patients with a variety of predominantly benign gastrointestinal disorders demonstrated occasional POA concentrations greater than 20 μg/mL. Approximately half the patients with pancreatic carcinoma had POA serum concentrations greater than 20 μg/mL. The high number of false negative and false positive values made this test unsuitable as a single screening test for pancreatic carcinoma.

The partial purification of a similar pancreatic oncofetal protein (POP) was reported by Mihas (1978) (Table 1), who raised antisera in rabbits against fetal pancreas, and absorbed the antisera with normal tissues. The antigen showed α_1–α_2 mobility in immunoelectrophoresis and was present on fetal pancreas and pancreatic carcinoma, but was not detected on adult pancreas or other fetal tissues. The antigenic activity of POP was destroyed by trypsin and chymotrypsin digestion, but was unaffected by neuraminidase treatment. No further biochemical, clinical, or tissue localization studies of this antigen were reported.

More recently, Knapp (1981) (Table 1), reported the partial characterization of an oncofetal pancreatic antigen (OPA) believed to be identical to the antigen described previously from that laboratory by Banwo (1974). Antiserum from rabbits hyperimmunized with fetal pancreas was rendered specific by absorption with glutaraldehyde insolubilized homogenates of normal adult pancreas, normal adult plasma, and a hepatoma patient's serum. This antiserum produced a single band of α_2 mobility when tested in crossed immunoelectrophoresis with fetal pancreas and pancreatic tumor homogenates, but did not react with fetal or adult liver, lung, stomach, colon, esophagus, nor with adult pancreas or serum. Tissue localization studies using an immunoperoxidase technique indicated that this antigen was expressed on adult pancreas. No other tissues were reported tested. The OPA was detected in serum from pancreatic carcinoma patients and was purified to an estimated > 90% purity by passing these sera over a column of antibody conjugated to Sepharose 4B. Albumin was a reported contaminating protein at a concentration of less than 6% of the total protein content. Purified serum OPA was resistant to DNase, RNase, and neuraminidase treatment, but was inactivated by trypsin, pepsin, and papain digestion. The molecular mass of OPA was estimated to be 40,000 daltons by SDS-PAGE. Thus, the molecular weight and molecular properties of this antigen are similar to the PaA antigen of Loor et al. (1981). The purified antigen preparation was used to develop a quantitative rocket immunoelectrophoresis assay which could also be used to evaluate serum samples from patients with a variety of disorders. Normal (nondiseased) individuals of different ages demonstrated serum OPA concentrations of less than 6 μ/mL, therefore this value was selected as an arbitrary diagnostic cut-off value. Using this parameter, 88% of sera from patients with pancreatic carcinoma were positive for elevated OPA levels. There was a much smaller but significant incidence (5–18%) of false positive OPA levels in patients with many other malignant and nonmalignant disorders. Other disorders, however, did not demonstrate increased serum OPA levels. Prospective studies determining OPA serum levels on nine patients with pancreatic carcinoma showed that: OPA levels dropped to normal ranges on one resected patient whose disease did not recur; OPA levels initially decreased in another resected patient, but afterwards increased until the patient died of metastatic disease; and OPA levels increased over time in patients with unresectable disease. Although data is not presented, and discrepancies in the reported characteristics exist, Knapp states in the discussion of this paper that collaborative work among Gelder et al. (1978), Arndt et al.

(1979), and himself indicated that the pancreatic antigens studied by these labs are immunologically identical.

2.3. Polyclonal Antibodies Elicited to Pancreatic Tumors

Other investigators have immunized animals with pancreatic tumors to try to detect tumor-associated antigens (Table 2). Kuntz and Archer (1979) immunized rabbits with saline extracts of pancreatic tumors or normal pancreas. Following absorption of these antisera with normal erythrocytes, lymphocytes, and pancreatic tissue, only the antitumor serum reacted in gel diffusion tests with tumor antigen extract, but not normal pancreas extract. The antigen was eluted in the void volume of a Sephadex G-200 column, and therefore probably had a molecular mass in excess of 380,000 daltons. No further characterization of this antigen has been reported.

Shultz and Yunis (1979) immunized rabbits with the pancreatic carcinoma cell line MIA PaCa-2 (grown in vitro and as tumors in nude mice), or with pancreatic tumor tissue, then absorbed the antisera with normal human pancreas tissue and various undiseased tissues from nude mice. Some of these sera defined an antigen with a molecular mass of approximately 900,000 daltons, with α_2–β_1 mobility in immunoelectrophoresis, which was sensitive to perchloric acid digestion. This antigen was not cross-reactive with CEA or alphafetoprotein and was expressed on the nuclear membrane of MIA PaCa-2 cells, fetal pancreas, and pancreatic tumors. The antigen could not be detected by Ouchterlony immunodiffusion in established melanoma and breast carcinoma cell lines, or in normal human liver, colon, lung, or pancreas. The antigen could be detected by counterimmunoelectrophoresis in the sera of a high percentage (65–70%) of patients with pancreatic carcinoma, and in a lower percentage (10–40%) of sera from patients with other malignant and nonmalignant disorders. The antigen was not found in 16 sera from nondiseased donors.

In addition to the PaA normal cell antigen previously discussed, Chu et al. (1977) have also described other antigens associated with pancreatic tumors. One antigen had a molecular mass of 185,000 daltons with a high carbohydrate content (45%). The antigen was purified from ascites fluid of a patient with pancreatic adenocarcinoma by perchloric acid extraction followed by successive chromatography, gel filtration, and gel electrophoresis. The purified antigen cochromatographed with purified radiolabeled CEA on a Sephadex G-200 column, but was distinct from different CEA preparations by amino acid and carbohydrate composition analyses. Rabbit antisera against this antigen absorbed with normal serum, liver, lung, and kidney did not cross-react with CEA. A second antigen was isolated by chromatography from ascitic fluid of a patient with

Table 2
Characteristics of Antigens Defined by Polyclonal Rabbit Antisera to Human Pancreatic Tumors

| Antigen | Reference | Immunizing material | Molecular weight | Antigen epitope | | Characteristics |
				Affected by	Unaffected by	
Pancreatic TAA	Kuntz and Archer, 1979	Pancreatic tumor extract	3.8×10^5	NR[a]	NR	Does not cross-react with CEA. Approximately 14% carbohydrate
Anti-MIA PaCa-2	Shultz and Yunis, 1979	Pancreatic carcinoma cell line	9.0×10^5	NR	NR	Elevated levels in sera of patients with pancreatic and other malignancies; found on fetal pancreas, pancreatic tumors
Ascites fluid glycoprotein	Chu et al., 1977	Fractionated ascites protein	1.85×10^5	NR	NR	Distinct from CEA; detected in pancreatic adenocarcinoma ascites; 45% carbohydrate
PCAA	Shimano et al., 1981	Absorbed ascites	$>1.6 \times 10^6$	Trypsin, pepsin, carboxypeptidase B, KSCN, lithium, diiodosalicylate, percholoric acid, 57°C for 10 min	Neuraminidase, β-glucosidase	Elevated serum levels in pancreatic and other adenocarcinoma patients; found on pancreas, colon, lung, breast, ductal epithelium of pancreatic, colonic, and gastric carcinomas; 20% carbohydrate

[a]Not reported

pancreatic adenocarcinoma as part of an immune complex with IgM (Harvey et al., 1978). The dissociated antigen had a molecular mass of approximately 160,000 daltons and was partially cross-reactive with CEA. No further biochemical data was presented nor was the molecule compared to the 185,000 mol wt antigen just described.

A third antigen described by this group (Shimano et al., 1981), was termed the pancreas cancer-associated antigen (PCAA). This antigen was prepared from pancreatic carcinoma patients' ascites by first passing the fluid over an antinormal human plasma immunoabsorbant column. The nonbinding material was pooled, concentrated, and injected into rabbits. The resulting antiserum and later second generation antisera were absorbed with normal human plasma and used to monitor purification of the PCAA by chromatography. The molecular mass of PCAA was greater than 1×10^6 daltons, of which 20% was carbohydrate. The antigen activity was stable following treatment with neuraminidase and β-glucosidase, but was diminished by treatment with trypsin, pepsin, carboxypeptidase B, KSCN, lithium diiodosalicylate, and perchloric acid and heating to 57°C for 10 min. An ELISA was developed for detecting PCAA in serum and tissue extracts. The antigen was detected in several normal tissues including pancreas, colon, lung, and breast. Serum concentrations of PCAA ranged from 0.1 μg/mL to 22.5 μg/mL in healthy individuals. Elevated PCAA concentrations were found in 67% of pancreatic adenocarcinoma patients, 27% of colorectal cancer, 30% of lung carcinoma, and 16% of breast carcinoma patients. The antigen, if present, was at concentrations of less than 0.1 μg/mL in pancreatic secretions from pancreatic adenocarcinoma patients. The serum PCAA concentration in pancreatic adenocarcinoma patients was evaluated according to disease stage and was found to be elevated in 78% of cases with liver metastases; elevated in 67% of patients with no liver metastases, but with unresectable disease; and elevated in 29% of patients with resectable disease. Later, as reported in an abstract, this group examined paraffin-embedded sections of pancreatic and nonpancreatic neoplasms, and nonneoplastic pancreatic leisons by immunoperoxidase staining (Nadji et al., 1982). They reported the presence of PCAA in 95% of 45 pancreatic carcinomas; none of 12 benign pancreatic disorders; and 29% of 49 colonic and gastric carcinomas.

A rather novel immunization protocol was reported by Grant and Duke (1981), who took serum from nude mice bearing primary human pancreatic tumor xenografts or human pancreatic carcinoma cell line tumor xenografts and used it to immunize immunocompetent hairy littermates. Following absorption with CEA, the resulting antisera showed reactivity by indirect immunofluorescent staining with malignant and normal adult and fetal pancreatic ductal epithelial cells. The sequential absorption of some of the antisera with two bladder, one breast, and one colon carcinoma cell lines and normal pancreas tissue reduced anti-body binding to pancreatic carcinoma cells to 16% of the preabsorption value in a radioimmunoassay. Comparable absorptions of the antisera with pancreatic tumor cells completely abolished their reactivity. These investigators stated that hybridoma antibodies were being generated from spleens of the immunized mice; however, these results have not yet been published.

3. Pancreatic Antigens Defined by Monoclonal Antibodies

3.1. Monoclonal Antibodies Elicited to Normal Pancreatic Cell Antigens

There have been few reported monoclonal antibodies against pancreatic antigens. Parsa (1982) prepared hybridomas from mice immunized with human undiseased cadaveric pancreatic cells, and selected antibody se-creting clones that were positive by indirect immunofluorescence for acinar cells or for pancreatic epithelia. A monoclonal antibody was isola-ted that reacted with acinar cells, but was negative for ductal, centroacinar, islet, and interstitial pancreatic cells. No other normal tis-sues were tested and no other tissue distribution or antigen characteriza-tion data were reported. This group then treated undiseased cadaveric pancreatic explants in organ culture with methylnitrosourea. These cells, after 12 wk of growth, were injected into nude mice and 14 resulting tumors were established as cell lines in primary tissue culture. These cell lines were not reported to be cloned. Of the 14 cell lines studied, only one was reported to be positive by immunofluorescence with the anti-acinar cell antibody. This cell line, unlike the others, had morphological features of acinar cells. These included prominent microvilli, a tendency to form acinar structures, and zymogen granule formation. Thus, this monoclonal could be detecting a human acinar cell-specific antigen. A more detailed specificity study has not yet been reported, but is warranted.

A second monoclonal antibody selected for positive im-munofluorescence activity against pancreatic ductal cells (HP-DU-1) was also reported by Parsa et al. (1982). This antibody reacted by immunofluorescence with cells lining main and interlobar pancreatic ducts in normal adult and 12–20 wk fetal pancreas tissue. The antibody did not react with acinar, endocrine, and connective tissue of normal adult pancreas. HP-DU-1 was positive on six of seven primary pancreatic tumors and was present on both the CAPAN 1 and CAPAN 2 pancreatic adenocarcinoma cell lines. No biochemical data for this antigen has been reported and again, specificity studies were limited by the few normal and tumor tissue samples studied.

3.2. Monoclonal Antibodies Reactive with Pancreatic Tumor-Associated Antigens

3.2.1. Pancreatic Tumor-Reactive Monoclonals Elicited to Nonpancreatic Tumors

There have been no published studies of monoclonal antibodies elicited to pancreatic tumor cells other than those from our laboratory. However, some monoclonal antibodies which were generated to nonpancreatic tumors have shown strong reactivity with carcinomas of the pancreas. Although some of these antibodies may be reviewed in other chapters, we would like to discuss briefly two of these antigen-antibody systems here because of their molecular similarities and possible relationships to the DU-PAN-2 antigen to be discussed in the next section.

The best characterized of these antigens is the 19-9 antigen defined by a monoclonal antibody (19-9) elicited to cultured SW116 colorectal carcinoma cells (Herlyn et al., 1979). An immunoperoxidase technique was employed to analyze tissue distribution of this antigen in normal and malignant tissues (Atkinson et al., 1982). In normal tissue, the antigen was distributed on the epithelium of the gall bladder, bronchial glands, large ducts of salivary glands, prostate, some breast ducts, and 14–17 wk fetal bowel. By this technique, the antigen was found to be present on approximately 85% of pancreatic and gastric carcinomas, but on only 59% of colon and 42% of gall bladder and lung adenocarcinomas. The antigen could also be found on some adenocarcinomas from other organ sites, but in many cases the number of samples studied was small.

The antigenic epitope defined by the 19-9 antibody is a sialylated Le^a-active pentasaccharide that is located on a ganglioside in the SW116 cells (Magnani et al., 1981). An indirect radioimmunoassay (RIA) was developed for the 19-9 antigen and was used to examine the levels of this antigen in serum from patients with benign and malignant disease and from healthy donors. The antigen was found in low concentrations in the sera of healthy individuals and most patients with benign disease, but was elevated in 79% of sera from patients with pancreatic adenocarcinoma, 50% of serum from patients with gastric, and 46% of sera from advanced colorectal cancer (Herlyn et al., 1982). Recently this group has isolated the antigen detected by 19-9 antibody in the serum of pancreatic and colorectal carcinoma patients. Interestingly, the serum form of the antigen has the properties of a mucin rather than a monosialoganglioside (Magnani et al., 1983). The antigen is found in salivary mucin of individuals of the Le (a+b−) or Le (a−b+) blood group, but not individuals of the Le (a−b−) blood group, who lack the fucosyltransferase necessary to construct the antigen epitope.

Recently, a monoclonal antibody (OC 125) was elicited to an ovarian carcinoma cell line (Bast et al., 1981) and was shown to be detecting an epitope (CA 125) on a high molecular weight glycoprotein that is expressed on certain epithelial cells of the coelomic cavity (Kabawat et al., 1983). A radioimmune assay was developed by Bast and his colleagues for the CA 125 antigen and this assay was used to monitor serum levels of this antigen (Bast et al., 1983). Similar to the assay results for 19-9 antigen, CA 125 antigen was present at low levels in all sera of healthy individuals and 94% of patients with nonmalignant disease. However, 82% of patients with ovarian carcinoma, 59% of patients with pancreatic carcinoma, and 22% of patients with colorectal carcinoma had elevated serum antigen levels. Some patients with carcinomas from other organ sites also had elevated serum levels. In serial studies of ovarian cancer patients, rising or falling serum levels often correlated with progression or regression of disease (Bast et al., 1983).

3.2.2. Monoclonal Antibodies Elicited to Pancreatic Tumors

In this section we will summarize the specificity, antigen characterization, and clinical studies of the DU-PAN monoclonals produced and characterized at Duke University. We have generated five murine monoclonal antibodies (DU-PAN-1, -2, -3, -4, and -5) against human pancreatic adenocarcinoma cells (Metzgar et al, 1982). These antibodies were elicited to a pancreatic adenocarcinoma cell line (HPAF-I) that was established from ascitic fluid of a patient with pancreatic adenocarcinoma. HPAF-I cells had an in vitro lifespan of only 20–30 population doublings. However, a spontaneopus variant of these cells, HPAF-II, demonstrated unlimited replicative capability. When injected subcutaneously into nude mice, both cell lines produced tumors which histologically resembled a liver metastasis of the patient from whom they were derived. The DU-PAN monoclonals were elicited to HPAF-I cells, but all of the antigens could be detected on HPAF-II cells. The DU-PAN antibodies were selected with an ^{125}I-antiglobulin binding assay from fusions of spleen cells of Balb/c mice immunized with HPAF-I cells and either P3 or NS1 myeloma cells. The isotypes of the monoclonal antibodies were determined by immunodiffusion and immunofluorescence to be: DU-PAN-1 and -3, IgG_2; DU-PAN-4 and -5, IgG_1; DU-PAN-2, IgM.

The cloned DU-PAN antibodies were tested by indirect immunofluorescence for reactivity with a variety of transformed human cell lines of pancreatic and other tumor origins (Table 3). The tissue distribution of the DU-PAN antigens was also examined by an indirect immunoperoxidase test on a variety of frozen sections of human tumors (Table 4), normal fetal tissues (Table 5), and normal adult tissues (Table

Table 3

Immunofluorescence Reactivity of DU-PAN Monoclonal Antibodies with Tissue Culture Cell Lines

Cell line type	Monoclonal antibodies				
	DU-PAN-1	DU-PAN-2	DU-PAN-3	DU-PAN-4	DU-PAN-5
Pancreatic adenocarcinoma	4/5[a]	4/5	5/5	5/5	1/5
Lymphoblastoid (T and B cell)	0/6	0/6	0/6	0/6	0/6
Fibrosarcoma	0/1	0/1	0/1	NT[b]	1/1
Melanoma	0/4	0/4	2/4	4/4	0/4
Lung carcinoma	0/2	1/2	2/2	2/2	0/2
Stomach carcinoma	0/1	0/1	NT	NT	0/1
Renal carcinoma	0/1	0/1	0/1	0/1	0/1
Colon carcinoma	0/4	2/4	2/4	2/4	2/4
Normal skin fibroblast	0/1	0/1	0/1	0/1	1/1

[a]Number positive/total number tested.
[b]Not tested.

6). We have also characterized, to differing degrees, the physicochemical properties of four of the five DU-PAN antigens (Table 7). The information in Tables 3–7 will be discussed in more detail in the sections devoted to the individual antigens. A clinical study measuring serum levels of DU-PAN-2 antigen will be discussed separately.

3.2.2.1. DU-PAN-1 Antigen. The DU-PAN-1 antigen has been partially purified from spent tissue culture media of HPAF-I cells (Table 7). The antigen was biosynthetically radiolabeled with ^{3}H-leucine and ^{3}H-glucosamine, indicating a glycoprotein composition. This glycoprotein migrated as a rather wide band between 30,000 and 35,000 daltons on 10% SDS polyacrylamide gels, suggesting that several intermediate glycosylation forms of the antigen were detected by the antibody.

DU-PAN-1 has been detected on four of five pancreatic carcinoma cell lines, but not on cell lines of other orgins (Table 3). This antigen was seen on a low percentage (<25%) of breast and ovarian carcinomas, a high percentage (>50%) of pancreatic, prostatic, and bladder tumors, but was not seen on most other tumor types (Table 4). In normal human fetal tissues, the antigen was found in low to moderate levels in some cells of the trachea, pancreas, esophagus, small intestine, bladder, and duodenum; it was not found on cells of many other organs or tissues (Table 5). In normal adult tissue, DU-PAN-1 antigen was found on goblet cells of

Table 4
Immunoperoxidase Reactivity of DU-PAN Monoclonal Antibodies with
Human Tumor Sections[a]

Tumor tissue origin	Monoclonal antibodies				
	DU-PAN-1	DU-PAN-2	DU-PAN-3	DU-PAN-4	DU-PAN-5
Pancreas (primary)	5/6[b]	21/22	6/6	3/3	6/6
Pancreas (liver metastasis)	2/3	2/3	2/3	NT[c]	2/3
Pancreas (lymph node metastasis)	2/2	2/2	2/2	NT	2/2
Lung	0/3	4/14	0/3	2/2	1/3
Breast	2/8	5/22	1/8	2/2	1/5
Stomach	0/2	0/2	0/2	NT	0/2
Ovary	3/14	29/53	3/14	NT	2/9
Kidney	0/9	1/15	0/9	NT	2/9
Testes	0/2	0/2	0/2	NT	NT
Colon	1/4	6/14	2/4	3/3	1/4
Rectum	0/1	0/1	0/1	NT	0/1
Spleen	0/1	0/1	0/1	NT	0/1
Lip	0/1	0/1	0/1	NT	0/1
Lymphoma	0/3	0/3	0/3	0/2	0/3
Adrenal	0/1	0/1	0/1	NT	0/1
Liver	0/1	0/1	0/1	NT	1/1
Prostate	3/26	3/26	6/26	NT	6/6
Bladder	6/10	3/10	4/10	2/2	1/9
Melanoma	0/2	0/2	0/2	2/2	0/2
Schwanoma	1/1	1/1	1/1	NT	1/1
Tetratocarcinoma	0/1	1/1	0/1	NT	1/1

[a]DU-PAN-2 data is compiled from both frozen and formalin fixed paraffin-embedded sections. Data on all other DU-PAN monoclonals is from frozen sections only.
[b]Number positive/total number tested.
[c]Not tested.

the ileum, jejunum, stomach, colon, bronchus, esophagus, trachea, and on some epithelial cells of the appendix, gall bladder, thymus, bladder, prostate, and breast, but was absent from many other organs and tissues (Table 6).

3.2.2.2. DU-PAN-2 Antigen.　The antigen defined by the DU-PAN-2 monoclonal antibody is the most studied of the DU-PAN antigens. The antigen was found to be heat stable and the epitope appeared to be a carbohydrate moiety which was still reactive with the antibody after formalin fixation and paraffin embedding. This provided us with access to more and different tumors and normal tissues for specificity studies. In addition, an indirect radioimmune assay (RIA) was established using par-

Table 5
Immunoperoxidase Reactivity of DU-PAN Monoclonal Antibodies with
Normal Human Fetal Tissues

Tissue	Monoclonal antibodies				
	DU-PAN-1	DU-PAN-2	DU-PAN-3	DU-PAN-4	DU-PAN-5
Colon	$-^a$	+	+	+	+
Small intestine	+	++	−	+	+
Stomach	++	++	++	++	++
Lung	−	−	−	−	−
Kidney	−	−	−	−	−
Liver	−	−	−	++	++
Salivary gland	−	++	−	−	−
Thyroid	−	−	−	−	−
Thymus	−	−	−	−	−
Blood vessel	−	−	−	−	−
Trachea	+	+	+	+	+
Pancreas	++	++	++	+++	+++
Esophagus	+	++	++	+	+++
Duodenum	+	++	+	+	+
Bladder	+++	+	+	++	NT^b

^{a}Intensity of immunoperoxidase stain with − being no staining, and +++ being the strongest staining.
^{b}Not tested.

tially purified soluble antigen from ascites of patients with pancreatic carcinoma. Competitive inhibition of the RIA was then used to monitor the antigen during its further isolation and purification and for the clinical studies to be described later.

DU-PAN-2 antigenic activity was eliminated by digestion with neuraminidase, but was quantitatively unaffected by digestion with collagenase, pronase, glucose oxidase, hyaluronidase, chondroitinase A, B, or C, endoglycosidase D, H, or endo-β-galactosidase (Table 7). The antigen was stable following heating to 100°C for 15 min, and was soluble in 50% ammonium sulfate and 1.0N perchloric acid. The pI for DU-PAN-2 ranges from pH 3.5 to 4.75. Gel filtration on Sepharose CL-2B revealed an antigenic profile of a sharp peak of activity in the void volume (fractions 32–44) and a broad peak that eluted in fractions 48–90. (Fig. 1). This profile was unaffected by pretreatment of DU-PAN-2 antigen with collagenase, hyaluronidase, chondroitinase A, B, or C, endoglycosidase D or H, endo-β-galactosidase, or when gel filtration was performed in 6M guanidine hydrochloride or 8M urea + 0.1% SDS + 65 mM dithiothreitol. Proteolytic digestion of DU-PAN-2 with pronase, however, eliminated the antigen peak at the void volume. We have been unable to prepare an acceptable immunoaffinity column with DU-PAN-2 antibody since the antibody shows markedly decreased antigen binding

Table 6

Immunoperoxidase Reactivity of DU-PAN Monoclonal Antibodies with Normal Adult Tissues

Tissue	Monoclonal antibodies				
	DU-PAN-1	DU-PAN-2	DU-PAN-3	DU-PAN-4	DU-PAN-5
Ileum	+[a]	+	−	NT[b]	+
Jejunum	+	+	NT	NT	NT
Stomach	+	+	+	+	+
Colon	+	+	+	−	+
Liver	−	−	−	−	−
Pancreas	−	+	+	+	−
Small intestine	−	+	−	−	+
Appendix	+	+	−	NT	+
Gall bladder	+	+	+	NT	+
Breast	−	−	−	+	−
Ovary	−	−	−	+	−
Prostate	+	−	+	+	+
Testes	−	−	−	+	−
Bladder	+	−	−	−	−
Kidney	−	−	−	+	+
Uterus	−	−	−	NT	−
Cervix	−	−	−	NT	−
Lymph node	−	−	−	−	−
Thymus	+	+	−	+	+
Tonsil	−	−	−	+	−
Smooth muscle	−	−	−	−	−
Skeletal muscle	−	−	−	−	−
Lung	−	−	−	+	−
Bronchus	+	+	+	NT	+
Trachea	+	+	+	NT	+
Parotid gland	−	+	−	+	+
Blood vessels	−	−	−	+	−
Fat	−	−	−	−	−
Endometrium	−	−	−	+	−
Esophagus	+	+	+	−	+
Adrenal	−	−	−	+	−

[a]+ = positive; − = negative.
[b]Not tested.

when coupled to an insoluble matrix. The antigen, therefore, has been purified by ammonium sulfate fractionation, multiple gel filtrations, pronase digestion, and ion exchange chromatography followed by affinity chromatography on immobilized wheat germ agglutinin. Carbohydrate analysis of the purified material revealed a composition consistent with that of a non-salivary mucin (Fernsten, 1984). The DU-PAN-2 antibody does not bind to the ganglioside defined by the 19-9 monoclonal antibody

Table 7
Molecular Properties of DU-PAN-1, -2, -3, and -5 Antigens

Antigen	Molecular weight	Composition	Antigen epitope	
			Affected by	Unaffected by
DU-PAN-1	30,000–35,000	Glycoprotein	NR[a]	NR
DU-PAN-2	>200,000	Glycoprotein	Neuraminidase	100°C for 15 min; 1.0N perchloric acid; collagenase; pronase; glucose oxidase; hyaluronidase; chondroitinase A, B, C; endo-β-galactosidase
DU-PAN-3	70,000	Nonglycosy-lated protein	NR	NR
DU-PAN-5	110,000	Glycoprotein	NR	NR

[a]Not reported

of Magnani et al. (1981), to five other sialogangliosides of similar structure, or to other ganglioseries gangliosides, including GM_4, GM_3, GM_2, GM_{1b}, GM_1, GD_{1a}, GD_{1b}, GT_{1a}, and GQ_{1b} (personal communication, Dr. Sen-itiroh Hakomori).

Studies using DU-PAN-2 antigen that was partially purified by ammonium sulfate fractionation and chromatography on Cibacron blue F3G-A sepharose indicated that the antigen could enter and be detected by electrophoresis in 0.5 or 1% agarose (personal communication, Michael Lan). When a sample of the partially purified antigen was applied onto 0.5% agarose gel in Tris-EDTA-acetic acid buffer, run for 4 h at 100 V and stained with Coomassie Blue, two major and one minor bands were seen. Transfer of these proteins to nitrocellulose and immunoblotting with DU-PAN-2 antibody showed that the specific DU-PAN-2 activity resided in two broad bands. However, since the DU-PAN-2 molecule is heavily glycosylated, the molecular size cannot be estimated by this technique. Recent studies have also shown that the two distinct bands demonstrated by immunoblotting could also be detected by radioimmune precipitation of DU-PAN-2 antigen metabolically labeled with various radioactive monosaccharides and sulfates (unpublished data). The ability of the DU-PAN-2 antigen to enter a gel electrophoretically offers new approaches to DU-PAN-2 antigen isolation and assessment of purity.

DU-PAN-2 antigen has shown a somewhat restricted expression pattern on human cell lines, being found on most of those derived from pancreatic adenocarcinomas and some lines from lung and colon carcinomas

(Table 3). Analysis of tissue sections of tumors indicated that DU-PAN-2 was expressed on almost all pancreatic, gall bladder, bile duct, and stomach adenocarcinomas, and was occasionally seen in malignancies of the breast, ovary, kidney, colon, liver, prostate, and bladder (Table 4). In pancreatic adenocarcinomas, DU-PAN-2 was present in primary lesions as well as liver and lymph node metastases. One primary sarcoma involving the pancreas did not bind DU-PAN-2 antibody (Table 4). Highly differentiated adenocarcinomas showed lumenal immunoperoxidase staining of tumor glands and intralumenal secretory material. Poorly differentiated adenocarcinomas generally showed individual intracellular reactivity. Usually there was marked heterogeneity of antigen expression within a single tumor. This included areas of tumor that did not react with DU-PAN-2 antibody in an otherwise positive lesion and individual cellular variations in antigen expression in cells that exhibited no detectable morphologic differences. Interestingly, in areas of some tumors that had a surrounding stromal inflammatory reaction, aggregates of macrophages were observed that were positive for DU-PAN-2 antigen. The antigen-positive adenocarcinomas of nonpancreatic origin showed reactivity patterns similar to pancreatic adenocarcinomas. In one of two signet ring adenocarcinomas of the stomach, the intracellular mucin droplet was positive for DU-PAN-2 antigen (Borowitz et al., 1984).

Among fetal tissues tested, DU-PAN-2 was found on stomach, trachea, pancreas, colon, esophagus, small intestine, duodenum, and bladder (Table 5). The distribution of DU-PAN-2 on normal adult tissues (Table 6) included pancreas, ileum, jejunum, stomach, colon, small intestine, appendix, gall bladder, thymus, bronchus, trachea, salivary gland, and esophagus. In normal adult pancreas, gall bladder, and bile duct, DU-PAN-2 was expressed only on ductal epithelial cells. In the stomach, small intestine, and colon, however, the lumenal surface of only a few gastric epithelial cells were antigen-positive. This was in contrast to malignancies of these organs, which contained a large number of antigen-positive cells (Borowitz et al., 1984). In general, the DU-PAN-2 expression on normal tissues was limited to certain glandular epithelial cells in some areas of the gastrointestinal and the upper respiratory tract, and this distribution was consistent with that of a mucin molecule.

3.2.2.3. DU-PAN-3 Antigen.   The antigen defined by the DU-PAN-3 monoclonal antibody appears to be a nonglycosylated protein molecule, based on the observation that radiolabeled carbohydrate precursors are not incorporated into the molecule. The analysis of DU-PAN-3 radioimmunoprecipitates of ^{125}I-labeled CAPAN 2 cell line lysates revealed a 70,000-dalton protein antigen (Table 7).

The DU-PAN-3 antigen was expressed on a larger number of human cell lines than were DU-PAN-1 and DU-PAN-2, including pancreatic carcinoma, melanoma, lung carcinoma, and colon carcinoma cell lines

(Table 3). This antigen was detected on almost all pancreatic adenocarcinomas, and was found on a low poercentage of breast, ovarian, prostate, and bladder tumors (Table 4). Human fetal tissues expressing DU-PAN-3 included stomach, trachea, pancreas, colon, esophagus, small intestine, duodenum, and bladder (Table 5). Normal adult tissues containing cells which expressed DU-PAN-3 antigen included stomach, colon, pancreas, ductal epithelium, gall bladder, prostate, bronchus, trachea, and esophagus (Table 6).

3.2.2.4. DU-PAN-4 Antigen.

The DU-PAN-4 antigen shows the broadest reactivity of the five monoclonals we have generated. This antigen was present on most human cell lines (Table 3), and on many normal adult (Table 6) and fetal (Table 5) tissues. Although the DU-PAN-4 antigen tissue distribution was not ubiquitous, there were no readily discernable patterns of reactivity that would make this antigen useful for studying or classifying malignancies. We have been unable to identify the molecular nature of the DU-PAN-4 antigen by conventional immunoprecipitation or immunoblotting techniques using a variety of antigen extraction and labeling procedures from various potential antigen sources.

3.2.2.5. DU-PAN-5 Antigen.

The DU-PAN-5 antigen immunoprecipitated from ^{125}I-labeled HPAF-I and HPAF-II cell lysates, appeared as a 110,000-dalton protein on SDS-PAGE gels (Table 7). This antigen was expressed on HPAF cells, but was not found on four other human pancreatic carcinoma cell lines. DU-PAN-5 was expressed on some colon carcinoma and fibrosarcoma cell lines (Table 3). The antigen has been found on a high percentage of primary pancreatic tumors and prostatic tumors, and was found in a lesser incidence on lung, breast, ovarian, renal, colon, hepatic, and bladder tumors (Table 4). The antigen was more widely distributed on normal fetal and adult tissues than DU-PAN-1, -2, and -3 antigens (Tables 5 and 6). It is interesting to note that the DU-PAN-5 antigen could not be detected on HPAF tumors growing in nude mice. The broad normal tissue distribution of this antigen, like DU-PAN-4, makes it less exciting for tumor diagnostic or classification purposes than DU-PAN-1, -2, and -3 antibodies. However, the antigens defined by both DU-PAN-4 and -5 monoclonal antibodies may be interesting markers of secretory epithelial cells and could be helpful in understanding their differentiation or transformation.

3.2.2.6. Clinical Studies with DU-PAN-2 Monoclonal Antibodies.

An RIA was initially developed for monitoring the presence of soluble DU-PAN-2 antigen during isolation and purification procedures. A completion or inhibition modification of this assay has been adapted for use in detecting and monitoring DU-PAN-2 antigen levels in the serum and ascites of patients with malignant and non-malignant disease (Metzgar et al., 1984). The antigen preparation used as target antigen and for the standard inhibition curves in this assay was prepared from ascites fluid of the patient from whom the HPAF cell lines were derived. The antigen was partially purified by salt precipitation, Cibacron Blue F3GA Sepharose CL-6B chromatography, and perchloric acid extraction. The standard antigen was stable for at least one yr when stored at $-20°C$. Instead of expressing RIA results as percent inhibitions and titer, the DU-PAN-2 antigen concentration in a sample was expressed as arbitrary U/mL based on the partially purified standard antigen reference sample. The amount of DU-PAN-2 antigen in 20 µL of a 1:500 dilution of the standard antigen preparation was designated as 100 U/mL. The results of plotting percent inhibition in the RIA versus U/mL was linear from 0 to 200 U/mL, and was highly reproducible. Body fluid samples tested in this manner were examined in serial twofold dilutions and U/mL were determined by multiplying the units calculated times the dilution, which gave between 30 and 80% inhibition.

The unfractionated ascites used for the standard antigen preparation contained greater than 50,000 DU-PAN-2 U/mL. Ascites from four other patients with pancreatic adenocarcinoma had 750 U/mL or more, with two samples having values greater than 20,000 U/mL. Ascites from patients with leukemia, lymphoma, and chronic renal failure had DU-PAN-2 levels of less than 10 U/mL, whereas patients with colon and lung carcinoma had concentrations of 150 U/mL and less than 100 U/mL, respectively. Interestingly, cyst fluid from a patient with a mucinous cystadenocarcinoma of the pancreas had greater than 100,000 U/mL, whereas fluids from two pseudo cysts from patients with pancreatitis had less than 50 U/mL.

Sera from normal volunteers and from patients with pancreatic carcinoma, colorectal carcinoma, gastric carcinoma, melanoma, a variety of pediatric cancer patients, and pancreatitis were evaluated for DU-PAN-2 concentrations (Table 8). All of the nonpancreatic tumor patients studied had active disease at the time of testing, but some of the pancreatic cancer patients were receiving therapy and were classified as having stable or minimal disease at the time of testing. The mean DU-PAN-2 concentrations for sera from normal, melanoma, ovarian, and pediatric cancer patients was 81, 92, 119, and 127 U/mL respectively, with all values less than 400 U/mL. Sera from 68 of 89 pancreatic adenocarcinoma patients and eight of 20 gastric adenocarcinoma patients had antigen concentrations greater than 400 U/mL, with mean values of 4888 U/mL and 861 U/mL, respectively. Only eight of 76 colorectal carcinoma patients and three of 58 patients with benign GI tract disease had DU-PAN-2 serum concentrations greater than 400 U/mL, with mean values of 303 U/mL and 223 U/mL, respectively. These findings largely parallel the immunoperoxidase distribution of DU-PAN-2 antigen. However, patients with ovarian carcinoma, whose tumors expressed DU-PAN-2 antigen,

Table 8
DU-PAN-2 Serum Antigen Levels by Competition RIA

Diagnosis	Number of patients tested	Mean serum DU-PAN-2, U/mL
Normal	126	81
Benign GI tract diseases	58	223
Melanoma	19	92
Pediatric solid tumors and lymphomas	22	127
Nasopharyngeal carcinoma	21	89
Pancreatic carcinoma	89	4888
Gastric carcinoma	20	861
Colorectal carcinoma	76	303
Ovarian carcinoma	55	119

had no detectable DU-PAN-2 antigen in serum taken at the time of surgery.

Serial serum samples from two pancreatic adenocarcinoma patients were available for retrospective studies of DU-PAN-2 serum concentrations. The first patient had mildly elevated antigen levels (380 U/mL) as well as elevated bilirubin concentrations when initially seen for a common bile duct obstruction. Following a surgical bypass operation, the DU-PAN-2 and bilirubin levels declined to normal ranges. Later, the hepatic duct became obstructed and was accompanied by increased bilirubin levels and DU-PAN-2 levels (1400 U/mL). When the obstructed duct was relieved, liver function improved and DU-PAN-2 levels reverted to normal values. Throughout this period, the patient was not on therapy and her tumor burden did not appear to change.

The second patient demonstrated a decrease in DU-PAN-2 U/mL from 992 to 1900 by the third day following surgical resection of his primary pancreatic tumor. The patient was clinically stable for one year with normal DU-PAN-2 serum concentrations, but thereafter was found to have recurrent progressive disease with increased DU-PAN-2 serum values. The patient died 1 month later, with DU-PAN-2 serum values of 1216 U/mL. There was no correlation in this patient between DU-PAN-2 concentration and bilirubin/alkaline phosphatase levels. Taken together, these results imply that some increased DU-PAN-2 values may reflect antigen shedding from tumor and perhaps be a reflection of tumor burden (Patient 2), whereas in other patients with impaired liver function (Patient 1), the serum levels may be a reflection of the impaired ability of the patient to catabolize the antigen. The influence of liver function on the serum CEA levels has previously been noted (Zamcheck and Kupchik, 1980).

Recently we have been able to detect elevated levels of DU-PAN-2 antigen in pancreatic duct fluid taken from patients at the time of surgery. The levels of the antigen in juice obtained directly from the duct of two pancreatic cancer patients were both > 2000 U/mL and were higher than their serum antigen levels. Pancreatic duct fluid from a patient with a nongastrointestinal tract malignancy was 83 U/mL. Thus, endoscopy or ERCP samples are now being evaluated for DU-PAN-2 levels. The clinical studies to date are preliminary but the data suggest that DU-PAN-2 antigen determinations in body fluids may provide useful diagnostic or clinical management information and thus should be evaluated in a larger prospective study.

4. General Discussion

The work summarized in this chapter reveals that the differentiation-related antigenic constituency of the exocrine pancreas and related tumors is poorly defined primarily because of a lack of high titered monospecific antibodies to characterize the molecules. Hybridoma technology has provided an approach to resolve this reagent problem by production of monoclonal antibodies. The plethora of these reagents to hematopoietic cell antigens has advanced our knowledge of lymphoid and myeloid cell differentiation. However, to date, few antibodies have been characterized to the point of making a significant impact in our knowledge of secretory epithelial cell transformation or differentiation.

Among the antigens characterized by polyclonal rabbit antisera to normal adult and fetal pancreas, and pancreatic tumors, the undesignated antigen of normal adult pancreas described by Nerenberg et al. (1980) and listed in Table 1 differs from the other antigens by molecular mass $(2.25 \times 10^5$ daltons) and antigen epitope sensitivity to neuraminidase. The remaining antigens listed in Tables 1 and 2 are insensitive to neuraminidase, but are sensitive to protease treatment. The PaA antigen of Loor et al. (1982) and the OPA antigen described by Knapp (1981) show molecular masses of approximately 4×10^4 daltons, whereas the POA of Gelder et al. (1978), the anti-MIA-PaCa of Shultz and Yunis (1979), and possibly the pancreatic TAA of Kuntz and Archer (1979) are reportedly larger at 7–9×10^5 daltons. The PCAA of Chu et al. (1977) is still larger at $> 1.6 \times 10^6$ daltons. Knapp states that his OPA is cross-reactive with Gelder's POA and another antigen described by Arndt (1979), presumably by double immunodiffusion analysis. The noted similarities in molecular properties among these antigens suggest that some of the laboratories may be examining the same antigen. However, unequivocal proof of this must be demonstrated by cross-absorption or immunoprecipitation experiments; certification of monospecificity of the antisera by techniques more sensitive than immunodiffusion; and by extensive tissue distribution analyses. The examination of an antigen's tissue distribution by immunodiffusion or immunoelectrophoresis is not sufficiently sensitive to certify a negative result. Current immunohistological procedures such as immunoperoxidase and immunofluorescence provide a better assessment of this parameter at the cellular level.

With the exception of the antigen described by Nerenberg et al. (1980) that is untested on tumors, all of the polyclonal antisera-defined antigens are expressed on pancreatic malignancies. Of these, PaA, OPA, POA, anti-MIA-PaCa, and PCAA have been tested for serum levels in patients with pancreatic cancer and certain other malignancies (generally of gastrointestinal tract or breast origin), and are detected at elevated concentrations compared to normal individuals. Only PCAA has been evaluated according to disease stage, and the results showed that a somewhat disappointing 29% of patients with early resectable pancreatic disease had elevated serum antigen concentrations. Though these results are interesting and possibly useful for prognostic and diagnostic information, no single polyclonal antiserum studied to date has demonstrated the necessary sensitivity and specificity required for an early pancreatic cancer detection assay.

With the possible exception of the antibodies to pancreatic duct mucin described by Gold et al. (1983), none of the antigens defined by polyclonal rabbit antibodies appear to be the same as the antigens defined by the murine monoclonal DU-PAN antibodies (Table 7). There were some similarities between the pancreas-specific antigen of Nerenberg et al. (1980) and DU-PAN-2, but the sensitivity of the former antigen to trypsin and perchloric acid distinguishes it from DU-PAN-2. Most of the other high molecular weight antigens differed from DU-PAN-2 by their insensitivity to neuraminidase. The biochemical and tissue distribution characteristics of the DU-PAN-2 antigen suggest that this molecule is a mucin. It has long been suspected that patients with some adenocarcinomas have elevated concentrations of mucin in their serum (Hakkinen and Virtanen, 1967; Runge and Pour, 1980). This is supported by the DU-PAN-2 and anti-colorectal monoclonal antibody 19-9 clinical studies on detection of their antigens in serum. The 19-9 antigen has been shown to be a sialylated lacto-N-frucopentaose II epitope that appears on cell lines and tumor cells as a ganglioside, but in serum as a mucin (Magnani et al., 1983). Reagent exchange, biochemical properties, and binding studies indicate that the molecules and epitopes recognized by the 19-9 and OC 125 monoclonals are different from that seen by DU-PAN-2 (unpublished data). The provocative antiserum absorption work of Gold et al. (1983) suggests that mucins secreted by pancreas, colon, and possibly an ovarian cystadenocarcinoma display both cross-reacting nontissuespecific and distinct tissue-specific antigenic determinants. This hypothesis is supported by observations from other labs, including that of Kim who has shown that the exposed carbohydrate moieties (detected by lectin binding studies) differ for colonic epithelium at various stages of differentiation and/or transformation to malignancy (Boland et al., 1982). It may be that monoclonal antibodies generated to tumors from different organ sites will also be capable of distinguishing tissue-specific epitopes on similar mucin molecules. The development of such monoclonal antibodies against tissue-specific antigenic determinants on circulating mucin molecules could be of great value in the diagnosis, classification, and clinical monitoring of the various mucin-producing adenocarcinomas. Consequently, our lab is developing second generation monoclonal antibodies to purified DU-PAN-2 antigen in an effort to detect tissue-specific and other epitopes on this molecule.

Further progress in understanding malignant and normal secretory epithelial cell differentiation will be made when panels of monoclonal antibodies with restricted tissue specificities are available for testing against body fluid and tissue samples. A comparison of the available tissue reactivities of the DU-PAN antibodies (Tables 5 and 6) supports this idea. For example, only three of the tissues tested thus far (stomach, trachea, and esophagus) expressed DU-PAN-1, -2, and -3 antigens in both fetal and adult tissues. Adult colon expressed DU-PAN-1, but fetal colon did not. Fetal pancreas and small intestine expressed DU-PAN-1, but this reactivity was lost on adult tissue. Fetal thymus did not express any DU-PAN antibody reactivity whereas adult thymus reacted with DU-PAN-1, -2, -4, and -5 antibodies. In general, DU-PAN-1, -2, and -3 were found on certain gastrointestinal organs and tissues containing secretory epithelium; however, the tissue distribution for each individual antigen was distinctly different. DU-PAN-5 showed a somewhat broader distribution in these tissues than either DU-PAN-1, -2, or -3 individually, and additionally was found on fetal liver and adult kidney. The DU-PAN-4 antigen tissue distribution was extensive. Interestingly, some DU-PAN antigen-positive tumors originated in tissues that were antigen-negative in the normal fetus and adult.

Immunoperoxidase tissue screening studies with the DU-PAN antibodies are continuing. Based on the results obtained thus far, it appears that existing DU-PAN monoclonals may have a more relevant clinical application in the classification of adenocarcinomasa rather than in diagnosis *per se*.

Thus far, we have not been successful in developing RIA or ELISA tests for detection of soluble DU-PAN antigens other than DU-PAN-2. This may be due to the biological properties of the monoclonals or the limited amount of antigen present in membrane extracts or body fluids of patients with pancreatic disease. We are currently continuing conventional purification techniques and have begun using recombinant DNA technology to address this goal. The recombinant techniques may be especially well suited for production of the 70,000-dalton DU-PAN-3 antigen, which is apparently nonglycosylated and is readily precipitated by the monoclonal antibody.

Preliminary studies indicate that DU-PAN-1 antibodies show in vivo localization in the nude mouse–human tumor xenograft model and are effective in preventing or delaying tumor formation in this model system. It may be that the monoclonals that show the least promise as serum diagnostic reagents will be the best prospects for localization and therapeutic studies since a limited amount of free or shed antigen would not interfere with in vivo binding to tumor cells.

In addition to developing new monoclonal antibodies to fetal and malignant pancreas tissue, we are analyzing pancreatic adenocarcinomas for oncogene products that may be expressed as transformation- or differentiation-related antigens. Preliminary work from our laboratory (unpublished results) and others (Pulciani et al., 1982; Cooper et al., 1984) has indicated that pancreatic adenocarcinomas express oncogenes that can be detected in the NIH 3T3 transfection assay. Our current research scheme involves using recombinant DNA techniques in conjunction with the development of monoclonal antibodies against proteins that become expressed in NIH 3T3 or other cell types when these cells are transfected with pancreatic adenocarcinoma DNA.

Though an early diagnosis test for pancreatic adenocarcinoma remains elusive, it is hoped that persistence in applying new immunological and molecular biology techniques combined with innovative experimental designs will ultimately yield a useful solution to the problems of detection and management of patients with pancreatic malignancies.

Acknowledgments

The authors gratefully acknowledge the following researchers from Dr. Metzgar's laboratory at Duke University who provided data and observations on the DU-PAN antigens and antibodies so that this chapter would be as current as possible: Olja Finn, Michael Lan, Nancy Zeleznik, Vicki Daasch, Phil Fernsten, Melissa Gaillard, Frank Tuck, and Karen Connor. The advice and editorial comments of Olja Finn, Michael Borowitz, and James Moore were deeply appreciated. We especially wish to thank Kathy Greenwell and Teresa Hylton who were patient and helpful in the preparation of this manuscript.

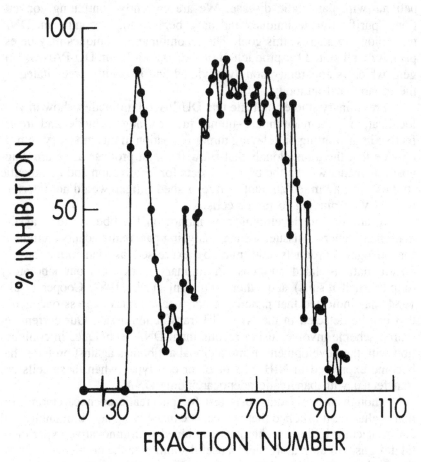

Fig. 1.   Fractionation of DU-PAN-2 antigen preparation on Sepharose CL-2B. Antigen activity was detected by competitive inhibition in a radioimmune assay. Digestion with pronase eliminated antigen activity in fractions 30–45.

References

Arndt, R., K. Nishida, W. M. Becker, and H. G. Thiele (1979), 6th Meeting Int. Soc. Oncodevel. Biol. Med. abstract, 229.

Atkinson, B. F., C. S. Ernst, M. Herlyn, Z. Steplewski, H. F. Sears, and H. Koprowski (1982), *Cancer Research* **42,** 4820.

Banwo, O., J. Versey, and J. R. Hobbs (1974), *Lancet* **1,** 643.

Bast, R. C. Jr., M. Feeney, H. Lazarus, L. M. Nadler, R. B. Cobrin, and R. C. Knapp (1981), *J. Clin. Invest.* **68,** 1331.

Bast, R. C. Jr., T. L. Klug, E. St. John, E. Jenison, J. M. Niloff, H. Lazarus, R. S. Berkowitz, T. Leavitt, C. T. Griffiths, L. Parker, V. R. Zurawski, and R. C. Knapp (1983), *New England J. Med.* **309,** 883.

Boland, C. R., C. K. Montgomery, and Y. S. Kim (1982), *Proc. Natl. Acad. Sci. USA* **79**, 2051.

Borowitz, M. J., F. L. Tuck, W. F. Sindelar, P. D. Fernsten, and R. S. Metzgar (1984), *JNCI* **72**, 999.

Chu, T. M., E. D. Holyoke, and H. O. Douglass (1977), *Cancer Research* **37**, 1525.

Cohn, I. (1976), *Cancer* **37**, 582.

Cooper, C. S., D. G. Blair, M. K. Oskarsson, M. A. Tanisky, L. A. Eoder, and G. F. Van de Woude (1984), *Cancer Research* **44**, 1.

Fernsten, P. D. (1984), *Dissertation Abstracts International* **44**, 3034-B.

Filly, R. A. and A. K. Fieimanis (1970), *Radiology* **96**, 575.

Fukumoto, K., M. Nakajama, K. Murakami, and K. Kawai (1974), *Am. J. Gastroent.* **62**, 210.

Gelder, F. B., L. J. Reese, A. R. Moosa, T. Hall, and R. Hunter (1978), *Cancer Research* **38**, 313.

Gold, D. V., P. Hollingsworth, T. Kremer, and D. Nelson (1983), *Cancer Research* **43**, 235.

Gold, D. V. and F. Miller (1978), *Tissue Antigens* **11**, 362.

Grant, A. G. and D. Duke (1981), *Br. J. Canc.* **44**, 388.

Greene, E. L., S. P. Halbert, and D. Kiffer (1975), *Int. Arch. Allergy Appl. Immunol.* **48**, 764.

Hakkinen, I. and S. Virtanen (1967), *Clin. Exp. Immunol.* **2**, 669.

Harvey, S. R., L. R. Van Dusen, H. O. Douglass, E. d. Holyoke, and T. M. Chu (1978), *JNCI* **61**, 1199.

Herlyn, M., Z. Steplewski, D. Herlyn, and H. Koprowski (1979), *Proc. Natl. Acad. Sci. USA* **76**, 1438.

Herlyn, M., H. F. Sears, Z. Steplewski, and H. Koprowski (1982), *J. Clin. Immunol.* **2**, 135.

Hirayama, T., J. A. W. Waterhouse, and J. F. Fraumeni (1980), *UICC Technical Report Series* **41**, 78.

Kabawat, S. E., R. C. Bast, A. K. Bhan, W. r. Welch, R. C. Knapp, and R. B. Cobrin (1983), *Lab. Invest.* **48**, 42A (abstract).

Knapp, M. L. (1981), *Ann. Clin. Biochem.* **18**, 131.

Kuntz, D. J. and S. J. Archer (1979), *Oncology* **36**, 134.

Loor, R., M. Kuriyama, M. L. Manzo, H. Inaji, H. O. Douglass, R. Berjian, J. J. Nicolai, G. N. Tytgat, and T. M. Chu (1981), *Clin. Chim. Acta.* **117**, 251.

Loor, R., N. J. Nowak, M. L. Manzo, H. O. Doublass, and T. M. Chu (1982), *Clinics in Laboratory Med.* **2**, 567.

Loor, R., T. Shimano, M. L. Manzo, L. Van Dusen, L. D. Papsidero, J. J. Nicolai, G. N. Tytgat, and T. M. Chu (1981), *Biochem. et Biophysic. Acta.* **668**, 222.

Magnani, J. L., M. Brockhaus, D. F. Smith, V. Ginsburg, M. Blaszczyk, K. F. Mitchell, Z. Steplewski, and H. Kropowski (1981), *Science* **212**, 55.

Magnani, J. L., Z. Steplewski, H. Koprowski, and V. Ginsburg (1983), *Cancer Research* **43**, 5489.

Metzgar, R. S. (1964a), *J. Immunol.* **93**, 176.

Metzgar, R. S. (1964b), *Nature* **203**, 660.

Metzgar, R. S. (1980), *Transplant. Proc.* **12,** 122.

Metzgar, R. S., M. T. Gaillard, S. J. Levine, F. L. Tuck, E. H. Bosen, and M. J. Borowitz (1982), *Cancer Research* **42,** 601.

Metzgar, R. S., N. Rodriguez, O. J. Finn, M. S. Lan, V. N. Daasch, P. D. Fernsten, W. C. Meyers, W. F. Sindelar, R. S. Sandler, and H. F. Seigler (1984), *Proc. Nat. Acad. Sci. USA* **81,** August 1984 (in press).

Mihas, A. (1978), *JNCI* **60,** 1439.

Mikal, S. (1965), *Ann. Surg.* **161,** 395.

Nadji, M., P. Ganjei, T. Shimano, and T. M. Chu (1982), *Lab. Invest.* **60,** A.

Nerenberg, S. T., R. Prasad, L. D. Pederson, and N. S. Biskup (1980), *Clin. Chem.* **26,** 209.

Parsa, I. (1982), *Cancer Lett.* **15,** 115.

Parsa, I., A. L. Sutton, C. K. Chen, and C. Dellridge (1982), *Cancer Lett.* **17,** 217.

Pulciani, S., E. Santos, A. V. Lauver, L. K. Long, S. A. Aaronson, and M. Barbacid (1982), *Nature* **300,** 539.

Runge, R. G., and P. Pour (1980), *Cancer Lett.* **10,** 351.

Shimano, T., R. M. Loor, L. D. Papsidero, M. Kuriyama, R. G. Vincent, T. Nemoto, E. D. Holyoke, R. Berjian, H. O. Douglass, and T. M. Chu (1981), *Cancer* **47,** 1602.

Shultz, D. R. and A. A. Yunis (1979), *JNCI* **62,** 777.

Sorabella, P. A., W. L. Campbell, and W. B. Seman (1974), *Radiology* **112,** 737.

Suzuki, T., K. Uchida, T. Tani, and I. Honjo (1974) *Am. J. Roentg.* **122,** 398.

Wave, M. (1975), *Br. Med. J.* ii, 354.

Witebsky, E. (1929), *Die Naturewissen* **40,** 771.

Witebsky, E., N. R. Rose, and H. Nadel (1960), *J. Immunol.* **85,** 568.

Zamcheck, N. and H. Z. Kupchik (1980), *Manual of Clinical Immunology Second Edition,* Ed. Noel R. Rose and Herman Friedman, American Society for Microbiology, Washington, DC, p. 919.

Chapter 13

Monoclonal Antibodies to Human Prostate Cancer-Related Antigens

T. MING CHU

*Diagnostic Immunology Research and Biochemistry Department,
Roswell Park Memorial Institute, Buffalo, New York*

1. Introduction

Hybridoma-derived monoclonal antibodies potentially useful in immuno-diagnosis and immunotherapy of human prostate cancer is the subject of this chapter. These monoclonal antibodies are directed primarily against protein components of malignant and normal prostate. The protein component or its derivative is thus defined operationally as antigen. As in other human tumors, prostate tumor specific antigen is yet to be identified even with the recently developed somatic cell hybridization technology. Several groups of investigators have produced monoclonal antibodies that recognize prostate cancer-associated antigenic components, or are directed to chemically well-defined organ-site cell-type specific proteins of the prostate, such as prostate specific antigen and prostatic acid phosphatase. At this stage of development, only monoclonal antibodies of murine origin are well described. Production and characterization of these antibodies are the major topic of this review. Experimental application of monoclonal antibodies to prostate antigen and prostatic acid phosphatase as serodiagnostic and immunohistologic reagent for prostate cancer is also described.

For the purpose of review, this chapter is presented in sections according to the source of the antigenic component that is used as the immunogen to generate monoclonal antibody.

2. Cell Surface Antigens of Established
Prostate Tumor Lines

Murine monoclonal antibodies to human prostate adenocarcinoma membrane antigens were generated by Starling et al. (1982) by fusing
P3x63/Ag8 mouse myeloma cells with spleen cells from BALB/c mice
immunized with the human prostate tumor line DU-145 intact cell suspension. Glutaraldehyde-fixed DU-145 cells were used as target antigens
in screening hybridoma culture fluid for antibodies by a solid-phase
radioimmunoassay. The injection of a single suspension of DU-145 cells,
so called "primary" immunization, into mice resulted in no production
of detectable antibody. A "hyperimmunization" protocol, i.e., "primary" plus one "booster," yielded one promising monoclonal antibody
83.21. The binding specificity of antibody 83.21 was characterized by
three additional techniques, membrane immunofluorescence and complement-dependent cytotoxicity as well as quantitative adsorption, using
various established human cell lines as the targets.

Among 44 cell lines examined, solid-phase radioimmunoassay revealed that antibody 83.21 bound strongly to the DU-145 human prostate
tumor cell line, a metastatic prostate adenocarcinoma to the brain, three
primary bladder tumor lines and one human embryonic lung cell line
transformed by cytomegalovirus isolated from a normal prostate (CMV-
Mj-HEL-1). The three other techniques demonstrated a strong binding activity of 83.21 against the above-mentioned cell lines, and additionally,
to the PC-3 cell line, a metastatic prostate adenocarcinoma to the bone.
PC-3 showing a low binding activity, if any, to the 83.21 antibody in the
radioimmunoassay, was revealed to possess a significant reactivity with
the antibody in membrane immunofluorescence, complement-dependent
cytotoxicity assay, and quantitative adsorption analysis. The results suggest the importance of using more than one antibody-binding activity assay in screening the antibody binding specificity of monoclonal antibody.
Monoclonal antibody 83.21 appears to be directed to a prostate and bladder cancer-associated antigen.

By means of quantitative adsorption, the reactivity of the antibody
83.21 to crude membrane preparation of a few human tissues was examined. One primary prostate carcinoma showed high reactivity. A secondary liver metastasis of this prostate carcinoma also was highly reactive. In
fact, based upon protein concentration of crude membrane, the metastatic
tumor demonstrated a higher reactivity. Normal liver and benign prostate
hyperplasia (BPH) were negative, whereas a normal prostate and two
prostate carcinomas showed a reduced adsorption activity.

The 83.21 monoclonal antibody is of IgM (k) isotype and directed
against a mol wt (M_r) 180,000 surface glycoprotein. It showed no cross-

reactivity with α-fetoprotein, carcinoembryonic antigen, HLA, fibronectin, prostate antigen, or prostatic acid phosphatase by a direct-binding or an inhibition assay. Therefore, antibody 83.21 is not directed against these well-known human tumor cell marker proteins. The strong reactivity with DU-145, PC-3 prostate tumor cell lines, and three transitional cell carcinomas of the urinary bladder cell lines would suggest that antibody 83.21 is directed against a urogenital differentiation antigen that is reexpressed upon malignant transformation. The positive reactivity of 83.21 with a cytomegalovirus-transformed human embryonic lung cell line and negative with a normal human embryonic lung cell line provided additional evidence to this suggestion. The antibody 83.21 could be a useful probe for the study of possible link between cytomegalovirus and transformation of prostate malignancy.

Recently, this same group of workers (Wright et al., 1983) also reported a monoclonal antibody P6.2, which was produced with a similar procedure as that of 83.21 by using PC-3 human prostate tumor cell line as the immunogen and the NS-1 mouse myeloma line as the fusion partner. Antibody P6.2 also is of IgM isotype. Although no detailed binding reactivity was described, data on the use of P6.2, along with 83.21, in immunohistochemical localization of the antigens reactive with these two monoclonal antibodies, were reported.

Using avidin–biotin immunoperoxidase assay and conventionally prepared formalin-fixed paraffin-embedded tissue sections, a variety of human malignant, benign, and normal tissues were examined on their reactivities with these two antibodies. P6.2 stained positively with 74% (14/19) of the primary prostate tumors, whereas 58% (11/19) were positive with 83.21. It is interesting that both 83.21 and P6.2 antibodies stained more strongly with poorly differentiated and undifferentiated tumors (83 and 92% of 12 tumors) than with well to moderately differentiated tumors (14 and 43% of seven tumors). In a limited number, six, of metastatic prostate tumors tested, 83.21 and P6.2 stained one and four, respectively. Again, more undifferentiated tumors were stained positively than well differentiated ones; the sites of metastases included regional lymph nodes, skin, liver, and urinary bladder. None of BPH, normal prostate, benign bladder, or normal bladder was stainable by either antibody, although a small number of breast, pancreas, and lung tumors showed a positive stain only with P6.2. Both antibodies, however, exhibited positive staining in proximal convoluted tubules of normal kidney, which was the only normal tissue showing the positive reactivity among 32 nonprostate normal tissues tested. These data are extremely encouraging on at least two points: the lack of or limited reactivity with normal human tissues and the reactivity with poorly differentiated and undifferentiated prostate tumors. To date, these are the only antibodies, along with αPro3 antibody (to be discussed next), associated with prostate cancer, either polyclonal or monoclonal, that exhibit the latter characteristics.

Ware et al. (1982) produced a monoclonal antibody, αPro3, by fusing splenocytes of mouse immunized with PC-3 prostate tumor cell (one primary and one booster) with the nonimmunologlobulin-secreting myeloma cell line SP2/0-Agl4. Radioactive protein A assay for cell surface target antigen was used in the screening of hybridoma antibody. Three separate fusions resulted in 1000 hybridomas, 30–55% of which recognized the PC-3 tumor cells as well as a human colon tumor cell line LoVo. Ten to 18% of these hybridomas showed, however, a preferential binding to the surface of PC-3 cells. αPro3, one of the clones, was characterized in detail.

αPro3 monoclonal antibody is of the IgG_{2a} isotype. Cell surface binding assay revealed that αPro3 also binds a human breast tumor cell line MDA-MB-231 and a normal human fibroblast cell line IMR90 more than a DU145 prostate tumor cell line (50, 30, and 20% as well as it binds PC-3, respectively). Absorption analysis with extract of various human tissues demonstrated that the reactivity of αPro3 to PC-3 cells can be abolished effectively by primary prostate tumor as expected. Poorly differentiated prostate carcinomas exhibited a more effective blocking activity than well-differentiated prostate carcinomas. Although BPH also showed reduced inhibitory effect, αPro3 was able to discriminate the blocking activity between prostate tumor and BPH, indicating that the antigen(s) recognized by αPro3 is quantitativly more in prostate tumor than in BPH. Extracts of normal human tissue, kidney carcinoma, bladder carcinoma, and ovarian carcinoma all exhibited a reduced inhibitory activity (greater than BPH). Only the extract of the testicular tumors showed greater inhibitory effect, to the same degree as that of prostate tumors. Therefore, αPro3 appears to recognize an antigen expressed equally well by both prostate and testicular tumors.

The antigenic molecule carrying the determinant as recognized by αPro3 is of 175,000 M_r under nonreducing condition. Upon reduction, the antigen has an apparent subunit M_r of 54,000 (designated P54). It is of interest to note that serum from prostatic cancer patients competes with αPro3 for binding to P54 of primary prostate tumor extract. This observation appears to be specific, since neither the normal human sera nor the sera of other nonprostatic urologic diseases exhibit a binding activity. No data were presented from sera collected from patients with testicular tumors. If the naturally occurring "immunoglobulin" can be shown as an antitumor antibody, αPro3 will be an invaluable probe to elucidate the pathobiology of prostate cancer.

Using a similar technique and a mixture of three established human prostate tumor cell lines (DU145, PC3, and LNCaP) as the immunogen, Webb and Ware (1983) produced a monoclonal antibody, αPro13, exhibiting restricted reactivity against prostate tumor cells. Unlike αPro3, αProl3 reacts with both PC-3 and DU145, and does not react with other cell lines of bladder, kidney, and pancreatic cancer origin, nor with cultured human fibroblast. By immunoperoxidase technique, αPro13 stained ductal epithelia of both malignant and benign prostatic hyperplastic tissues. The antigen(s) that is recognized by αPro13 is shown to be a M_r 140,000 protein under nonreducing condition, which contains a major M_r 30,000 and a minor M_r 17,000 component. No further information regarding αProl3 monoclonal antibody was reported.

In addition to αPro3 and αPro13 monoclonal antibodies, Webb and Ware and their associates (1983) produced another antibody, αPro5, by fusing spleen cells of mouse immunized with PC-3 cells with SP2/0-Ag14 mouse myeloma line, an identical procedure as that for αPro3 production. Indirect evidence as obtained from prostate tissue (normal, benign, carcinoma) adsorption and sequential immunoprecipitation of PC-3 xenograft tumor extract and of radiolabeled PC-3 cell surface proteins suggest that αPro5 and αPro3 are directed against two different epitopes on the same P54 antigen molecule. Although direct proof will require experiments when P54 is purified, a series of results were presented to show the inherent stability of P54 on the PC-3 cell surface and the cell surface interaction of αPro3 and αPro5 with P54 moiety.

Experiments on biosynthetic labeling of PC-3 culture with ^{14}C-glucosamine and radioiodination of spent culture fluid revealed that P54 is biochemically a glycoprotein and is not readily shed from the PC-3 cell surface. Although intact P54 remains on cell membrane of PC-3, a nonglycosylated protein of 50,000 M_r was detected in culture medium that is immunoprecipable with αPro3. Similarly, this protein also is detected in prostatic cancer patients serum. It appears that upon interaction with antibody αPro3 or αPro5 (an IgG_{2b} isotype) P54 is not readily shed from the PC-3 cells. Data also were presented to suggest that PC-3 cell surface-bound (via P54 binding) antibody is lost by internalization of antibody αPro3 and P54 antigen complex or by dissociation of antibody from the cell surface after internalization of P54 antigen alone.

Of additional interest is the observation that at higher concentration of αPro3 antibody, "capping" or modulation of PC-3 does occur, apparently by endocytosis of αPro3-P54 immune complex, as defined by an indirect immunoassay. However, such phenomena of modulation and endocytosis of αPro5 antibody are not detectable, except when a direct binding assay is employed. Furthermore, a combination of αPro3 and αPro5 demonstrate a greater endocytosis of the antibody-antigen complexes than either antibody alone, i.e., synergistic effect of αPro3 and αPro5 on endocytosis. Additionally, viability of PC-3 cell remains unchanged upon the manipulation with monoclonal antibodies.

These are very interesting and potentially important data. Two prostate cancer-associated monoclonal antibodies apparently directed to the same antigen molecule expressed on an established prostate tumor cell line have been obtained. Extensive in vitro analysis for the effect of monoclonal antibody in the biological behavior of tumor cells can be designed and executed. Mechanism of antibody and antigen interaction is readily obtainable. This model is potentially a valuable tool in immunotherapy and immunodiagnosis of prostate cancer.

3. Prostate Membrane-Associated Antigens

Frankel et al. (1982a) reported the production of murine monoclonal antibodies by fusing splenic lymphocytes of mouse immunized with membrane-enriched fraction of human BPH with mouse myeloma line N5-1. Antibody screening was performed by solid-phase radioimmunoassay directed against enriched membrane preparation of BPH. Thirteen monoclonal antibodies were obtained from 580 primary hybrids. These 13 hybridoma-derived monoclonal antibodies were found, by a competitive blocking assay, to bind with seven different antigenic components (sites) in the membrane preparation. Further examination on enriched membrane prepared from various human tissues by radioimmunoassay, and on frozen tissue sections by immunoperoxidase revealed that these antibodies can be separated into two major groups: five reacted specifically with epithelium element of the prostate and others, such as breast and salivary gland, and two specifically with stroma, although authors indicated that two antibodies of the former group are prostate specific.

By a direct binding assay on five established human cell lines, DU145 and PC-3 prostate carcinomas, T24 bladder carcinoma, CALU lung carcinoma, and CMV-HEL embryonic lung cell, as that reported by Starling et al.(1982), no activity was found with the two stroma specific antibodies. The epithelium specific monoclonal antibodies exhibited differential binding activities; two (antibodies 24 and 25) reacted with PC-3 alone; one (antibody 35) reacted with both PC-3 prostate and T24 bladder carcinomas; another reacted with all but CMV-HEL, whereas the last one reacted with all five cell lines tested. It appears that the cell binding activity of antibody 35 is similar to that of αPro3 as determined from this limited number of cell lines. Whether antibody 35 also directs to the P54 antigenic moiety of αPro3 remains to be seen.

All these seven antibodies are not reactive with prostate antigen (Wang et al., 1979) or prostatic acid phosphatase (Chu et al., 1978 and Lee et al., 1978). The authors debated whether the antibody 35 could be of direct use in the treatment of prostate cancer patients refractory to conventional therapy, although no evidence was presented to support this suggestion.

4. Prostate Antigen

Human prostate specific antigen (PA) was first reported by Wang et al., (1979). PA is a chemically definable glycoprotein with a mol wt of 34,000, an isoelectric point of 6.9, and a sedimentation coefficient of 3.1S. It is present only, in isomeric forms, in human prostate and seminal plasma (Wang et al., 1982a,b). Detailed amino acid (97%) and carbohydrate (3%) composition of PA were reported recently (Wang et al., 1983). Using rabbit monospecific polyclonal antibodies to PA, PA has been established as a serodiagnostic marker for prostate cancer (Kuriyama et al., 1980, 1981), a marker for human prostatic epithelial cells (Papsidero et al., 1981) and as an immunohistologic marker for prostate neoplasms (Nadji et al.,1981). Physical, chemical, and immunological characteristics of PA (Wang et al., 1982a,b, 1983,), including N-terminal amino sequence and tryptic peptide mapping (Chu et al., unpublished), have shown clearly that PA is a distinct protein from prostatic acid phosphatase, the most well-known secretory enzyme of the human prostate.

Several murine monoclonal antibodies directed to PA have been reported by three groups of investigators (Frankel et al., 1982b; Papsidero et al., 1983; Myrtle et al., 1983). All were prepared using purified PA (Wang et al., 1979) as the immunogen.

Frankel et al. (1982b) produced three monoclonal antibodies against PA by fusing splenocytes of mice immunized with PA with the NS-1 mouse myeloma cell line. A solid-phase radioimmunoassay using PA as target antigen was used to screen hybridoma antibody. From 160 primary hybrids secreting antibodies reactive with PA, three monoclonal antibodies, 1C5, 2G7, and 1F3, were finally obtained. All were of IgG$_1$ isotype. By cross-binding and cross-blocking experiments on PA, 1F3 was shown to direct one antigenic site, while both 1C5 and 2G7 were directed another site that was different from the determinant recognized by 1F3. Also, only one site per PA molecule is present. Additional data ascertaining the binding of these monoclonal antibodies to PA were provided by two-dimensional gel electrophoresis experiments. Analysis of two-dimensional gel electrophoresis of the radiolabeled immunoprecipitate confirmed the antigen M_r of 34,000 and the average isoelectric po int of 6.8 from three charged species of immunoreactive PA.

Immunoperoxidase staining of formalin-fixed and paraffin-embedded tissue sections with these three monoclonal antibodies revealed cytoplasmic stain in prostatic epithelial cells of both benign and malignant prostate. Among other sections examined, including colon, pancreas, stomach, and kidney, only the renal tissue was stained. Normal renal tubules, but not glomeruli, stained significantly by all three antibodies. However, no PA was detected by the absorption and sandwich type immunoassay tests using these antibodies. It is suggested that a nonidiotypic binding between murine monoclonal immunoglobulin and a receptor on renal tubular-epithelium is the cause for this observation. It is also noted that frozen sections of BPH demonstrate weak, nonspecific staining, perhaps due to washout or loss of PA in unfixed specimens. None of the antibodies reacted with a variety of human tissue membrane preparations, including those of prostate origin. A sandwich radioimmunoassay using 2G7 antibody to coat the plate and ^{125}I-labeled 1F3 to detect 2G7-bound PA was developed to quantitate PA. Elevated serum PA (>5 ng/mL) was detected only in prostate cancer.

Papsidero et al. (1983) also produced a monoclonal antibody, F5, by fusing mouse immune spleen cells with mouse myeloma cell line P3X63Ag8.653. A solid-phase enzyme immunoassay employing plastic tube-coated PA as target antigen was used to screen hybridoma antibody. Monoclonal antibody F5 is of IgG$_1$ subclass. F5 reacted only with prostate tissue extract among various human tissues examined (heart, urethra, pancreas, lung, kidney, spleen, and bladder) by a competitive inhibition enzyme immunoassay. Using purified and radiolabeled PA, an affinity constant of 2.5×10^{10} L/M was determined, indicating that F5 is a high-affinity monoclonal antibody to PA.

Specificity of F5 antibody was examined by an indirect immunoperoxidase assay, similar to that by Frankel et al. (1982b), in a large panel of formalin-fixed paraffin-embedded human tissue sections, both normal and carcinoma. Among normal tissues examined, including prostate, urinary bladder, seminal vesicles, testes, kidney, colon, pancreas, liver, brain, breast, uterus, myocardium, salivary gland, vas deferens, urethra and lymph nodes, only prostate, five out of five specimens, stained positively and significantly. It is of interest to note that none of two kidney normal specimen sections stained, a different observation from those of Frankel et al. Thus, F5 appears to be distinct from 1F3, 1C5, and 2G7 antibodies. Apparently, the F5 determinant and F5 mouse immunoglobulin, although also of IgG$_1$ isotype, are different from those determinants and mouse immunoglobulins as reported by Frankel et al. (1982b).

A large panel of malignant tissue sections also were examined by F5 antibody staining, including carcinomas of the prostate, colon, breast, pancreas, stomach, uterus, ovary, lung, esophagus, transitional cell carcinoma of the bladder, testis, kidney, malignant melanoma, and lymphosarcoma and mesothelioma. Only prostate adenocarcinomas were stainable by F5 antibody. Both primary (25/25) and metastatic (7/7) prostate adenocarcinomas expressed F5 epitope recognized as cytoplasmic stain by the antibody. Stain intensity and percentage of stained cells varied among the specimens, i.e., heterogeneity of F5 immunoreactive cells was observed. Positive stain is most intense in well-differentiated tumors and appears to be related to the grade (Gleason) of the tumors.

The detection of F5 epitope in metastatic prostate tumors will provide an invaluable tool for differential diagnosis of metastasis with unknown primary, as similarly reported previously using rabbit polyclonal antibodies to PA (Nadji et al., 1981).

Myrtle et al. (1983) also produced two murine monoclonal antibodies against purified PA and developed an immunoradiometric assay for PA. Since these two antibodies, as reported, are directed against two separate, sterically distinct PA determinants, one is immobilized on a solid phase plastic bead, and another is radiolabeled with ^{125}I served as a measurable parameter. The immunoradiometric assay results in a dose-response curve of 2–100 ng/mL and sensitivity of 0.4 ng/mL. A normal range of less than 3 ng/mL is obtained from this assay, a range similar to that reported by Kuriyama et al. (1980) using rabbit polyclonal antibodies (Wang et al., 1979) in an enzyme-linked immunosorbent assay. No clinical data were described by Myrtle et al. in their brief report.

Although not directly related to the subject of monoclonal antibody to PA, it is interesting to review a recent report by Chu et al. (1984) describing a naturally occurring immunoglobulin that is shown to bind PA in circulation, named prostate antigen-binding globulin (PABG). Elevated PABG is found only in patients with advanced stage of prostate cancer, and has been purified from serum. By immunoprecipitation techniques, PABG is reactive with PA, anti-PA xenoantibody and antihuman IgG. By immunoperoxidase procedure, PABG positively stains prostatic ductal epithelial cells, and negatively with all other human tissues examined. In circulation PABG exists in both free form and complexed with PA. These results suggest that PABG is an auto-antibody, and also imply that generation of hybridoma-derived monoclonal antibodies of human origin, directed to PA, is experimentally possible by fusing patients' B-lymphocytes and an appropriate mutant myeloma cell partner.

Such an approach to the generation of human monoclonal antibody has been demonstrated to be experimentally feasible by Glassy et al. (1983). A human IgM secreting hybrid, MHG7, is produced by fusing lymphocytes of cancer regional lymph nodes and a 6-thioguanine resistant human lymphoblastoid B cell line, UC729-6. MHG7 binds LNCaP and PC-3 prostate tumor cell lines and a panel of other tumor cells. If prostate metastatic lymph nodes are used for lymphocyte isolation, and, if needed, fortified by PA in vitro sensitization, along with the use of PA as target for antibody screen, a human monoclonal antibody directed to PA can be easily generated.

5. Prostatic Acid Phosphatase

Prostatic acid phosphatase (PAP) is the most well-known marker protein for prostate cancer (Chu et al., 1982). PAP is one of the oldest tumor markers, as it has been employed as a laboratory aid in association with metastatic prostate cancer since the 1930's. Biochemically, PAP is a glycoprotein of 100,000 mol wt, consisting of two subunits, 50,000 each, and of 13% carbohydrates and 87% peptides. Amino acid content and carbohydrate composition of PAP has been reported (Lin et al., 1983a). Additionally, amino-terminal sequence, with lysine as the N-terminal amino acid, of PAP is now known (Lin et al., 1983b; Taga et al., 1983). As discussed previously, peptide map of PAP (Lin et al, 1983a) is different entirely from that of PA. Simultaneous determination of both PA and PAP has been reported to yield additive clinical value in serodiagnosis of prostate cancer (Kuriyama et al., 1982).

Generation of murine monoclonal antibodies to PAP has been reported primarily by two groups of investigators (Choe et al., 1982a; Lee et al., 1982), although immunologic reagents of monoclonal anti-PAP antibody are also available from commercial source. However, specificity characterization of anti-PAP monoclonal antibodies has been reported only by Choe et al. and Lee et al.

By a conventional hybridoma technique using purified PAP isolated from seminal plasma as immunogen, Choe et al. produced 12 clones of hybrid secreting anti-PAP antibodies, eight of which were further characterized and also used in characterization of antigenic sites of PAP. PAP was first mildly digested with submaximal protease to yield three fragments with M_r of 22,000 (Sp-1), 16,000 (Sp-2) and 11,000 (Sp-3). By competitive antigen binding assay, i.e., PAP was saturated with 12 monoclonal antibodies, followed by reacting briefly with six ^{125}I-labeled monoclonal antibodies for competitive binding, three distinct groups of antibodies were detected, representing three nonidentical and non-overlapping antigenic determinants on the intact PAP molecule. A direct binding assay revealed that all monoclonal antibodies were bound exclusively to the largest $(M_r$ 22,000) Sp-1 fragment.

It deserves to be mentioned that another interesting aspect of the work reported by Choe and his associates (1982b) is their identification of a common cross-reacting antigen determinant on the smallest Sp-3 fragment of protease digestion by its binding reactivity with rabbit unfractionated anti-PAP polyclonal antibodies and anti-lysosomal acid phosphatase polyclonal antibodies. Further, upon binding to anti-PAP polyclonal antibodies, Sp-3 fragment exhibited a small, yet significant, acid phosphatase catalytic reactivity, suggesting Sp-3 contains the enzyme active site of PAP and one common antigenic site for, perhaps, all acid phosphatases. The identification of four antigenic determinants by polyclonal antibodies, three of which by monoclonal antibodies, seems to confirm a previous report by Lee et al. (1980).

Lee and associates (1980) partially hydrolyzed purified PAP with trypsin, which resulted in three fragments $(M_r$, I, 65,000; II, 25,000 and

III, 11,000, respectively). By using goat polyclonal anti-PAP antibodies, only fragment III was precipitable by immunoprecipitation techniques (e.g., immunodiffusion and immunoelectrophoresis) suggesting at least two sites are present in the fragment III. An indirect binding assay (double antibody radioimmunoassay) detected two additional antibody binding sites, one each on fragments I and II. Thus, the results suggested that the entire molecule of PAP possesses a minimum of four different antibody-binding sites, as examined by goat polyclonal anti-PAP antibodies. It is interesting to note that the same number of antigenic determinants were identified independently by these two groups of investigators using differently prepared antibody reagents and entirely different approaches/techniques. These results certainly do not imply that antigenic determinants as reported by Lee et al. and by Choe et al. are identical.

Lee et al. (1982) also have produced murine monoclonal antibodies to purified PAP. A rapid and effective technique was used to screen hybrid culture fluid for anti-PAP antibody by using PAP coupled-sheep red blood cells as target cells in an immune hemolytic method (Jou and Bankert, 1981). A total of 156 hybrids (150 IgG_1, 2 IgG_1, 2 IgG_{2a}, 1 IgG_3, 2 IgM) secreting anti-PAP monoclonal antibodies were obtained from three fusion experiments. Four antibodies, one each from IgG1, IgG_{2a}, IgG_3, and IgM, were selected for further characterization. By a solid-phase quantitative binding assay with excess amount of ^{14}C-labeled monoclonal antibodies against PAP, three antigenic determinants of PAP were identified. IgG_1 and IgM antibodies reacted with two different nonblocking antigenic sites of the PAP molecule, whereas IgG_{2a} and IgG_3 antibodies bind to an identical or two partially overlapping determinants. Thus, PAP molecule contains a minimum of three different epitopes as revealed by these four monoclonal antibodies.

The immunological specificity of these monoclonal anti-PAP antibodies was characterized by a competitive-inhibition assay between PAP and acid phosphatases prepared from other human tissues. Monoclonal anti-PAP IgG_1 and IgM antibodies were shown to exhibit a higher degree of specificity for PAP than for other nonprostatic acid pbosphatases in comparison with monoclonal anti-PAP IgG_{2a} or IgG_3 antibody, and a goat xenoantiserum. These relative specificities were further confirmed by an immunocytochemical procedure on various formalin-fixed and paraffin-embedded human tissue sections. IgG_1 and IgM both expressed an intense cytoplasmic stain in benign prostatic hypertrophy and primary, as well as in metastatic, prostate carcinomas, whereas IgG_{2a} and IgG_3 showed only moderately intense stain in these prostate specimens. Monoclonal IgG_1 and IgM antibodies failed to stain tissue sections of nonprostate origin, except a weak or questionable peroxidase stain was found in the spleen, pancreas, and kidney. IgG_{2a} and IgG_3 antibodies, however, demonstrated an unequivocal stain with all normal tissues examined. These monoclonal antibodies appear to be useful probes in the characterization of antigenic structure of PAP molecule, and in the immunocytochemical examination of PAP and various acid phosphatases. It is noted that using rabbit polyclonal antibodies against PAP purified from prostate tumor and absorbed by normal female serum (Chu et al., 1978), Nadji et al. (1980) have shown that PAP antibody reagent is a potentially useful histologic marker for prostate cancer.

Recently, Lin et al. (1983c), using the monoclonal anti-PAP IgG$_1$ antibody alone as characterized by Lee et al. (1982), developed a simple quantitative assay for circulating PAP. Upon binding to antibody, PAP-anti-PAP IgG$_1$ complexes were precipitated by 7.5% polyethylene glycol and PAP activity was measured. Of special interest regarding this assay is the use of a single monoclonal anti-PAP antibody and the application of polyethylene glycol as precipitant of immune complexes and sensitivity enhancer of PAP measurement. Initial serum evaluation showed that this assay is a simple and effective procedure for PAP immunoassay.

A PAP assay kit developed by a commercial firm with two monoclonal anti-PAP antibodies and an immunoradiometric technique also has been reported (Davies and Gochman, 1983).

Another potential application for monoclonal anti-PAP antibody is its use in antibody-directed radioimaging and chemotherapy of prostate cancer, as reported recently by Lee et al. (1983). In in vivo experiment with LNCaP human prostate tumor xenograft in nude mice, radiolabeled anti-PAP IgG$_1$ was shown to localize the tumor, superior to similarly prepared goat polyclonal anti-PAP antiserum. In addition, monoclonal anti-PAP antibody was conjugated to an antitumor drug, 5-fluorouracil deoxyriboside. Immunological and pharmacological reactivities of the antibody-drug remained as tested in an in vitro system using LNCaP as the target. The growth of xenografted prostate tumor also was greatly inhibited by drug and monoclonal antibody conjugate in comparison with the controls (drug, antibody alone, or a mixture of antibody and drug without coupling). This experimental animal work with monoclonal antibody certainly will provide useful information toward the possible addition of new modalities to prostate cancer.

6. Summary

Murine monoclonal antibodies directed to human prostate cancer-related antigens are reviewed. These antibodies are produced against established human prostate tumor lines, namely DU-145 and PC-3, membrane-enriched preparation of human prostate, and against two chemically defined prostate organ-site and cell-type specific glycoproteins: prostate-specific antigen and prostatic acid phosphatase.

Five monoclonal antibodies reactive with cell surface components of human prostate tumor lines are available, 83.21, P6.2, αPro3, αPro5 and αPro13. Antibody 83.21 appears to be prostate and bladder cancer-associated and is directed against a 180,000 mol wt glycoprotein. It also reacts with a cytomegalovirus-transformed human embryonic lung cell line, and thus could be a useful probe for the study of a possible link between cytomegalovirus and transformation of prostate malignancy. Both antibodies 83.21 and P6.2 react more strongly with poorly differentiated and undifferentiated prostate tumors, primary and metastatic, than with well to moderately differentiated tumors. No normal human tissues, including prostate and urinary bladder, is reactive with either antibody, except proximal convoluted tubules of normal kidney. αPro3 antibody is primarily associated with prostate and testicular cancers. Both αPro3 and αPro5 recognize two separate determinants of an antigenic component (P54) of a 175,000 mol wt glycoprotein on the surface of PC-3 tumor cells. P54 is not readily shed from PC-3 cell surface, although a nonglycosylated protein of 50,000 mol wt is detectable in spent culture medium. PC-3 cells can be modulated by αPro3-P54 and αPro5-P54 immune complexes by mechanism of endocytosis. A combination of both antibodies demonstrate a greater endocytosis, i.e., synergistic effect, of the antigen-antibody complexes than either antibody alone. This model is potentially a valuable immunotherapeutic tool. αPro13 antibody recognize an antigen of 140,000 mol wt and reacts with ductal epithelia of both malignant and benign prostate.

Seven monoclonal antibodies directed to plasma membrane-enriched fraction of benign human prostate have been generated, five of which are reported to be reactive specifically with the epithelium element of the prostate (and breast and salivary gland), and two specifically with stroma. One antibody in the former group appears to be similar to αPro3 antibody in its cell-binding activity against prostate and bladder tumor lines, and it is suggested that it could be useful in the treatment of prostate cancer patients.

Six monoclonal antibodies have been reported to react with purified human prostate specific antigen, a chemically and histologically well-defined prostatic epithelial cell marker. Three antibodies, 1C5, 2G7, and 1F3, recognize two separate nonblocking determinants on prostate antigen, one per molecule (one with 1F3, and another with 2G7 and 1C5). Specificity of antibodies is confirmed by immunostaining and adsorption procedures. All three antibodies are reactive only with human prostate, although normal renal tubules are also stainable, which is caused by a nonidiotypic binding between mouse immunoglobulin and a receptor on renal tubular epithelium. A sandwich radioimmunoassay is developed using 1F3 and 2G7 antibodies. Elevated serum prostate antigen is detected only in prostate cancer. Another monoclonal, F5, is shown to be unequivocally prostate epithelium-specific. Unlike the above three antibodies, F5 does not stain normal kidney. F5, a high affinity monoclonal antibody, is shown to be especially useful in localizing tumor cells of prostate origin in secondary metastasis. Heterogeneity of F5 immunoreactive stain cells has been observed as most intense in well-differentiated tumors and appears to be related to the grade of the tumors. Two other monoclonal antibodies, reportedly to recognize two separate, sterically distinct epitopes, have been used in a commercially available immunoradiometric assay for quantitation of serum prostate antigen.

More than 100 hybrids secreting monoclonal antibodies to prostatic acid phosphatase, one of the oldest tumor markers, are available. Using some of these antibodies, a miniumum of three distinct determinants especially associated with prostatic acid phosphatase have been identified independently by two groups of investigators. Since carbohydrate content, amino acid composition and partial amino-terminal sequence of prostatic acid phosphatase are known, antigenic structure of this enzyme can be worked out with these monoclonal antibodies in the not too distsnt future. This will provide useful information in the molecular biology of prostatic acid phosphatase. Two additional applications have been developed in the use of monoclonal antibodies to prostatic acid phosphatase. Using one single monoclonal antibody, a simple immunoenzyme assay has been developed. An assay kit with two antibodies and an immunoradiometric technique is also available commercially. Initial experimental animal work has shown the potential application of monoclonal antiprostatic acid phosphatase antibody in radioimaging and immunochemotherapy (antibody-drug conjugate) of prostate cancer.

References

Choe, B. K., H. S. Lillehoj, M. K. Dong, S. Gleason, M. Baron, and N. R. Rose (1982a), *Ann. NY Acad. Sci.* **390**, 16.

Choe, B. K., M. K. Dong, D. Walz, S. Gleason, and N. R. Rose (1982b), *Proc. Natl. Acad. Sci. USA* **79**, 6052.

Chu, T. M., M. C. Wang, W. W. Scott, R. P. Gibbons, D. E. Johnson, J. S. Schmidt, S. A. Loening, G. P. Prout, and G. P. Murphy (1978), *Invest. Urol.* **15**, 319.

Chu, T. M., M. C. Wang, C. L. Lee, C. S.Killian, and G. P. Murphy (1982), in *Biochemical Markers for Cancer* (T. M. Chu, ed.), Marcel Dekker, p.117.

Chu, T. M., M. Kuriyama, E. A.Johnson, L. D. Papsidero, C. S. Killian, G. P. Murphy, and M. C. Wang (1984), *Tranplantation Proc.* **16**, 481.

Davies, S. N. and N. Gochman (1983), *Am. J. Clin. Pathol.* **79,** 114.

Frankel, A. E., R. V. Rouse, and L. A. Herzenberg, (1982a), *Proc. Natl. Acad. Sci. USA* **79,** 903.

Frankel, A. E., R. V. Rouse, M. C.Wang, T. M. Chu, and L.A. Herzenberg (1982b), *Cancer Res.* **42,** 3714.

Glassy, M. C., H. Handley, D. Stayer, H. Lowe, R. Astarita, and I. Royston (1983), *Fed. Proc.* **42,** 402 (abstract).

Jou, Y. H. and R. B. Bankert (1981), *Proc. Natl. Acad Sci. USA,* **78,** 2492.

Kuriyama, M., M. C. Wang, L. D. Papsidero, C. S. Killian, T. Shimano, L. A. Valenzuela, T. Nishiura, G. P. Murphy, and T. M. Chu (1980), *Cancer Res.* **40,** 4658.

Kuriyama, M., M. C. Wang, C. L. Lee, L. D. Papsidero, C. S. Killian, H. Inaji, N. S. Slack, G. P. Murphy, and T. M. Chu (1981), *Cancer Res.* **41,** 3874.

Kuriyama, M., M. C. Wang, C. L. Lee, C. S. Killian, L. D. Papsidero, H. Inaji, R. M. Loor, M. F. Lin, T. Nishiura, N. H. Slack, G. P. Murphy, and T. M. Chu (1982), *J. Natl. Cancer Inst.* **68,** 99.

Lee, C. L., M. C.Wang, G. P. Murphy, and T. M. Chu (1978), *Cancer Res.* **38,** 2871.

Lee, C. L., G. P. Murphy, and T. M. Chu (1980), *Fed. Proc.* **39,** 413 (abstract).

Lee, C. L., C. Y. Li, Y. H. Jou, G. P. Murphy, and T. M. Chu (1982), *Ann. NY Acad. Sci.* **390,** 52.

Lee, C. L., E. Kawinski, S. S. Leong, J. S. Horoszewicz, G. P. Murphy, and T. M. Chu, (1983), *Fed. Proc.* **43,** 682 (abstract).

Lin, M. F., C. L. Lee, S. L. Li, and T. M. Chu (1983a), *Biochem.* **22,** 1055.

Lin, M. F., C. L.Lee, F. S. Sharief, S. L. Li, and T. M. Chu (1983b), *Cancer Res.* **43,** 3841.

Lin, M. F., C. L. Lee and T. M. Chu (1983c), *Clin. Chim. Acta.* **130,** 263.

Myrtle, J. F., W. Schackelford, R. M. Bartholomew, and J. Wampler (1983), *Clin. Chem.* **29,** 1216 (abstract).

Nadji, M., S. Z. Tabei, A. Castro, T. M. Chu, and A. R. Morales (1980), *Am. J. Clin. Pathol.* **73,** 735.

Nadji, M., S. Z. Tabei, A. Castro, T. M. Chu, M. C. Wang, G. P.Murphy, and A. R.Morales (1981), *Cancer* **48,** 1229.

Papsidero, L. D., M. Kuriyama, M. C.Wang, J. S.Horoszewicz, S. S. Leong, L. A. Valenzuela, G. P. Murphy, and T. M. Chu (1981), *J. Natl. Cancer Inst.* **66,** 37.

Papsidero, L. D., G. A.Croghan, M. C. Wang, M.Kuriyama, E. A.Johnson, L. A. Valenzuela, and T. M. Chu (1983), *Hybridoma* **2,** 139.

Starling, J. J., S. M. Sieg, M. L. Beckett, P. F. Schellhammer, L. E. Ladagan, and G. L. Wright, Jr. (1982), *Cancer Res.* **42,** 3084.

Taga, E. M., D. L. Moore and R. L. Van Etten (1983), *Prostate,* **4,** 141.

Wang, M. C., L. A. Valenzuela, G. P.Murphy, and T. M. Chu (1979), *Invest. Urol.* **17,** 159.

Wang, M. C., M. Kuriyama, L. D. Papsidero, R. M. Loor, L. A. Valenzuela, G. P. Murphy, and T. M. Chu (1982a), in *Methods of Cancer Research* (H. Busch and L. C. Yeoman, eds.) Academic Press, **19,** 179.

Wang, M. C., L. A. Valenzuela, G. P. Murphy and T. M. Chu (1982b), *Oncology* **39,** 1.

Wang, M. C., R. M. Loor, S. L. Li, and T. M. Chu (1983), *IRCS Med. Sci.* **11,** 327.

Ware, J. L., D. F. Paulson, S. F. Parks and K. S. Webb (1982), *Cancer Res.* **42,** 1215.

Webb, K. S. and J. L. Ware (1983), *Fed. Proc.* **42,** 630 (abstract).

Webb, K. S., J. L. Ware, S. F. Parks, W. H. Briner and D. F. Paulson, (1983), *Cancer Immunol. Immunotherap.* **14,** 155.

Wright, G. L., Jr., M. L. Beckett, J. J. Starling, P. F. Schellhammer, S. M. Sieg, L. L. Ladaga, and S. Poleskic (1983), *Cancer Res.* **43,** 5509.

Chapter 14

Monoclonal Antibodies to Renal Cancer Markers

NEIL H. BANDER[1,2] AND
CARLOS CORDON-CARDO[3]

*James Buchanan Brady Foundation, Division of Urology, New York
Hospital-Cornell Medical Center, New York, New York[1]; Laboratory of
Human Cancer Immunology[2] and Laboratory of Immunopathology[3],
Memorial Sloan-Kettering Cancer Center, New York, New York[2]*

1. Introduction

Seventeen thousand Americans develop renal cancer annually. At the time of diagnosis, 30% have metastatic disease demonstrable by conventional radiologic or nuclide imaging techniques. Of the remaining patients who are ostensibly surgically curable, about 40% have micrometastatic disease that will later manifest itself. Currently no effective method exists for detection of micrometastatic disease. Likewise, no effective systemic therapy exists and these patients will die of their disease.

Potentially great benefit would be derived if markers were available to: (1) screen for renal cancer; (2) monitor the course of disease; (3) identify those patients at increased risk of having micrometastatic disease; (4) permit detection and localization of disseminated disease while still at a microscopic level; and (5) provide targets for treatment of disease at these levels when potential for cure is greatest.

Although such markers of renal cancer have been diligently sought in the past, none have been shown to be of clinical value. However, the advent of hybridoma technology is allowing the dissection of the complex cancer cell into its molecular components. Monoclonal antibodies (Mab) are identifying components not previously detected or definable. This, in turn, is allowing us to refine our level of cancer classification and comprehension from the microscopic to the molecular level. The greater precision of molecular subclassification will allow better understanding of natural history and prognosis and, therefore, enhance our therapeutic decision-making. Indeed, it should allow better understanding of basic cancer cell biology.

This chapter discusses four Mabs that demonstrate both utility as markers for renal cancer as well as early indications of potential clinical application. They were generated by immunization of (C57BL6 X BALB/c)F$_1$ mice with viable renal cancer cells from lines established in the Laboratory of Human Cancer Serology at the Memorial Sloan-Kettering Cancer Center (Ueda et al., 1981). These Mabs were characterized by a detailed specificity analysis and by immunoprecipitation of the defined antigens (Ag) from metabolically labeled cell lysates. Further analysis has included study of the in vivo specificity of these Mabs by applying immunohistologic techniques to frozen sections of normal adult, fetal and neoplastic tissues (Finstad et al., in press).

2. Mab S$_4$

Mab S$_4$ immunoprecipitates a 160 kilodalton glycoprotein (gp 160) from metabolically labeled cell lysates of SK-RC-7, the immunizing cell line. This cell line was derived from a localized (stage I), well-differentiated renal cancer in 1976. In vitro expression of gp160 is restricted to some renal cancers and all normal kidney lines (Table 1). A single

Table 1
Immunochemical and Serological Characterization
of Four Renal Monoclonal Antibodies

Mab	Ig Subtype	Immunochemistry, (M_r)	Cultured cells
S$_4$	Gamma 2A	gp 160,000	Normal kidney Renal carcinoma Choriocarcinoma
S23	Gamma 1	gp 120,000	Normal kidney Renal carcinoma
S6	Gamma 1	gp 120,000	Normal kidney Fibroblasts Renal, bladder, colon, lung carcinomas Astrocytomas
S22	Gamma 1	gp 115,000	Normal kidney Renal and ovarian carcinoma

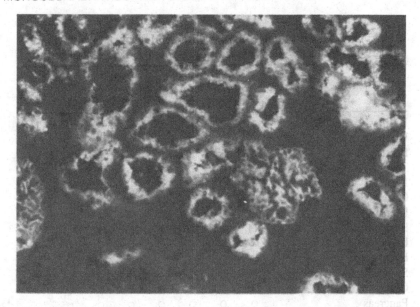

Fig. 1.   Monoclonal antibody S_4 binds to the renal glomerulus and proximal tubule. Neighboring distal tubules do not fluoresce ($\times$ 128).

neuroblastoma line SK-NMC represents the only nonrenal derived line that is gp160$^+$ (W. Rettig, unpublished observations) in a panel of over 100 cell lines.

Immunofluorescence and immunoperoxidase assays of Mab S_4 on frozen sections of normal adult kidney reveal staining of the glomerulus and proximal tubular epithelium (Cordon-Cardo et al., 1984). (Fig. 1). Mab $S_4$$^+$ staining is not detectable on any normal tissue outside the kidney (Table 2). Thirty-one of 56 (55%) renal cancer specimens were gp160$^+$. This includes 25/44 (57%) and 6/12 (50%) lesions derived from primary or metastatic sites, respectively. All 39 nonrenal cancers studied were gp160$^-$ (Table 3).

3. Mab S_{22}

Mab S_{22} was derived from a fusion using SK-RC-7 as the immunizing line. This IgG$_1$ antibody immunoprecipitates a 115,000 molecular weight glycoprotein from serologically positive cell lines. Direct cell-binding assays reveal gp115 to be expressed by a subset of renal cancers (titer: 10^{-4}–10^{-7}), all normal kidney cultures (titer: 10^{-3}), and one ovarian cancer line, SK-OV-3 (titer: 10^{-2}).

Immunohistologic assays fail to reveal any normal adult or fetal tissues which are gp115$^+$. However, 20/56 (36%) renal cancer specimens are gp115$^+$. Again, the proportion of gp115$^+$ primary (14/44) and metastatic (6/12) lesions is not significantly different.

Table 2
Immunohistologic Analysis of Four Renal Monoclonal Antibodies
on Frozen Sections of Fetal and Adult Human Normal Tissues[a]

Tissues	S4		S23		S6		S22	
	F	A	F	A	F	A	F	A
Kidney	●	●	●	●	●	●	○	○
Urothelium	○	○	○	○	○	○	○	○
Prostate	NT	○	NT	●	NT	●	NT	○
Testis	○	○	○	○	○	○	○	○
Breast	NT	○	NT	●	NT	○	NT	○
Ovary	○	○	○	○	○	○	○	○
Uterus	○	○	○	○	○	○	○	○
Placenta	NT	○	NT	●	NT	●	NT	○
Lung	○	○	○	○	○	○	○	○
Esophagus	○	○	○	○	○	○	○	○
Stomach	○	○	○	○	○	○	○	○
Colon	○	○	●	●	○	○	○	○
Pancreas	○	○	○	○	○	○	○	○
Liver	○	○	○	○	○	○	○	○
Skin	○	○	○	○	○	○	○	○
Brain	○	○	○	○	○	○	○	○
Adrenal	○	○	○	○	○	○	○	○
Thyroid	NT	○	NT	○	NT	○	NT	○
Lymph node	○	○	○	○	○	○	○	○
Spleen	○	○	○	○	○	○	○	○
Thymus	○	NT	○	NT	○	NT	○	NT
Heart	○	○	○	○	○	○	○	○
Soft tissues	○	○	○	○	○	○	○	○
Blood vessels	○	○	○	○	○	○	○	○
Interstitial matrix	●	●	○	○	○	○	○	○

[a] ● = Presence or ○ = Absence of antigenic reactivity by immunofluorescence and immunoperoxidase techniques. F = Fetal; A = Adult; NT = Not tested or tissue not available.

4. Mab S_{23}

Mab S_{23} immunoprecipitates a glycoprotein of 120 kilodaltons. This antigen is restricted to renal-derived tissue in vitro. It is designated gp120r to distinguish it from a nonrestricted epitope detected by Mabs$_6$ (vide infra). gp120r is expressed by 16/33 renal cancer cell lines and all normal kidney cultures. All nonrenal lines are gp120r⁻.

Frozen sections of normal kidney demonstrate staining of the proximal tubule (Fig. 2) and occasionally a short segment of the descending loop of Henle. Normal prostate, breast and colon and 5 of 39 nonrenal cancers expressed gp120r by immunohistologic assays. Of 56 renal carcinoma specimens, 27 (48%) were gp120r⁺.

Table 3
Immunopathology of Four Renal Monoclonal Antibodies on Frozen
Sections of Nonrenal Human Tumors[a]

Tumors	S4	S23	S6	S22
Transitional carcinomas				
Kidney	0/2	0/2	0/2	0/2
Ureter	0/2	0/2	0/2	0/2
Bladder	0/6	0/6	0/6	0/6
Prostatic adenocarcinomas	0/2	2/2	2/2	0/2
Breast carcinomas	0/5	0/5	0/5	0/5
Colon adenocarcinomas	0/5	3/5	0/5	0/5
Lung carcinomas	0/5	0/5	0/5	0/5
Teratocarcinomas	0/3	0/3	0/3	0/3
Astrocytomas	0/3	0/3	0/3	0/3
Melanomas	0/3	0/3	0/3	0/3
Lymphomas	0/3	0/3	0/3	0/3
Total:	0/39	5/39	2/39	0/39

[a]Number of positive cases/total number of cases studied:
Positivity = Presence of antigenic reactivity by immunofluorescence and immunoperoxidase techniques

5. Mab S$_6$

Mab S$_6$ also precipitates a 120,000 molecular weight glycoprotein. Because it is not restricted to renal derived lines in vitro, the defined antigen
is designated gp120nr. Unlike the previous Mab that subset renal tumors

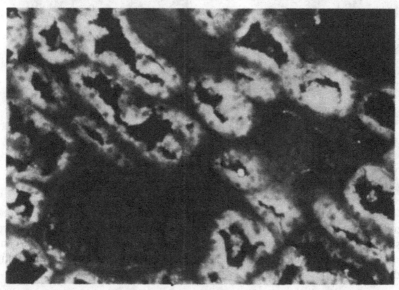

Fig. 2. Monoclonal antibody S$_{23}$ localizes to the proximal tubular cells.
Glomeruli and distal tubules are negative ($\times$ 128).

in vitro (based on presence or absence of their defined Ag), all renal cancer lines are gp120nr$^+$. All normal kidney cultures and approximately one-quarter of nonrenal lines also express gp120nr.

Frozen sections of normal kidney demonstrate S_6 staining of the proximal tubule and a short segment of the descending limb of Henle's loop (Fig. 3). Outside the adult kidney, only prostatic glands were gp120nr$^+$. Similarly, among 39 nonrenal cancer specimens, only 2 prostatic adenocarcinoma were positive. Of 56 renal cancers, 52 (93%) were gp120nr$^+$.

6. Use as Markers of Proximal Tubular Cells

Three of these four antigens (gp160, gp120r, gp120nr) are expressed by cells of the normal nephron. As noted in Fig. 4, the area of overlap of these markers is the proximal tubule. The restricted specificity of these Mab both in vivo and in vitro make them good markers for cells of the proximal nephron.

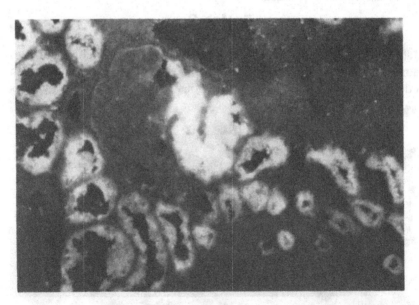

Fig. 3.   Monoclonal antibody S_6 localizes to the proximal tubule and descending loop of Henle. A, While the glomerulus and distal tubules are unstained, the proximal tubule as it exits Bowman's space is brightly fluorescent ($\times$ 200); B, In the juxtamedullary area, the loops of Henle bind monoclonal antibody S_6 ($\times$ 256).

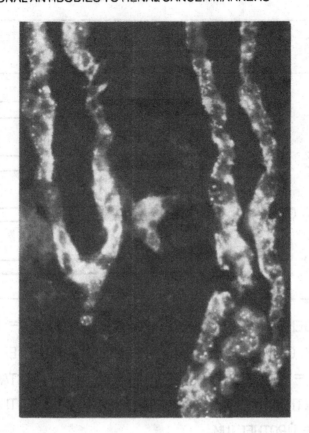

7. Ability to Discriminate Renal from Nonrenal Cancers

Immunopathological analysis reveals that 93% (52/56) of renal cancers are gp120nr$^+$. Conversely, only 5% (2/39) of nonrenal cancers tested express gp120nr. This single marker, therefore, provides significant accuracy in differentiating renal from nonrenal cancers. Furthermore, because of the restricted nature of these markers, expression of a combination of two or more of them (gp120nr plus gp160 and/or gp115) make renal origin of a tumor a virtual certainty.

8. Subclassification of Renal Cancer

Perhaps the most interesting feature of these Mab is that they allow subclassification of renal cancers based on antigen expression. This subclassification occurs at two distinct levels.

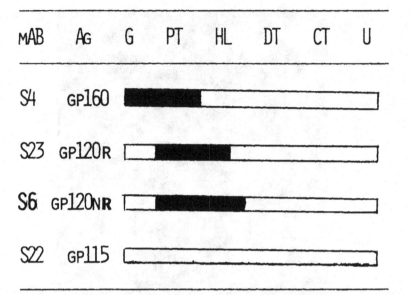

LEGEND: MAB = MONOCLONAL ANTIBODY; AG = ANTIGEN;
G = GLOMERULUS; PT = PROXIMAL TUBULE EPITHELIUM;
HL = HENLE'S LOOP EPITHELIUM; DT = DISTAL TUBULE
EPITHELIUM; CT = COLLECTING TUBULE EPITHELIUM;
U = UROTHELIUM

Fig. 4.   Distribution of antigen expression along the nephron.

8.1. gp120nr

Expression of gp120nr appears to be pivotal. As previously noted 52/56 (93%) renal cancers are gp120nr$^+$ (Fig. 5). Of these, 42/52 (81%) expressed at least one additional proximal tubular antigen (i.e., gp160 and/or gp120r). Conversely, 4/56 (7%) specimens were gp120nr$^-$ (Table 4). Amongst these four neoplasms, none express a single proximal tubular antigen. The incidence of the gp120nr$^-$/gp120r$^-$/gp160$^-$/gp115$^-$ phenotype to the absolute exclusion of other possible gp120nr$^-$ phenotype is statistically significant ($p < 0.001$). These findings are consistent with expression of gp120nr being pivotal in marking differentiation of proximal tubular cells. When gp120nr is not expressed, other known proximal tubular markers (e.g., gp160 and gp120r) are coordinately · repressed.

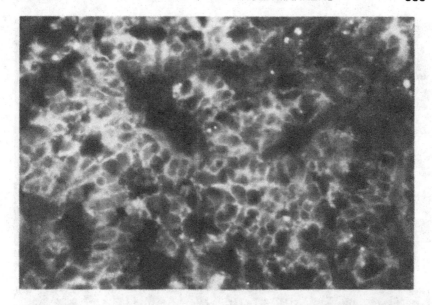

Fig. 5.   A

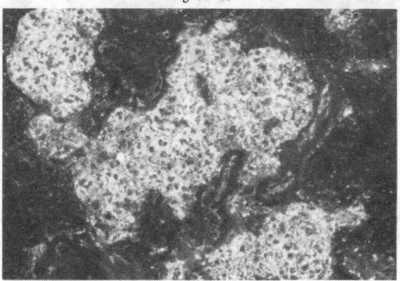

Fig. 5.   B

Fig. 5.   Examples of immunofluorescent reactivity of monoclonal anti-bodies on sections of renal cancer of differing histologic types: A, monoclonal antibody S_6—clear cell carcinoma ($\times$ 256); B, monoclonal antibody S_6—granular cell carcinoma ($\times$ 128); C, monoclonal antibody S_4—papillary adenocarcinoma ($\times$ 168).

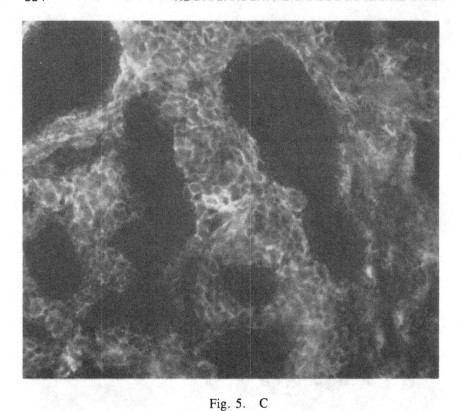

Fig. 5.   C

Table 4
Phenotypes of 56 Renal Cancers: gp120nr/gp120r/gp160/gp115

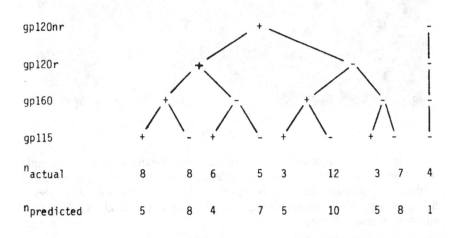

gp120nr			+					−
gp120r		+				−		−
gp160	+		−		+		−	−
gp115	+	−	+	−	+	−	+	−	−
n_{actual}	8	8	6	5	3	12	3	7	4
$n_{predicted}$	5	8	4	7	5	10	5	8	1

Absence of gp120nr from these four renal cancers could be explained by derivation of these tumors either from cells other than the proximal tubule or from a point along the differentiation pathway prior to gp120nr expression. It is interesting to note that in the original immunopathological study of renal cancer by Wallace and Nairn in 1972, ten of their eleven specimens were positive for a brush border (proximal tubule) antigen. The one cancer that was brush border negative was found to express Tamm-Horsfall protein that is derived from the ascending loop of Henle and distal tubule. They attributed this finding to the ability of "neoplastic cells to differentiate along other pathways". Since gp120nr can be demonstrated on cells of the metanephrogenic blastema (Finstad, et al., in prep.), the earliest embryonic form of the adult kidney, we believe that the evidence is most consistent with the hypothesis that these tumors arise from cells outside the proximal tubule.

Two of the four gp120nr⁻ tumors in the present series were oncocytomas. The origin of oncocytomas is controversial and has variously been ascribed to the proximal tubule (Johnson et al., 1979; Pearse and Houghton, 1979), ascending loop of Henle (Chaudhry et al., 1979), distal tubule (Bannasch et al., 1978), or collecting tubule (Sakar et al., 1979). Possible sites of origin within the kidney are currently being explored with mAbs specific for other segments of the nephron.

8.2. Subclassification of gp120nr⁺ Renal Cancers

The hypothesis that gp120nr⁺ tumors are derived from the proximal tubule is consistent with earlier immunological by Wallace and Nairn (1972) and ultrastructural data (Oberling et al., 1960; Seljelid and Ericsson, 1965). Among the gp120nr⁺ tumors, a second level of subclassification is apparent. Presence or absence of any of 3 Ag (gp120r, gp160, gp115) defines eight possible antigenic phenotypes. Indeed, among the 52 gp120nr⁺ tumors, all eight phenotypes are seen. In addition, the distribution into these eight subsets is that which would be anticipated if these three Ag are expressed independently of one another. This finding differs from the coordinate expression (or lack of expression) seen in the gp120nr⁻ group (where gp160, gp115, and gp120r are coordinately repressed) or in the studies of lymphopoietic tumors and melanomas (Houghton, et al., 1982). In these latter two examples, tumors express only selected phenotypes, which in turn correspond to stages along their respective differentiation pathways. The tumor phenotype presumably marks the point along the pathway where the tumor arises.

The variance of renal cancer from the pattern seen in the previously defined systems is significant if only in that it represents a somewhat different tumor model. The cause of this phenomenon may be explained either by loss of antigen expression related to neoplastic transformation or

Table 5
Extent of Disease vs Antigen Expression

	gp160$^+$	gp115$^+$	gp120$^+$
Localized	20/24	10/24	18/24
Disseminated	11/28	10/28	9/28
	$p < 0.001$		$p < 0.001$

perhaps development of cancer in cells that never fully or normally differentiated. Further study will be required to answer this question.

9. Correlation of Antigenic Phenotypes and Clinical Parameters

Identification of lymphopoietic tumor subsets has been shown to correlate with different clinical characteristics. We sought to determine whether this was also the case with the subsets we had defined amongst renal cancers. Comparison of tumor histology, the majority of which were mixed clear and granular cells, with antigenic phenotype revealed no correlation. Tumor grade, however, did appear to correlate. Low grade (more differentiated) tumors more closely expressed the full complement of proximal tubular markers. Conversely, high grade, anaplastic tumors tended to be marker-negative.

Comparison of the patient's age with the phenotype of the tumor revealed that those patients with gp120nr$^+$/gp120r$^-$/gp160$^-$ tumors represented a younger subgroup (mean 46.5 yr) than the remaining patients (mean 57.1 yr). Furthermore, although these patients presented at an earlier age, their tumors tended to be larger (mean diameter 8.5 vs 6.1 cm).

In this series with followup of limited duration (median 24 months, range 10–32 months), we compared phenotype to stage—currently the best available prognostic indicator. Although gp115 typing did not demonstrate any correlation, gp160$^+$ or gp120r$^+$ tumors were significantly ($p < 0.001$) more likely to be low stage (I or II-localized) cancers, whereas gp160$^-$ or gp120r$^-$ tumors tended to be high stage (disseminated) cancers ($p < .001$; Table 5). This correlation becomes even more pronounced when the combined gp160/gp120r phenotype is scored. Fourteen of 16 (88%) gp160$^+$/gp120r$^+$ were localized ($p < 0.001$). Of the ten gp160$^-$/gp120r$^-$ tumors, seven were disseminated at presentation. The remaining three patients with gp160$^-$/gp120r$^-$ tumors developed metastatic disease after brief followup (median less than 3 mo) ($p < 0.001$; Table 6). Reciprocal expression, that is gp160$^+$/gp120r$^-$ or gp160$^-$/gp120r$^+$, appeared to offset each other equally as a signifficant trend no longer existed.

Table 6
Extent of Disease vs gp160/gp120r Phenotype

	$+/+$	$+/-$	$-/+$	$-/-$
Localized	14/24	6/24	4/24	0/24
Disseminated	2/28	9/28	7/28	10/28
	$p < 0.001$			$p < 0.001$

Lastly, the natural history of renal cancer is widely appreciated to be quite variable. Some patients present with huge localized tumors and are surgically cured whereas others have small but disseminated and incurable cancers. In addition, other clinically recognized "syndromes" occur. For example, oncocytomas (which represent about 5% of renal cancers) are virtually always benign. Another 5% of patients have humoral hypercalcemia of malignancy (HHM). When patients' tumors in this series were studied, the two with oncocytomas were both $gp120nr^-/gp120r^-/gp160^-/gp115^-$ and all three with the HHM syndrome were $gp120nr^+/gp120r^-/gp160^-/gp115^-$. Whereas this small number of cases of known renal cancer "syndromes" precludes definitive conclusions, the fact that they were each of the same molecular subsets is suggestive that molecular subclassification may indeed define subgroups of tumors with similar natural histories.

10. Summary

These four Mabs define markers that allow discrimination of renal from nonrenal cancers. In addition, one marker (gp120nr) appears to distinguish two major subsets of renal cancer. Those that are $gp120nr^+$ (93%) appear to derive from the proximal tubule. Those that are $gp120nr^-$ (7%) probably arise elsewhere in the nephron. Amongst the $gp120nr^+$ tumors are at least eight more subsets. There appears to be biological significance to these subsets as demonstrated by correlation with several parameters.

These markers appear to have clinical utility. It would be appropriate to substratify, according to antigenic phenotype, patients involved in experimental treatment protocols. This would allow identification of a particular subgroup of renal cancers responding to a particular form of therapy that might otherwise go unnoticed if results are applied to renal cancers in general. Substratification for phenotype should eventually allow significantly increased precision in treatment decisions.

Subclassification by phenotype will also enhance our understanding of the potentially variable natural history, risk, and etiologic factors associated with these subgroups. Identification of those patients at high risk $(gp120r^-/gp160^-)$ might alter management of these patients. One might consider further diagnostic modalities and closer follow-up for this subgroup of patients. In addition, these patients would be prime candidates for adjuvant therapy when this is available.

Potential future application of these markers is currently being investigated regarding their use as targets for immunolocalization and immunotherapy. The ability to currently identify those at high risk will hopefully soon be compounded by the ability to identify microscopic sites of tumor as well as to treat them when they are most amenable to eradication.

Acknowledgments

The authors wish to acknowledge Ms. Connie Finstad as a significant contributor to this work. Willet F. Whitmore, Jr., Myron Melamed, Herbert Oettgen, and Lloyd Old provided helpful discussions and support. Rosemarie Ramsawak and Maryanne Corbino provided expert technical assistance and Soledad Salome excellent secretarial assistance.

References

Bannasch, P., Krech, R., Zerban, H. (1978) Z. Krebsforsch 92, 87.

Chaudhry, A. P., Satchidanand, S. K., Gaeta, J. F., Slotkin, E., Shenoy, S. and Nickerson, P. A. (1979) Urology, 14, 392.

Cordon-Cardo, C., Bander, N. H., Fradet, J., Finstad, C., Lloyd, K., Whitmore, W., Melamed, M., Oettgen, H., and Old, L.: (1984) J. Histochem. Cytochem, 32, 1035.

Finstad, C., Bander, N. H., Cordon-Cardo, C., Whitmore, W., Melamed, M., Oettgen, H., and Old, L. (1984) PNAS, USA, in press.

Finstad, C., Cordon-Cardo, C., Bander, N. H., Whitmore, W., Melamed, M., Oettgen, H. and Old, L. manuscript in preparation.

Houghton, A., Eisinger, M., Albino, A., Cairncross, J. and Old, L. (1982) J. Exp. Med. 156, 1755.

Johnson, J. R., Thurman, A. E., Metter, J. B. and Banniyan, G. A. (1979) Urology 14, 181.

Oberling, C., Riviere, M., and Haguenau, F. (1960) Nature 186 402.

Pearse, H. and Houghton, D. (1979) Urology 13, 74.

Sakar, K., Ejeckam, G. C., MaCaughey, W. T. E. and Tolnai, G. (1979) Lab Invest. 40, 282.

Seljelid, R. and Ericsson, J. (1965) Lab Invest 14, 435.

Ueda, R., S. Ogata, D. Morrissey, C. Finstad, J. Szkudlarek, W. Whitmore, H. Oettgen, K. Lloyd, and L. Old. (1981) PNAS, USA 78, 5122.

Wallace, A. C. and Nairn, R. C. (1972) Cancer 29, 977.

Chapter 15

Immunochemistry of Human Teratocarcinoma Stem Cells

PETER W. ANDREWS[1] AND IVAN DAMJANOV[2]

The Wistar Institute of Anatomy and Biology, Philadelphia, Pennsylvania[1] and Hahnemann University School of Medicine, Philadelphia, Pennsylvania[2]

1. Introduction

The recent development of monoclonal antibodies to tumor-associated markers of human teratocarcinomas is a logical continuation of the research along two major avenues of investigation. On the one hand, the present work is a continuation of the efforts to improve the diagnostic techniques for immunochemical detection of germ cell tumors in a clinical setting. Some of the recent advances in this field have been reviewed by Lange (1982), Stigbrand and Engvall (1982), Moon et al. (1983). On the other hand, the work on human teratocarcinoma-derived cell lines represents an extension of similar studies performed on murine teratocarcinomas, which have culminated in detailed immunochemical characterization of mouse teratocarcinoma stem cells and their derivatives (Solter and Knowles, 1978; Stern et al., 1978; Muramatsu et al., 1978; *see also* Appendix in Silver et al., 1983).

The identification of tumor markers of teratocarcinoma stem cells has been considerably facilitated by the recent advances in somatic cell hybridization and monoclonal antibody production (reviewed by Damjanov and Knowles, 1983). This approach seems to be particularly suitable for the immunochemical analysis of heterogeneous cell populations and tumors composed of diverse tissue components. Since teratocarcinomas usually contain multiple different tissues, each of which

339

could bear distinct cell surface epitopes, monoclonal antibodies represent the only practical approach for sorting out those potentially useful markers restricted in their expression to teratocarcinoma stem cells from all other widely distributed and less specific antigenic determinants. In this article we shall briefly review our present knowledge of the biochemistry of human teratocarcinomas, particularly concentrating on the results obtained with monoclonal antibodies and presenting them as they contribute to our understanding of the nature of the teratocarcinoma stem cells and their unique characteristic—their ability to differentiate into multiple somatic and extraembryonic tissues.

2. Stem Cells of Human Teratocarcinomas

Teratocarcinomas are complex tumors composed of developmentally pluripotent malignant stem cells and more differentiated cell types corresponding to various embryonic, fetal, and adult somatic tissues and components of extraembryonic membranes. The developmentally pluripotent stem cells of teratocarcinomas have been called embryonal carcinoma (EC) cells. Like all other stem cells (Leblond, 1981), the EC cells form a self renewing, clonogenic pool of cells that, under appropriate conditions, undergo differentiation to give rise to biologically, morphologically, and immunochemically distinct derivatives (Pierce, 1980). In most instances the differentiated descendants of EC cells have a limited growth potential and are biologically benign. Occasionally, however, the EC cells do differentiate into cells of a different phenotype which still retain all the features of malignancy (Fig. 1). This event accounts for yolk sac

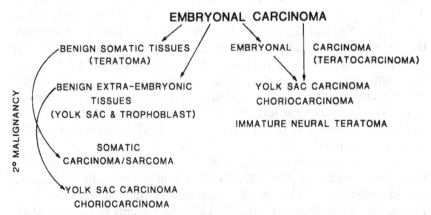

Fig. 1. Terminally differentiated and secondary malignant stem cells originating from embryonal carcinoma. Terminal differentiation of EC into benign tissues is indicated on the left and the formation of malignant stem cells by retention of the malignant potential of EC is shown on the right side. The terminally differentiated cells can undergo secondary malignant alteration, *de novo*, as indicated by curved arrows on the left side.

carcinomas, choriocarcinomas, or immature neural tumors evolving in teratocarcinomas. Alternatively there is sufficient evidence to suggest that some of the "benign" differentiated descendants of EC cells undergo malignant alteration and thus give rise to a distinct secondary malignancy. This accounts for the various somatic forms of cancer, such as squamous cell carcinoma or rhabdomyosarcoma, which occur most frequently in benign, well-differentiated ovarian teratomas. However, the malignant tumors evolving in either case are clinically and biologically distinct from typical teratocarcinomas. Furthermore, these tumors contain stem cell populations that are distinct from EC cells, the typical stem cells of teratocarcinomas. In some cases these secondary malignant stem cell populations can be easily distinguished from EC cells because they resemble neuroblasts or sarcoma cells. On the other hand, the distinction of EC cells from closely related yolk sac carcinoma cells and various cells corresponding to the intermediary cell forms marking the differentiation of normal embryonic cells is not so easy, and is frequently impossible by standard morphological approaches (Damjanov, 1984).

Since teratocarcinomas may contain, in addition to EC cells, other malignant stem cell populations, any work on precise phenotypic characterization of malignant stem cell populations is contingent on the identification and immunochemical analysis of the typical primordial, developmentally pluripotent EC cells. This includes delineation of their phenotype, identification of variants or subtypes, and their demarcation from other more developmentally restricted malignant cells in teratocarcinomas.

2.1. Human Embryonal Carcinoma Cells

A precise definition of the human EC cell phenotype has so far not been fully accomplished. First of all, as a result of their undifferentiated nature, these cells lack positive identification markers and morphologically resemble many other undifferentiated, or poorly differentiated tumor cells. Thus, pathologists have been empirically trained to recognize EC cells as the undifferentiated malignant cells with high nucleocytoplasmic ratio, prominent nucleoli, and indistinct cell borders (Andrews et al., 1983b). Distinction from other germ cell tumors such as dysgerminoma or yolk sac carcinoma remains subjective and is frequently arbitrary (Pugh and Cameron, 1976). Second, human EC occur in several histologic patterns, such as solid, acinar, tubular, and papillary (Mostofi, 1980). It is not known whether the cells forming these histologically distinct structures are at different stages of differentiation, whether all of them are pluripotent, or whether these represent normal variants determined by environmental conditions regulating their growth. Third, EC cells quite frequently undergo various forms of differentiation that can be fully appreciated only after the cells have reached a stage hallmarked by distinct morphologic or immunohistochemical characteristics. Thus, for example, yolk sac differentiation can be easily recognized in immunohistochemically stained slides using the alphafetoprotein (AFP) as a marker of terminal differentiation. However, immunohistochemical studies of germ cell tumors (Jacobsen and Jacobsen, 1983) clearly show that this terminal form of differentiation is preceded by one or several steps that at the present time cannot be exactly defined, but which most likely correspond to stages in the development of the normal yolk sac during embryogenesis. Fourth, developmentally pluripotent human EC cells have not been cloned in vitro until recently. However, even these cell lines, such as 2102Ep and NTera-2 (Andrews et al., 1982; 1983a,b; and 1984a; Matthaei et al., 1983) do not show the full spectrum of differentiation expected from a truly pluripotent EC cell line. Finally, as will be shown later, the data concerning human EC cells have been subject to conflicting interpretations in the past because of the assumption that human EC cells are biologically identical to mouse EC cells. This assumption, based on the initially discovered homologies between mouse and human EC has delayed the acceptance of species differences and the definition of the morphologic, immunologic, and biologic characteristics of human EC cells. However, all these obstacles are slowly being overcome and although a definitive consensus about a "universal" prototype of a developmentally pluripotent human EC cell has not yet been reached, we seem to be closer to this goal than ever before.

2.2. Surface Markers of Human EC Cells

The considerable similarity between human and mouse embryonal carcinoma cells (Martin, 1980) has prompted several investigators to use antisera raised against mouse EC cells to study human EC cells (Holden et al., 1977; Hogan et al., 1977). These initial attempts indicated considerable homology between mouse and human EC cells. However, soon after the first monoclonal antibodies to mouse EC were tested on clonally derived human EC cell lines, dramatic differences between human and mouse EC cells became evident (Andrews et al., 1982). Antibodies, such as that to the murine stage specific embryonic antigen one (SSEA-1) (Solter and Knowles, 1978), which react with undifferentiated mouse EC, but not with their immediate differentiated descendants, did not react with undifferentiated human EC cells, but did react with their differentiated descendants. On the other hand, antibodies recognizing other murine embryonic antigens, such as antibodies to SSEA-3 and SSEA-4, did not react with mouse EC cells, although they were strongly reactive with human EC cells (Shevinsky et al., 1982; Kannagi et al., 1983a). Since these antibodies to mouse embryonic antigens have so far been the most helpful in defining the human EC cell phenotype, a detailed description of the antigenic determinants recognized by these antibodies will follow.

2.2.1. SSEA-3 and SSEA-4

SSEA-3 is a cell-surface antigen defined by a monoclonal antibody that was obtained by the ''hybridoma'' technique from rats immunized with four-cell stage mouse embryos (Shevinsky et al., 1982). It is present on the cleaving embryos of most mouse strains, but after blastocyst formation, it disappears from the cells of the inner cell mass that go on to form the primitive ectoderm and embryo proper. Correspondingly, murine EC cells, that are thought to be developmentally equivalent to the primitive ectoderm, are SSEA-3-negative. Nevertheless, this antigen is present on cells of the primitive and visceral endoderm, but not the parietal endoderm (Fox et al., 1984). By contrast to murine EC cells, human EC cells are SSEA-3-positive. Shevinsky et al. (1982) demonstrated the presence of many SSEA-3-positive cells in several human teratocarcinoma cell lines, whereas Andrews et al. (1982) reported the strong expression of SSEA-3 by clonal human EC cells of the 2102Ep line, originally obtained from an explanted testicular germ cell tumor (Andrews et al., 1980; Wang et al., 1980). More recently Andrews et al. (1984a) observed the expression of SSEA-3 by pluripotent human EC cells of the Tera-2 line, which can differentiate into a variety of cell types including neurons (Andrews, 1984). Also, the general utility of SSEA-3 as a marker for human EC cells was confirmed by the immunohistochemical staining of germ cell tumor biopsies (Fig. 2) in which reactivity with antibody to

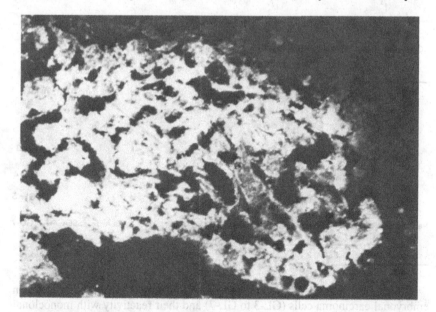

Fig. 2. Human teratocarcinoma. Immunofluorescent microscopy with the monoclonal antibody to SSEA-3 shows reaction only in the nest of EC cells.

SSEA-3 was restricted to histologically recognized EC cells (Damjanov et al., 1982). Of many human cells tested, including those from a large panel of diverse tumor-derived cell lines, only erythrocytes, in addition to EC cells, were found to express SSEA-3 (Shevinsky et al., 1982). The expression of this antigen by the early human embryo has not yet been examined. By analogy with murine embryos, one might expect that parts of the human yolk sac would also express SSEA-3 and so, therefore, might some human yolk sac tumors. However, the one cell line we have examined (1411H), which might correspond to yolk sac carcinoma, lacks SSEA-3 (Andrews et al., 1983a).

The SSEA-3 antigenic determinant is associated with both glycoproteins (Shevinsky et al., 1982) and glycolipids (Kannagi et al., 1983b) present on the surface of human EC cells. Little is known of the glycoproteins except that, among several specifically immunoprecipitated by anti-SSEA-3 antibody from 2102Ep human EC cells, there is a major polypeptide with an apparent molecular weight of 70,000 by SDS-polyacrylamide gel electrophoresis. More is known of the glycolipids. The major neutral glycolipids and one ganglioside found in extracts of 2102Ep cells were identified as belonging to an extended globoseries having the common core oligosaccharide, $Gal\alpha1\rightarrow4Gal\beta1\rightarrow4Glc\beta1\rightarrow$ ceramide (Fig. 3) (Kannagi et al., 1983b). SSEA-3 antibody was shown

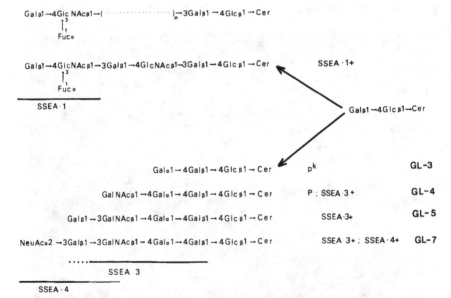

Fig. 3. Schematic presentation of major neutral glycolipids of human embryonal carcinoma cells (GL-3 to GL-7) and their reactivity with monoclonal antibodies raised to stage specific embryonic antigens SSEA-1, SSEA-3, and SSEA-4 and antibodies, to blood group antigens P and p^k. The structure of GL-6 is not given. GL-6 differs from GL-7 only in the terminal sugar, which is $Fuc\alpha2$ instead of the $NeuAc\alpha2$ found in GL-7 (Kannagi et al., 1983a,b).

to react strongly with GL-5 and GL-7 as well as less strongly with GL-4 (globoside) and weakly with the fucosylated derivative GL-6.

An antibody recognizing SSEA-4 was produced by a hybridoma that was derived from splenocytes of a mouse immunized with 2102Ep EC cells. SSEA-4 is present on human EC cells and has a similar cellular distribution to SSEA-3 (Kannagi et al., 1983a). However, antibody to SSEA-4 was found to react only with the GL-7 in the series of glycolipids from 2102Ep cells, and in addition with GM_{1b} ganglioside. Kannagi et al. (1983a) concluded that whereas the SSEA-3 epitope consisted of the internal core of the oligosaccharide, the SSEA-4 epitope consisted of the terminal residues:

GL-7: NeuAc α2 → 3Gal β 1 → 3GalNAc β 1 → 3Gal α 1 → 4Gal β 1 → 4Glc β 1 → Cer

SSEA-3

SSEA-4

Together, antibodies to SSEA-3 and SSEA-4 defined the GL-7 oligo-saccharide. As with SSEA-3, SSEA-4 antigenic determinants were also found associated with cell surface glycoproteins.

The globoseries glycolipids contain epitopes recognized as blood group antigens of the P blood group system. In particular, the p^k antigen is associated with the same glycolipid identified as GL-3 in 2102Ep cells, whereas the P antigen is associated with globoside (GL-4) that also carries SSEA-3 activity (Kannagi et al., 1983b). Accordingly, P and p^k antigens have been found on several human teratocarcinoma cell lines (Bono et al., 1981). Of practical significance is the fact that individuals with the rare p and p^k phenotypes lack the P antigen, presumably because they cannot synthesize globoside; we might, therefore, predict that EC cells of such individuals will also lack SSEA-3 and SSEA-4. So far, no data are available to test this possibility. It has been suggested that the high frequency of early abortions associated with the p phenotype, often, attributed to fetal-maternal incompatibility (Levine and Koch-Elisabeth, 1954), might be connected with a lack of expression of the SSEA-3/SSEA-4 antigens during early development (Kannagi et al., 1983b). However, no function has yet been attributed to these molecules and, at least during the cleavage stage of mouse development, it seems doubtful if they have a critical function since several mouse strains do not express SSEA-3 during early embryogenesis, although it appears later on other embryonic, fetal, and adult cell types (Shevinsky, personal communication).

2.2.2. Other Antigens Defined by Monoclonal Antibodies to Human EC Cells

Williams et al. (1982) described a monoclonal antibody, LICR.LON. FC10.2, that recognizes another antigen of restricted cell distribution expressed by human EC cells. This antibody was raised against formalin-fixed cells of the HT39/7 human EC line (Cotte et al., 1982). On a limited panel of human germ cell tumor-derived lines, reactivity with this antibody was observed only with cell lines judged to contain "undifferentiated" cells (HT39/7, Tera-1, and SuSa), but not with others judged to contain "more differentiated" cells (Tera-2, LICR.LON. HT$_3$B$_1$, PA-1). In sections of xenografted human germ cell tumors, as well as of clinical biopsies, the antigen was detected in association with the cell membrane, especially on luminal surfaces, of a variable proportion of EC cells, as well as in areas of endodermal differentiation in yolk sac tumors and intestinal differentiation in teratomas. Seminoma cells were unreactive. In human fetuses, reactivity was associated with the luminal surface of the intestine and bronchus. Apart from a few cells in three carcinomas of the small intestine, no reactivity with a wide variety of nongerm cell tumors was noted. Immunoprecipitation demonstrated that on HT39/7 human EC cells, the LICR.LON.FC10.2 antigen was associated with a glycoprotein with an apparent polypeptide molecular weight of 200,000. This polypeptide also carries receptors for the galactose-specific lectin, peanut agglutinin.

2.2.3. Major Histocompatibility Antigens

The class I major histocompatibility (MHC) antigens (HLA-A,B,C in humans; H-2K, D, and L in mice) are expressed by most nucleated cells in mammals, although with considerable quantitative variation (Brodsky et al., 1979). Cells that do not express these antigens include cells of the human trophoblast (Goodfellow et al., 1976) and murine EC cells (Artzt and Jacob, 1974; Morello et al., 1978). Since detailed experimental study of murine teratocarcinomas preceded that of human germ cell tumors, it was first assumed that human EC cells, like their murine counterparts, would lack class I MHC antigens. However, the data now available are consistent with the view that human EC cells do express these antigens, albeit at a low level. The significance of this is difficult to assess since expression is often variable, both within cell lines and between different cell lines.

Many human teratocarcinoma-derived cell lines express HLA-A,B,C antigens and the associated molecule β_2-microglobulin (β_2m). In different studies, these have been detected by alloantisera specific for polymorphic antigens of the HLA-A and HLA-B loci (Hogan et al., 1977; Bronson et al., 1980; Zeuthen et al., 1980), and by monoclonal antibodies specific for monomorphic antigens common to the HLA-A,B and C loci (Andrews et al., 1980; 1981; 1982; 1984a; Bronson et al., 1980; Avner et al., 1981). Further, in the case of 2102Ep cells, Andrews et al. (1983b) confirmed that the monoclonal anti-HLA-A,B,C that they used for their studies (W6/32, Barnstable et al., 1978) did indeed immunoprecipitate the expected 45,000 and 12,000 (β_2m) polypeptides from lysates of surface-radioiodinated cells. Also mRNA for the HLA heavy chain was detected in Tera-1 and PA-1 human teratocarcinoma cells (Morello and Avner, 1982) and in the clonal human EC cell line 2102Ep (Goodfellow et al., 1983).

In all cases, the expression of HLA-A,B,C antigens was weak when compared with other human cell types, and cells scored as HLA-positive and HLA-negative were usually found in the same cultures. Some authors suggested that the HLA-positive cells were differentiated derivatives of HLA-negative stem cells (Hogan et al., 1977), a view consistent with re-sults obtained with murine teratocarcinomas. However, flow cyto-fluorimetric analyses of several human teratocarcinoma cell lines revealed single, rather than bimodal, distributions of HLA-expression that overlapped the fluorescence distributions of the negative controls (An-drews et al., 1981). This suggested that the distinction between HLA-positive and negative cells was arbitrary, and that these cells belonged to the same population. Indeed, in an experiment with 2102Ep, cells from an EC culture were fractionated by fluorescence activated cell sorting into apparently HLA-A,B,C-positive and negative populations; when grown and reanalyzed 2 d later the same distribution of HLA expression was seen in both, indicating no stable difference between the two populations (Andrews et al., 1983b). Also, in some cultures of 2102Ep, characterized as containing mostly EC cells, almost 100% of the cells may be scored HLA-A,B,C-positive without any other evidence of differentiation (e.g., Andrews et al., 1984a). These data all suggest that human EC cells differ from murine EC cells by expressing low levels of MHC antigens, a con-clusion supported by the finding that somatic cell hybrids of human cells and murine EC cells, which continue to present an EC-like phenotype, also continue to express HLA-A,B,C genes although their murine H-2 genes remain inactive (Goodfellow et al., 1982; 1983). Nevertheless, even with well characterized human EC cell lines, results may vary con-siderably from one experiment to another. Thus, Cotte et al. (1982) noted that sometimes all the cells of the HT39/7 human EC cell line lacked β_2-microglobulin, whereas at other times, in excess of 80% of the cells were weakly positive. Likewise, we have found similar extreme varia-tions in HLA-A,B,C and β_2-microglobulin expression by the clonal pluripotent human EC cells (NT2/B9 and NT2/D1) derived from Tera-2 (Andrews et al., 1984a). The reasons for this variability remain unknown.

Whereas HLA-A,B,C antigens are weakly expressed by human EC cells, HLA-Dr antigens have not been detected. This has been demon-strated both by lack of reactivity with anti-HLA-Dr monoclonal antibod-ies (Andrews et al., 1980) and by the absence of detectable HLA-Dr mRNA (Goodfellow et al., 1983).

2.2.4. Alkaline Phosphatase

Human alkaline phosphatases (ALP) are membrane-bound enzymes consisting of at least three isozymes encoded by separate genetic loci: liver/bone/kidney ALP, intestinal ALP, and placental ALP (Fishman, 1974; Seargeant and Stinson, 1979). The placental ALP locus that encodes the isozyme found in second and third trimester fetal trophoblast is evidently the product of recent evolution and is found only in the higher primates (Goldstein and Harris, 1979). Apart from the placenta, placental-like ALP is commonly synthesized by a variety of miscellaneous tumors of nontrophoblast origin (Fishman et al., 1968; Jacoby and Bagshawe, 1971; Greene and Sussman, 1973; Benham et al., 1978) as well as being found at low levels in the endocervix (Goldstein et al., 1980) and testis (Chang et al., 1980).

Histochemical staining has demonstrated ALP in the EC cells of both murine and human teratocarcinomas (Damjanov et al., 1971 and 1977; Paiva et al., 1983). Similarly, in a number of cell lines derived from human teratocarcinomas, very high levels of ALP activity have generally been observed (Andrews et al., 1981; Zeuthen et al., 1980). In their study of eight human teratocarcinoma cell lines, Benham et al. (1981) found high levels in seven lines (the eighth line was identified as a differentiated, non-EC cell line though of teratocarcinoma origin) and that most of the activity (usually in excess of 90%) could be attributed to a form of ALP indistinguishable from the liver/bone/kidney isozyme. This conclusion was based upon heat lability of the enzyme, its inhibition by L-homoarginine, but only slight inhibition by L-phenylalanine, L-phenylalanylglycylglycine and L-leucine, and by its profile upon starch gel electrophoresis. Similarly, in the HT39/7 human EC cell line, high ALP activities were found, about 60% of which was heat labile and identified as the liver/bone/kidney isozyme (Cotte et al., 1982). Recently, Andrews et al. (1984b) found that two monoclonal antibodies (TRA-2-49 and TRA-2-54), raised to cell surface antigens of the 2102Ep cells, specifically recognized determinants associated with the liver/bone/kidney form of ALP. These reacted with more than 90% of the cells in cultures of 2102Ep.

In most human teratocarcinoma lines exhibiting high levels of ALP, a proportion of the activity was found to be heat stable, a hallmark of the placental isozyme. It was also found that this enzyme cross-reacts with antisera and monoclonal antibodies specific for placental ALP (Benham et al., 1981; Cotte et al., 1981; 1982). Benham et al. (1981) found that in most cases, less than 5% of the total ALP activity thus resembled placental ALP, though in one set of assays they recorded over 20% heat stable activity in the two human teratocarcinoma lines Tera-1 and 2102Ep. On the other hand, Cotte et al. (1981; 1982) reported 30% to 60% in the different panel of lines they studied. Despite similarities to true placental ALP, the heat stable ALP of the human teratocarcinoma cell lines differed with regard to its sensitivity to inhibition by phenylalanylglycylglycine (less sensitive than placental ALP) and by L-leucine (more sensitive than placental ALP). These differences suggested greater resemblance to the placental-like enzyme of normal testis than the placental isozyme (Benham et al., 1981). However, increased sensitivity to L-leucine has been observed for several ectopically synthesized placental-like ALP in various different tumors (Inglis et al., 1973). It is also a feature of the normal placental ALP found in placentae of individuals heterozygous for one of the rare allelic variants ('D' variant) at the placental ALP locus (Beckman and Beckman, 1968). Whether the teratocarcinoma cell lines express placental-like ALP ectopically, as in the case of some other tumors, whether it reflects normal expression of an embryonic form of ALP found in cells of the very early embryo, or whether it reflects continued expression of a gene active in normal testis cells, is unknown. Nevertheless, it is evident that there is considerable variation between different lines in their level of expression of this isozyme. In the case of defined clonal human EC cell lines, in different experiments, from 28 to 74% of the cells in cultures of 2102Ep were scored as reactive with monoclonal antibodies specific for placental ALP, a few cells staining very strongly, whereas no reactivity was found in cultures of clonal pluripotent EC cells of the NTera-2 lines (Andrews et al., 1984a).

Similar variability in the expression of placental or placental-like ALP has been noted in immunohistochemical studies of tumor biopsies. Thus, Uchida et al. (1981) failed to observe immunoreactive placental ALP in EC cells of human germ cell tumors. They, and also Wahren et al. (1979) observed reactivity in most, but not all, seminomas and proposed that this might be used diagnostically. On the other hand, Paiva et al. (1983) found that embryonal carcinoma cells in all of the human testicular teratocarcinomas that they studied did react with one or more monoclonal antibodies specific for placental ALP (Fig. 4). They classified the placental ALP expressed by these tumors according to whether reaction was observed with all six of a panel of antiplacental ALP monoclonal antibodies (placental ALP) or whether reaction was observed with only a subset of the monoclonal antibodies (placental-like ALP). Accordingly, placental ALP was observed in three EC-containing tumors, and placental-like ALP in the other four. However, it should be noted that this definition (according to immunoreactivity) is different from that used by Benham et al. (1981) (according to inhibitor sensitivity) in their in vitro study.

The variability in expression of ALP resembling placental ALP (both within cell lines and tumors, and between them) suggests that cau-

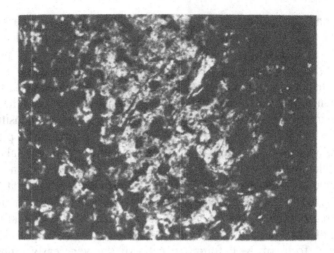

Fig. 4. Immunohistochemical demonstration of placental ALP in human embryonal carcinoma.

tion needs to be excercised in using the enzyme as a diagnostic marker. It could be that expression of placental-like ALP occurs in some particular subset of EC cells, perhaps according to their developmental or neoplastic potential. However, this is currently in the realm of speculation and more information is required. Nevertheless, the high level of expression of ALP activity of the liver/bone/kidney type, is a common feature of EC cells.

2.2.5. Cell Surface Carbohydrates

The EC cell marker oligosaccharides associated with the surface antigens SSEA-3 and SSEA-4 have already been discussed. Other carbohydrates potentially characterizing EC cells have been identified by biochemical means, as well as by reactivity with various lectins. Thus, just as complete pronase digestion of murine teratocarcinoma cells released unusually large glycopeptides thought to be associated with the cell surface (Muramatsu et al., 1978), several human teratocarcinoma cell lines (Tera-1, PA-1, Huttke, SuSa) were also found to carry large, surface associated glycopeptides (Muramatsu et al., 1979; Rasilo et al., 1980). Such large glycopeptides were not typically found associated with a variety of more "differentiated" tumors and, as in the murine case, they appeared to consist of a core of repeating galactose and N-acetyl-glucosamine units (Muramatsu et al., 1982). This core was fucosylated since it was metabolically labeled when the cells were cultured with ^{3}H-fucose, and it carried binding sites for the fucose binding protein (FBP) of *Lotus tetragonolobus*. This suggested a structure similar to the ABH blood group substances, but neither A nor B antigens nor the H-precursor substance were detected in any of these cells, with the possi-

ble exception of a subpopulation in cultures of the ovarian teratocarcinoma line, PA-1 (Bono et al., 1981).

The available data do not permit a conclusion as to whether the large
glycopeptides are associated with the EC cells or with more "differentiated" derivatives present in the cultures. The cell surface antigen
SSEA-1, the determinant of which is a fucosylated lactosamine structure
(see Fig. 3) such as that found in these large glycopeptides, is not expressed by human EC cells (Andrews et al., 1982; Damjanov et al., 1982;
Cotte et al., 1982) despite its expression by murine EC cells (Solter and
Knowles, 1978). SSEA-1 does, however, appear upon some types of differentiation which commonly occur spontaneously in cultured human
teratocarcinoma cells. Nevertheless, it is not known whether the large
glycopeptides that have been reported, necessarily carry SSEA-1
antigenic determinants, although lactosamine oligosaccharides covalently
bound to fibronectin synthesized by SSEA-1-positive differentiated
2102Ep cells (Cossu et al., 1983) evidently do not carry SSEA-1 activity
(Andrews, 1982).

In a study of six human teratocarcinoma cell lines (Tera-1, Tera-2,
SuSa, HX39/7, T_3B_1, and PA-1), McIlhinney (1981) noted that none
bound the fucose binding protein (FBP) from *Lotus tetragonolobus*, and
that all except T_3B_1 bound peanut agglutinin (PNA), which has a
specificity for terminal galactose residues. On the contrary, however,
Bono et al. (1981) found that Tera-1, Tera-2, SuSa, PA-1, and Huttke
cells did react with FBP although only 40% of Tera-2 cells and 25% of
PA-1 cells were positive. In agreement, they found that all were positive
for PNA reactivity. The reason for the discrepancy is unknown, but probably lies in the phenotypic variation that is common in human
teratocarcinoma cell lines, and which probably reflects the spontaneous
differentiation seen in well-defined clonal EC cell lines such as 2102Ep
(Andrews et al., 1982) or NTera-2 (Andrews et al., 1984a). The reactivity of these cells with PNA and FBP has not been studied, but from the
neutral glycolipid composition of 2102Ep EC cells and the known structure of SSEA-3, reactivity with PNA would be expected, particularly
with GL-5 (see Fig. 3). The defined human EC cell line HT-39/7 is PNA-
positive, as expected (Cotte et al., 1982). In this case it was found that
PNA reacted with a variety of glycoproteins including one (mol wt
200,000) which carried the antigenic determinant recognized by the
monoclonal antibody LICR.LON.FC.10.2 discussed earlier (McIlhinney
and Patel, 1981; Williams et al., 1982).

2.3. Intermediate Filaments

There is well known cell lineage specificity in the expression of intermediate filaments in different cell types (Osborn and Weber, 1983). Both the
2102Ep and HT39/7 human EC cells have been examined for their ex-

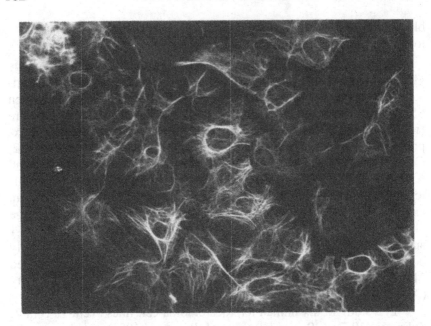

Fig. 5.   Immunohistochemical demonstration of intermediate filaments in human EC cells 2102Ep. The cells were stained with antibodies to keratin.

pression of intermediate filament proteins (Damjanov and Andrews, 1983; McIlhinney et al., 1983). In both studies cytoplasmic keratin could be demonstrated immunohistochemically (Fig. 5) and was particularly notable along the periphery of the cells. Interestingly, vimentin was absent in the HT39/7 cells, and found in only 15 to 20% of the 2102Ep EC cells. It was thought possible that the latter might represent spontaneously differentiated derivatives, although the possibility that they represented a subset of EC cells could not be ruled out. These observations are in striking contrast to murine EC cells in which vimentin is the predominant cytoskeletal protein (Paulin, 1981), rather than keratin, which appears only upon differentiation of EC cells into endodermal cells (Oshima, 1982).

3. Markers of Differentiation

3.1. The Nature of Differentiation

Cellular differentiation implies both a change in the spectrum of gene products synthesized by a cell and that the change is irreversible or, at least, not commonly reversed under normal conditions. In the context of developmental biology the first without the second is not usually considered as differentiation but may be termed phenotypic modulation. With regard to cellular differentiation as it occurs during embryogenesis, there is also the notion of progressive differentiation along diverging lineages to which cells become committed. Thus, it is commonly envisaged that embryogenesis occurs by cells making successive decisions to differentiate into one rather than another phenotype. A "more differentiated" cell may then be considered as having fewer options of cell phenotypes into which it can eventually differentiate than a "less differentiated" cell.

To follow the pathways of differentiation that occur in teratocarcinomas, as in embryos, cell autonomous products that can be assayed at the single cell level would serve as the most useful markers. As illustrated by studies of the immune system, cell surface antigens provide the most generally practical markers of this type, although other cytoplasmic components such as cytoskeletal proteins may also be used. The disadvantage of the latter is that they require fixation of the cell and so cannot be used if viable cells are being studied. Secreted products may be good indications of the presence of particular cell types in a heterogenous population, but may not permit the direct identification of those cells. Clearly, to be useful markers, any such products should only be produced by a subset of cell types, but not necessarily by one type alone; cell phenotypes may be classified by their pattern of expression of several markers. Evidence of the irreversible nature of the changes observed may be difficult to obtain, but the extent of the changes can provide a useful circumstantial indicator in the absence of definitive data. These can only come from the direct isolation of cells expressing the proposed differentiated phenotype and an assessment of their ability to regenerate an EC cell phenotype.

Differentiation of EC cells may be marked both by the disappearance of products that they characteristically express, or by the appearance of new products. The disappearance of EC markers is not always easily interpreted, however, because EC cells often persist amongst their differentiated derivatives and such markers may also be unexpectedly expressed by some types of derivative cells; in addition they might persist, due to slow turnover for some time after the gene activity responsible for their expression has been turned off and other changes have occurred. Appearance of new markers provides less ambiguous evidence of differentiation. Such products not expressed by EC cells can be classified either as commonly expressed by many other cell types (e.g., SSEA-1 or the ABH blood group antigens) or expressed only by certain well-characterized differentiated cell types such as neurons. The former can be used to indicate EC cell differentiation; the latter may be useful for indicating the direction that the differentiation takes.

Definitive evidence of cellular differentiation by clonal human EC cells has only recently been presented (Andrews et al., 1982; McIlhinney et al., 1983; Andrews et al., 1983a,b; 1984a; Andrews, 1984). Thus, few direct data are available concerning changes during human EC differentiation. However, from the phenotypes of cells that occur in human teratocarcinomas and are presumed to arise by differentiation of human EC cells, changes that would be expected to occur in experimental systems can be inferred.

3.2. The Disappearance of EC Cell Markers

SSEA-3 and SSEA-4 are so far the best characterized markers of human EC cells, as has been discussed already. Since they are absent from a variety of the cell types that are also found in teratocarcinomas (e.g., Shevinsky et al., 1982; Andrews et al., 1983a; Damjanov et al., 1982), they should be expected to disappear as EC cells differentiate. During the spontaneous differentiation of 2102Ep and NTera-2 EC cells in vitro, a reduction in the proportion of cells expressing SSEA-3 is usually observed, and in well-differentiated xenograft tumors of NTera-2 in nude mice, SSEA-3 is indeed restricted to morphologically recognizable EC cells (Andrews et al., 1982; 1984a). In culture, a more dramatic elimination of SSEA-3 expression is observed when NTera-2 EC cells are exposed to retinoic cid (Andrews, 1984). The initial cells produced in response to retinoic acid are almost entirely SSEA-3-negative. They have not been identified with any particular embryonic cell type, but they eventually give rise to various other cells that include neurons. Although a very few EC cells do persist in these cultures, it seems that most, if not all the SSEA-3-negative cells are unable to re-express the EC phenotype. SSEA-4 has not yet been examined in detail in these systems but from our knowledge of the structure of its epitope, it would be expected to follow the same pattern. Some data confirm this (Kannagi et al., 1983a; Andrews, unpublished observations), although it would not necessarily disappear if synthesis of the GM_{1b} ganglioside were to be induced. This raises another point; disappearance of SSEA-3 and SSEA-4 from the immediate differentiated derivatives of human EC cells does not preclude their reappearance in other differentiated cell types that may appear further along various pathways of differentiation although such SSEA-3 and SSEA-4-positive differentiated cells have yet to be observed. Indeed, this is all the more likely for antigens the epitope of which can be associated with several quite different molecules, such as SSEA-4.

Other markers that may disappear upon EC cell differentiation are alkaline phosphatase, the LICR.LON.F10.2 antigen, and reactivity with peanut agglutinin. Alkaline phosphatase activity, known to be high in EC cells, is certainly much lower in some other components of teratocarcinomas (e.g., Benham et al., 1981). During spontaneous differentiation of 2102Ep EC cells and NTera-2 EC cells in vitro, no significant changes have been observed (Andrews et al., 1982; 1984; Andrews, unpublished observations), but following exposure to retinoic acid, NTera-2 cells express lower levels of L-ALP (Andrews, 1984). McIlhinney et al. (1983) also observed a marked decrease in ALP activity in HT39/7 EC cells when they differentiated in response to TPA. However, they did not record whether both or only one of the two isozymes (liver and placental ALP) recognized in these cells (Cotte et al., 1982) was diminished. McIlhinney et al. (1983) also noticed that the number of cells expressing the 200,000 mol wt antigen, detected by their monoclonal antibody, LICR.LON.FC10.2, decreased markedly in culture of HT39/7 human EC cells exposed to TPA. Coincident with this they noted the disappearance of reactivity with the galactose-specific lectin, PNA, that reacted with the LICR.LON.F10.2 antigen amongst others associated with the surface of human EC cells (McIlhinney and Patel, 1983).

3.3. The Appearance of New Cell Markers

3.3.1. SSEA-1

SSEA-1 is a cell surface antigenic determinant defined by a monoclonal antibody reactive with murine EC cells and, in the early mouse embryo, with cells of the late morula, primitive ectoderm, and visceral endoderm (Solter and Knowles, 1978; Fox et al., 1981) In humans, a diverse variety of normal and neoplastic tissues were found to express SSEA-1 (Fox et al., 1983) but, in contrast to the mouse, studies of in vitro cell lines and tumor biopsies indicated that human EC cells are SSEA-1-negative (Andrews et al., 1980; 1982; 1984a; Damjanov et al., 1982; Cotte et al., 1982). Nevertheless, other components of human germ cell tumors, for example, some yolk sac carcinoma (Fig. 6) and choriocarcinoma cells, were found to express this antigen (Damjanov et al., 1982; Andrews et al., 1980; 1983a).

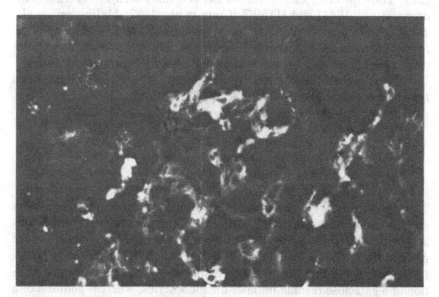

Fig. 6. Immunohistochemical demonstration of SSEA-1 in yolk sac components of a human teratocarcinoma.

When the clonal human EC cell line 2102Ep was examined, it was noticed that whereas cultures containing predominantly EC-like cells, judged by morphology and the expression of SSEA-3, contained few SSEA-1-positive cells, changes in culture conditions, particularly plating cells at a low density, led to the formation of many more SSEA-1-positive cells, as well as to fewer SSEA-3-positive cells (Andrews et al., 1982). At the same time, many of the cells also acquired a different morphology characterized by a larger, flatter appearance and, ultrastructurally, a more complex cytoplasm (Damjanov and Andrews, 1983). In addition, the extracellular matrix protein fibronectin, which was not produced by the EC cell cultures, began to be synthesized in large amounts (Andrews, 1982). By fractionating cells from such "differentiated" cultures by fluorescence-activated cell sorting, according to their expression of SSEA-1, it was shown that the fibronectin was synthesized by the SSEA-1-positive cells, and not by the persisting SSEA-1-negative EC cells. From these and other data, it may be hypothesized that differentiation in cultures of the 2102Ep EC cells occur along a pathway: SSEA-1^-/SSEA-3^+ → SSEA-1^+/SSEA-3^+ → SSEA-1^+/SSEA-3^- → SSEA-1^-/SSEA-3^-. Along the way, other genes, such as that for fibronectin, are activated and, in this case, at least some of the cells are thought to end up as trophoblastic giant cells synthesizing HCG (Damjanov and Andrews, 1983). It is not known at what stage, and indeed if ever, this sequence of events becomes irreversible. The appearance of SSEA-1, however, is clearly a common event in the early differentiation of human EC cells. Thus, in other clonal human EC cell lines such as NTera-2 (Andrews et al., 1984) and HT39/7 (Cotte et al., 1982; McIlhinney et al., 1983) induction of differentiation, by seeding at low cell density in the former case and by exposure to tetradecanoylphorbol acetate in the latter case, is accompanied by the appearance of cells expressing SSEA-1.

The structure of the SSEA-1 epitope has been shown to be a branched oligosaccharide (Gooi et al., 1981):

$$\text{Gal } \beta\ 1 \rightarrow 4\text{GlcNAc}\beta1\rightarrow$$
$$\uparrow\ {}^3_1$$
$$\text{Fuc}\alpha$$

This can evidently occur as part of an elongated polylactosamine chain such as has been isolated as a glycosphingolipid from human erythrocytes and murine EC cells (Kannagi et al., 1982) (*see* Fig. 3). Synthesis of the globoseries (SSEA-3-reactive) and lactoseries (SSEA-1-reactive) glycolipids begins with the common precursor lactosylceramide; further addition of a galactose residue initiates the globoseries, whereas addition of a glucosamine residue initiates the lactoseries (*see* Fig. 3). Since during differentiation in the early mouse embryo, as in differentiation of human

EC cells, initial SSEA-3 expression gives way to SSEA-1 expression, it has been suggested that a crucial site of regulation of these respective oligosaccharides is at this branch point; a change in activity of the two relevant glycosyltransferases could accomplish this (Kannagi et al., 1983; 1984). However, since the P-blood group antigen (globoside) seems to be more widely distributed than SSEA-3 (e.g., see Bono et al., 1981; Fellous et al., 1973; 1974; Shevinsky et al., 1982), it may be that expression of the SSEA-3 epitope is also regulated at a later point, perhaps by the addition of galactose to globoside to produce the strongly SSEA-3 reactive oligosaccharide. Similarly, other antigens not necessarily coexpressed with SSEA-1 (e.g., the I/i and ABH systems) depend on the polylactosamine core, and thus their expression may be also regulated at subsequent steps.

3.3.2. Appearance of Other Widely Distributed Antigens

The antigens of the ABH system are the only widely distributed antigens for which any data are available. Bono et al. (1981) reported that these were not expressed by three human teratocarcinoma cell lines (SuSa, Tera-1, and Tera-2), but they were expressed by a few cells of another teratocarcinoma-derived cell line (PA-1). However, the H-enzyme (2 α-L-fucosyltransferase), which adds fucose to the polylactosamine core to produce the H-antigen, was detected in all of these lines. Since each of these lines may contain EC cells (*see* Andrews, 1983), it seems likely that human EC cells, in general lack ABH antigens. This could correlate with their lack of SSEA-1 that is synthesized from the same precursor. So far, no additional studies have addressed the question of when the ABH group substances appear during differentiation. We might suppose, however, that the H antigen positive cells in the PA-1 line represented differentiated derivatives.

Although no other widely distributed antigens have been described as being absent from EC cells, there are antigens for which expression is very weak on EC cells, but much increased upon differentiation. One such antigen present on most human cells, was defined by a monoclonal antibody LICR.LON.FIB75.1 (McIlhinney et al., 1983). It is associated with a cell membrane glycopeptide with a mol wt of 19,000 and was detected, very weakly, on most cells of the human EC line HT39/7. When differentiation was induced by TPA, the resulting cells expressed this antigen much more strongly. The HLA-A,B,C antigens behaved similarly in this system. Although, in other cases, we have described disappearance of the weak HLA-A,B,C expression by some EC cells (Andrews et al., 1983b), in yet other cases, we have noted increased HLA-A,B,C expression: when NTera-2 EC cells were induced to differentiate with retinoic acid (Andrews, 1984), it was found that after 2–3 wk, many cells were expressing much higher levels of HLA-A,B,C than the EC cells from which they were derived (unpublished observation). In the case of

HLA-A,B,C, whether an increase or decrease in expression is observed may depend upon the lineage along which differentiation occurs.

3.3.3. Appearance of Antigens of Restricted Distribution

In view of the many cell types that occur in teratocarcinomas, it is likely that some cell- and tissue-specific antigens could be used to follow the differentiation of human EC cells along specific cell lineages. Thus, for example, the intestinal isozyme of alkaline phosphate is normally restricted to cells of the intestine. Reactivity of gland-like structures in xenograft tumors of the NTera-2 human EC cell line, with a monoclonal antibody recognizing this isozyme, was used to support the contention that these represented EC cell differentiation into primitive gut (Andrews et al., 1984a). Similarly, Heyderman (1978) has described CEA associated specifically with elements of human germ tumors that seemed to exhibit intestine-like differentiation. Hepatocellular differentiation in a testicular germ cell tumor was immunohistochemically substantiated with antibodies to α-1-antitrypsin and AFP (Cardoso de Almeida and Scully, 1983). Neuronal differentiation is commonly observed in teratocarcinomas, and has been induced in vitro by retinoic acid in cultures of the clonal human EC cell line NTera-2 (Andrews, 1984). In this case, the appearance of the neuronal-specific cell membrane-associated ganglioside that serves as the receptor for tetanus toxin was used to demonstrate the neuronal nature of the differentiated cells. This was confirmed by their reactivity with monoclonal antibodies specific for neurofilaments, intermediate filament proteins expressed only in neurons (Osborn and Weber, 1983). Such monoclonal antibodies were also used to confirm spontaneous neuronal differentiation in xenograft tumors of the NTera-2 cell line (Andrews et al., 1984a). The use of antibodies to neurofilaments illustrates the potential for the general use of the intermediate filament cytoskeletal proteins as markers with which to follow and characterize differentiation. So far, however, they have been put to only limited use in the investigation of human teratocarcinomas.

Muscle differentiation is also common in teratocarcinomas. Sera containing antibodies to a smooth muscle antigen (SMA) and to a striated muscle antigen (MGA) have been obtained from patients suffering from chronic active hepatitis and thymoma, respectively. They were used to study the presence of both types of muscle in a number of ovarian teratomas (Pertschuk, 1975). In that study, smooth muscle, but not striated muscle, reactive with these respective sera, was commonly found.

These few examples illustrate the potential for employing markers identified in other studies to follow particular types of differentiation in human germ cell tumors.

3.3.4. Secreted Products

Secreted molecules such as HCG and AFP (Javadpour et al., 1978; Talerman et al., 1977 and 1980) and pregnancy specific β-1-glycoprotein (SP1) (Tatarinov et al., 1974; Tatarinov, 1980) have all found clinical use as markers of human germ cell tumors. It seems unlikely that any are produced by EC cells, but rather by certain of their differentiated derivatives. HCG and SP1 indicate trophoblast differentiation (Stigbrand and Engvall, 1982) and AFP, yolk sac differentiation (Talerman et al., 1980). Few studies of the production of these markers by human teratocarcinoma cell lines in vitro have been reported. A number of gestational choriocarcinoma cell lines have been described that produce HCG (e.g., Pattillo and Gey, 1968; Pattillo et al., 1971), and Pierce et al. (1958) described a xenografted testicular choriocarcinoma that appeared to produce HCG. Cotte et al. (1981) noted transient production of HCG and CEA while they were establishing several lines from testicular germ cell tumors, but this property was subsequently lost. In their study of eight independent human testicular teratocarcinoma-derived cell lines, Andrews et al. (1980) detected traces of HCG in culture supernatant rom 833KE, 2102Ep, and SuSa, as well as traces of AFP produced by 2102Ep. However, neither AFP nor HCG was detected in culture supernatants from the cloned EC cells in cultures undergoing spontaneous differentiation at low density, although some cells contained immunoreactive HCG in their cytoplasm (Damjanov and Andrews, 1983). This was interpreted as indicating trophoblastic differentiation. In their human EC cell line, HT39/7, Cotte et al. (1982) also failed to detect HCG, AFP, or CEA production, and Andrews et al. (1984a) found no evidence of HCG or AFP production in their cloned EC sublines of Tera-2. These observations, therefore, serve to confirm that EC cells do not synthesize these markers, the production of which could therefore be taken to indicate differentiation.

With regard to yolk sac carcinomas, several studies have shown that xenografted lines produce AFP, as well as, in some cases, other serum proteins known to be produced by the normal fetal yolk sac (Yoshimara et al., 1978; Takeuchi et al., 1979; Hata et al., 1980; Kaneko et al., 1980). Vogelzang et al. (1983) have described a cell line, 1411H, that produces xenograft tumors with areas histologically consistent with both yolk sac carcinoma and embryonal carcinoma. It was also found to synthesize AFP. Bronson et al. (1983) have described an EC-like line, 1777N, that differentiated to give rise to both HCG- and AFP-producing cells in culture.

The extracellular matrix proteins, fibronectin and laminin, may also be useful markers for differentiation of human EC cells, which themselves appear to produce neither (Andrews, 1982; Andrews et al., 1983a and 1984a; McIlhinney and Patel, 1983). As already discussed, the

2102Ep cells differentiate in vitro into SSEA-1-positive cells that secrete fibronectin (Andrews, 1982) like the HT39/7 EC cells in response to TPA (McIlhinney and Patel, 1983). In both cases, the fibronectin synthesized has a higher molecular weight than fibronectin synthesized by fibroblasts. A similar observation was made in the case of fibronectin synthesized by two xenografted yolk sac carcinomas, when it was suggested that the fibronectin resembled that found in amniotic fluid from normal embryos (Ruoslahti et al., 1981). Part of the reason for the larger size of teratocarcinoma-associated fibronectin may be that it appears to carry covalently-bound chains of lactosaminoglycan and heparan sulfate (Cossu et al., 1983). In view of the bound lactosaminoglycan, it is of interest to note that, at least in the 2102Ep line (Andrews, 1982), the fibronectin does not carry SSEA-1 antigenic determinants though synthesized by SSEA-1 positive cells.

Laminin, though not synthesized by EC cells, has been reported to be synthesized by cell lines that appear to consist of, or contain elements of, yolk sac carcinoma (Andrews et al., 1983a; McIlhinney and Patel, 1983). Its appearance, however, could indicate differentiation into various endodermal cell types, not merely those corresponding to the extraembryonic endoderm. No strong evidence on human EC cells differentiating, in culture, into laminin-secreting cells has been forthcoming, although there was some suggestion that NTera-2 EC cells may occasionally differentiate into a minor population of such cells (Andrews et al., 1983a).

4. Conclusions

Monoclonal antibodies specifying antigens associated with human teratocarcinoma stem cells have proved to be extremely useful probes for the study of these, in many respects, unique tumor cells. Although many of the antigens recognized by the monoclonal antibodies appear to selectively recognize EC cells in complex teratocarcinomas, none of them was exclusively found on these tumor cells. Hence, on one side monoclonal antibodies have thus had relatively limited application in clinical practice. On the other hand, under defined conditions, they are some of the most reliable tools for identifying human EC cells and on following their differentiation. As identification markers, the antigenic determinants described in the present review will, we hope, serve as criterion to which all future studies on human germ cell tumors could refer, using the present data as an objective reference point.

Acknowledgments

The original work reviewed in this article was supported by USPHA research grants CA29894, CA 23097, and CA 38405 provided by the National Institute of Health. Secretarial help was provided by Ms. Jacklyn Powell.

References

Andrews, P. W. (1982), *Int. J. Cancer* **30,** 567.

Andrews, P. W. (1983), in *The Human Teratomas: Experimental and Clinical Biology* (Damjanov, I., B. B. Knowles and D. Solter, eds.), Humana Press, Clifton, NJ, p. 285.

Andrews, P. W. (1984), *Dev. Biol.* **103,** 285–293.

Andrews, P. W., D.L. Bronson, F. Benham, S. Strickland, and B. B. Knowles (1980), *Int. J. Cancer* **26,** 269.

Andrews, P. W., D. L. Bronson, M. V. Wiles, and P. N. Goodfellow (1981), *Tissue Antigens* **17,** 493.

Andrews, P. W., Goodfellow, L. Shevinsky, D. L. Bronson, and B. B. Knowles (1982) *Int. J. Cancer* **29,** 523.

Andrews, P. W., P. N. Goodfellow, and D. L. Bronson (1983a), In *Teratocarcinoma Stem Cells*, Cold Spring Harbor Conferences on Cell Proliferation, vol. 10 (Silver, L. M., G. R. Martin, and S. Strickland, eds.) Cold Spring Harbor, NY, p. 579.

Andrews, P. W., P. N. Goodfellow and I. Damjanov (1983b), *Cancer Surveys* **2,** 41.

Andrews, P. W., I. Damjanov, D. Simon, G. S. Banting, C. Carlin, N. C. Dracopoli, and J. Fogh (1984a) *Lab. Invest.* **50,** 147.

Andrews, P. W., L. J. Meyer, K. L. Bednarz, and H. Harris (1984b), *Hybridoma,* **3,** 33–39.

Artzt, K., and F. Jacob (1974), *Transplantation* **17,** 632.

Avner, P., R. Bono, R. Berger, and M. Fellous (1981), *J. Immunogenetics* **8,** 151.

Barnstable, C. J., W. F. Bodmer, G. Brown, G. Galfre, C. Milstein, A. F. Williams, and A. Ziegler (1978), *Cell* **14,** 9.

Beckman, L., and G. Beckman (1968), *Acta Genet. Stat. Med.* **18,** 543.

Benham, F. J., M. S. Povey, and H. Harris (1978), *Clin. Chem. Acta.* **86,** 201

Benham, F. J., P. W. Andrews, D. L. Bronson, B. B. Knowles, and H. Harris (1981), *Dev. Biol.* **88,** 279.

Bono, R., J. P. Cartron, C. Mulet, P. Avner, and M. Fellous (1981), *Blood Transfusion Immunohematol.* **24,** 97.

Brodsky, F.M., P. Parham, C. J. Barnstable, M. J. Crumpton, and W. F. Bodmer (1979), *Immunol. Rev.* **47,** 3.

Bronson, D. L., P. W. Andrews, D. Solter, J. Cervenka, P. H. Lange and E. E. Fraley (1980), *Cancer Res.* **40,** 2500.

Bronson, D. L., P. W. Andrews, R. L. Vessella, and E. E. Fraley (1983), in *Teratocarcinoma Stem Cells*, Cold Spring Harbor Conferences on Cell Proliferation, vol. 10 (Silver, L. M., G. R. Martin, and S. Strickland, eds.), p. 597.

Cardoso de Almeida, P. C., and R. E. Scully (1983), *Am. J. Surg. Pathol.* **7,** 633.

Chang, C. H., D. Angellis, and W. H. Fishman (1980), *Cancer Res.* **40,** 1506.

Cossu, G., P. W. Andrews, and L. Warren (1983), *Biochem. Biophys. Res. Comm.* **111,** 952.

Cotte, C. A., G. C. Easty, and A. M. Neville (1981), *Cancer Res.* **41**, 1422.
Cotte, C., D. Raghavan, R. A. J. McIlhinney, and P. Monaghan (1982), *In Vitro* **18**, 739.
Damjanov, I. (1984), *World I. Urol.* **2**, 12.
Damjanov, I., and P. W. Andrews (1983), *Cancer Res.* **43**, 2190.
Damjanov, I., and B. B. Knowles (1983) *Lab. Invest.* **48**, 510.
Damjanov, I., D. Solter, and N. Skreb (1971), *Z. Krebsforsch.* **76**, 249.
Damjanov, I., L. S. Cutler, and D. Solter (1977), *Am. J. Pathol.* **87**, 297.
Damjanov, I., N. Fox, B. B. Knowles, D. Solter, P. H. Lange, and E. E. Fraley (1982), *Am. J. Pathol.* **108**, 225.
Damjanov, I., B. B. Knowles, and D. Solter, eds. (1983) *The Human Teratomas: Experimental and Clinical Biology,* Humana Press, Clifton, NJ.
Fishman, W. H. (1974), *Am. J. Med.* **56**, 617.
Fishman, W. H., N. R. Inglis, S. Green, C. L. Anstiss, N. K. Ghosh, A. E. Reif, R. Rustigian, M. J. Krant, and L. L. Stolbach (1968), *Nature* **219**, 697.
Fox, N., I. Damjanov, A. Martinez-Hernandez, B. B. Knowles, and D. Solter (1981), *Dev. Biol.* **83**, 391.
Fox, N., I. Damjanov, B. B. Knowles, and D. Solter (1983), Cancer Res. **43**, 669.
Fox. N., I. Damjanov, B. B. Knowles, and D. Solter (1984), *Dev. Biol.* **103**, 263–266.
Goldstein, D. J., and H. Harris (1979), *Nature* **280**, 602.
Goldstein, D. J., L. Blasco, and H. Harris (1980), *Proc. Natl. Acad. Sci. USA* **77**, 4226.
Goodfellow, P. N., C. J. Barnstable, W. F. Bodmer, D. Snary, and M. J. Crumpton (1976), *Transplantation* **22**, 595.
Goodfellow, P. N., G. Banting, J. Trowsdale, S. Chambers, and E. Solomon (1982), *Proc. Natl. Acad. Sci. USA* **79**, 1190.
Goodfellow, P. N., F. Benham, P. W. Andrews, J. Trowsdale, J. Lee, and M. Quintero (1983), in *Teratocarcinoma Stem Cells,* Cold Spring Harbor Conferences on Cell Proliferation, vol. 10. (Silver, L. M., G,R. Martin, and S. Strickland, eds.), Cold Spring Harbor, NY, p. 439.
Gooi, H. C., T. Feizi, A. Kapadia, B. B. Knowles, D. Solter, and M. J. Evans (1981) *Nature* **292**, 156.
Greene, P. J., and H. H. Sussman (1973), *Proc. Natl. Acad. Sci. USA* **70**, 2936.
Hata, J.-I., Y. Ueyama, N. Tamaoki, A. Akatsuka, S. Yoshimura, K. Shimuzu, Y. Morikawa, and T. Furukawa (1980). *Cancer* **46**, 2446.
Heyderman, E. (1978) *Scand. J. Immunol.* **9**, suppl. 8, 119.
Hogan, B., Fellous, P. Avner, and F. Jacob (1977) *Nature* **270**, 515.
Holden, S., O. Bernard, K. Artzt, W. F. Whitmore, Jr., and D. Bennett (1977), *Nature* **270**, 518.
Inglis, N. R., S. Kirley, L. L. Stolbach, and W. H. Fishman (1973), *Cancer Res.* **33**, 1657.
Jacobsen, G. K., and M. Jacobsen (1983) *Acta. Pathol. Microbiol. Immunol. Scand. A* **91**, 165.
Jacoby, B., and K. D. Bagshawe (1971), *Clin. Chem. Acta.* **35**, 473.

Javadpour, N., K. R. McIntire and T. A. Waldmann (1978), *Natl. Cancer Inst. Monograph* **49**, 209.

Kaneko, M., T. Takeuchi, Y. Tsuchida, S. Saito, and Y. Endo (1980), *Gann*, **71**, 14.

Kannagi, R., E. Nudelman, S. B. Levery, and S.-I. Hakomori (1982) *J. Biol. Chem.* **257**, 14865.

Kannagi, R., N. A. Cochran, F. Ishigami, S.-I. Hakomori, P. W. Andrews, B. B. Knowles, and D. Solter (1983a) *EMBO J.*, **2**, 2355.

Kannagi, R., S. B. Levery, F. Ishigami, S.-I. Hakomori, L. H. Shevinsky, B. B. Knowles, and D. Solter (1983b), *J. Biol. Chem.* **258**, 8934.

Lange, P. H. 1982), in *Human Cancer Markers* (Sell, S. and B. Wahren, eds.), Humana Press, Clifton, NJ, p. 259.

Leblond, C. P. (1981), *Am. J. Anat.* **160**, 114.

Levine, P., and A. Koch-Elisabeth (1954), *Science* **120**, 239.

Martin, G. R. (1980), *Science* **209**, 768.

Matthaei, K., P. W. Andrews, and D. L. Bronson (1983), *Exp. Cell. Res.* **143**, 471.

McIlhinney, R. A. J. (1981), *Int. J. Androl. Suppl.* **4**, 88.

McIlhinney, R. A. J., and S. Patel (1983), *Cancer Res.* **43**, 1282.

McIlhinney, R. A. J., S. Patel, and P. Monaghan (1983), *Exp. Cell. Res.* **144**, 297.

Moon, T. D., R. L. Vessella, and P. H. Lange (1983), *J. Urol.* **130**, 584.

Morello, D. and P. Avner (1982) *Ann. Immunol. Inst. Pasteur* **133**, 121.

Morello, D., G. Gachelin, P. Dubois, M. Tanigaki, D. Pressman, and F. Jacob (1978), *Transplantation* **26**, 119.

Mostofi, F. K. (1980), *Cancer* **45**, 1735.

Muramatsu, T., G. Gachelin, J. F. Nicolas, H. Condamine, H. Jakob, and F. Jacob (1978), *Proc. Natl. Acad. Sci. USA* **75**, 2315.

Muramatsu, T., P. Avner, M. Fellous, G. Gachelin, and F. Jacob (1979), *Somatic Cell Genet.* **5**, 753.

Muramatsu, H., T. Muramatsu, and P. Avner (1982), *Cancer Res.* **42**, 1749.

Osborn, M., and K. Weber (1983), *Lab. Invest.* **48**, 372.

Oshima, R. G. (1982), *J. Biol. Chem.* **257**, 3414.

Paiva, J., I. Damjanov, P. H. Lange, and H. Harris (1983), *Am. J. Pathol.* **111**, 156.

Pattillo, R. A. and G. O. Gey (1968), *Cancer Res.* **28**, 1231.

Pattillo, R. A., A. Ruckert, R. Hussa, R. Bernstein and E. Delfs (1971), *In Vitro* **6**, 398.

Paulin, D, (1981), *Biochimie* **63**, 347.

Pertschuk, L. P. (1975), *Cancer Res.* **35**, 750.

Pierce, G. B. (1980), in *Cancer Markers—Developmental and Diagnostic Significance* (Sell, S., ed.), Clifton, NJ, p. 1.

Pierce, G. B., F. J. Dixon, and E. Verney (1958), *Cancer Res.* **18**, 204.

Pugh, R. C. B., and K. M. Cameron (1976), in *Pathology of Testis,* Blackwell Scientific, Oxford, p. 199.

Rasilo, M.-L., J. Wartiovaara, and O. Renkonen (1980), *Canad. J. Biochem.* **58**, 384.

Ruoslahti, E., H. Kalanko, D. E. Comings, A. M. Neville, and D. Raghavan (1981), *Int. J. Cancer* **27**, 763.

Seargeant, L. E., and R. A. Stinson (1979), *Nature* **281**, 152.

Shevinsky, L. H., B. B. Knowles, I. Damjanov, and D. Solter (1982), *Cell* **30**, 697.

Silver, L. M., G. R. Martin, and S. Strickland (eds.) (1983), *Teratocarcinoma Stem Cells*, Cold Spring Harbor Conferences on Cell Proliferation, vol. 10, Cold Spring Harbor, NY.

Solter, D., and I. Damjanov (1979), *Meth. Cancer Res.* **18**, 277.

Solter, D., and B. B. Knowles (1978), *Proc. Natl. Acad. Sci. USA* **75**, 5565.

Stern, P. K., K. Willison, E. Lennox, G. Galfre, C. Milstein, D. Secher, and A. Ziegler (1978), *Cell* **14**, 775.

Stigbrand, T. and E. Engvall (1982), *Human Cancer Markers* (Sell, S. and B. Wahren, eds.), Clifton, NJ, p. 275.

Takeuchi, T., M. Nakayasu, S. Hirohasi, T. Kameya, M, Kaneko, K. Yokomori and Y. Tsuchid (1979), *J. Clin. Pathol.* **32**, 693.

Talerman, A., W. B. van der Pompe, W. G. Haije, J. Baggerman and H. M. Boekenstein-Tjahjadi (1977), *Br. J. Cancer* **35**, 288.

Talerman, A., W. G. Haije, and L. Baggerman (1980), *Cancer* **46**, 390.

Tatarinov, Y. S. (1980), *Br. J. Cancer* **41**, 821.

Tatarinov, Y. S., N. V. Mesnyankina, D. M. Nikoulina, L. A Novikova, B. O. Toloknov, and D. M. Falaleeva (1974), *Int. J. Cancer* **14**, 548.

Uchida T., T. Shimoda, H. Miyata, T. Shikata, S. Iino, H. Suzuki, T. Oda, K. Hirano, M. Sugiura (1981), *Cancer* **48**, 1455.

Vogelzang, N. J., D. L. Bronson, D. Savino, and E. E. Fraley (1983), in *Teratocarcinoma Stem Cells*, Cold Spring Harbor Conferences, vol. 10 (Silver, L. M., G. R. Martin, and S. Strickland, eds.), p. 607.

Wahren, B., P. A. Holmgren, and T. Stigbrand (1979), *Int. J. Cancer* **24**, 749.

Wang, N., B. Trend, D. L. Bronson, and E. E. Fraley (1980), *Cancer Res.* **40**, 796.

Williams, L. K., A. Sullivan, R. A. J. McIlhinney, and A. M. Neville (1982), *Int. J. Cancer* **30**, 731.

Yoshimura, S., N. Tamaoki, Y. Ueyama, Y. Hata (1978), *Cancer Res.* **38**, 3474.

Zeuthen, J., J. O. R. Norgaard, P. Avner, M. Fellous, J. Wartiovaara, A. Vaheri, A. Rosen, and B. C. Giovanella (1980), *Int. J. Cancer* **25**, 19.

Chapter 16

Use of Monoclonal Antibodies in Neurobiology and Neurooncology

CAROL J. WIKSTRAND AND DARELL D. BIGNER

*Department of Pathology, Duke University Medical Center,
Durham, North Carolina*

1. Introduction

Neuroimmunology is a comparatively new field; the recent application
and widespread use of hybridoma methodology in the neurosciences has
contributed much by "uncovering" new biochemical moieties not previously defined by heteroantisera.

The production of hybridomas in both animal model systems and
protocols involving human cells as responder or immunogen have recently allowed the development of libraries of reagents that are enabling
neurobiologists to begin to define cell origins, relationships, and lineages. The proceedings of a workshop on monoclonal antibodies (Mabs)
against neural antigens (McKay et al., 1981) well summarize the early
efforts in the field. Perhaps the most ambitious work was that reported by
Franko et al. (1981) who developed a battery of over thirty murine
antimouse nervous system Mabs, and then systematically used these to
describe elements of the neuropil, neuronal cytoplasm, nuclei, axons,
astrocytes, and ependyma in mouse and hamster tissues and mouse, hamster, rat, and human cultured cell lines. Similar cell differentiation markers were defined by Hirn et al. (1982) and Lagenaur et al. (1980); by 1982
a systematic classification of both astroglial and neuronal maturation and
differentiation was well underway (Hawkes et al., 1982). This was perhaps the most significant advance in neuroimmunology, for it made possible the extension of research into markers of neuroectodermal tissue-

derived tumor cells, once the establishment of markers for normal nervous system development were available. This work is presently at a descriptive stage since the biochemical characterization of the antigens detected by such Mabs is still in its infancy.

Of most interest and potential significance are determination of the cell of origin of many nervous system tumors, and whether the markers determined to be characteristic of given tumors would be of prognostic significance, either to the natural disease course or response to various therapeutic modalities.

Immunohistology utilizing polyclonal antisera has been a staple of neuropathology; currently Mabs are being introduced as they become characterized and available. The advantages of specificity and consistency of reagent provided by Mabs is unquestioned (Bonin and Rubenstein, 1984; Trojanowski and Lee, 1983a). As shown recently by Hickey et al. (1983), however, there is no way to predict the sensitivity of a given Mab; in a well-controlled study of Mabs against myelin basic protein and neurofilament proteins, these investigators demonstrated a wide range in sensitivity of various Mabs, some of which were more, and some of which were less, sensitive than well-characterized polyclonal sera. The important observation, however, was that the increased specificity associated with Mabs need not be attained by compromising sensitivity, and that a panel or mixture of Mabs, the specificities and affinities of which are known and controllable, is potentially the best reagent for immunohistochemical diagnosis and in vivo localization (Bonin and Rubenstein, 1984; Bourdon et al., 1984a). The relative advantages or disadvantages of polyclonal versus monoclonal antibodies for immunohistochemical application in diagnostic neuropathology will be established as Mabs become available against GFAP, vimentin, neuron-specific enolase, S-100, and glutamine synthetase, for example.

2. Markers of Central and Peripheral Nervous System (PNS) Tumors Defined by Mabs

As summarized in Wikstrand and Bigner (1980), immunization of rodents, rabbits, or nonhuman and human primates with nervous system normal or tumor tissue results in the production of antibodies directed against a wide range of antigenic specificities. The capacity of hybridoma methodology to isolate the response of a single cell has allowed the concomitant delineation of unique antigenic specificities detected. Early animal model studies performed with the C1300 murine neuroblastoma model system utilized spleen cells from mice bearing C1300 neuroblastomas as the immune cell partner for hybridoma production (Revoltella et al., 1982). The Mabs produced defined "a spectrum of distinct alloantigenic specificities'' (ibid.) including an epitope of the Ia complex, fetal-neonatal antigens, and neuronal-restricted specificities. Initial results obtained from fusions involving immunization with human neuroectodermal tumor-associated antigens (HNTA) have been identical to those described with model animal tumor systems.

The antigens defined by anti-human HNTA Mab fall roughly into four categories: (1) biochemically defined markers [glial fibrillary acidic protein (GFAP), S-100, gangliosides]; (2) shared nervous system-lymphoid antigens (HLA-DR, CALLA, Thy); (3) cross-reactive neuroectodermal-oncofetal specificities, predominatly cell-surface in location; and (4) putatively tumor-type restricted markers. For ease of reference we have listed the major Mab-antigen systems in Table 1. This table is not meant to be comprehensive, but rather offers an outline of the types of markers detected.

2.2. Biochemically Defined Markers

Perhaps the best known specific marker within the human central nervous system (CNS) is glial fibrillary acidic protein (GFAP), the major component of glial filaments, the intermediate filaments expressed by astroglial cells (Eng et al., 1971). Problems defining the nature of this labile 51 Kd protein with polyclonal antisera were expected to be resolved by the production of anti-GFAP Mab. As outlined by Eng et al. (1983) and by Lee et al. (1984), the family of intermediate filament proteins [neurofilament (NF), vimentin, keratin, desmin, and GFAP] share highly immunogenic cross-reactive epitopes, readily detected even by Mab produced against gel-excised GFAP. However, Mabs specific for noncross-reactive epitopes of GFAP have been produced (Eng et al., 1983; Pegram et al., 1984); these Mabs, raised against partially purified bovine GFAP and selected by screening against the GFAP-positive human glioma cell line U-251 MG, recognize a phylogenetically conserved interspecies GFAP-restricted epitope common to human, nonhuman primate, canine, bovine, ovine, porcine, avian, murine, rat, rabbit, and guinea pig brain as determined by Mab absorption analysis. Neoplastic human, rat, and rabbit astrocytes also express this GFAP epitope as determined by immunoblot techniques. The utility of these Mabs that are specific for cells of astrocytic lineage is apparent; however, the ease and frequency with which Mabs reactive with shared intermediate filament epitopes were obtained indicate that independent immunochemical and immunohistochemical assays are necessary for precise characterization of Mabs in this system. Mabs such as these may well define the GFAP determinant most useful for diagnostic interpretation.

Mabs to the S-100 protein marker of the nervous system have recently been produced (Golden et al., 1984); the utility of this protein as a tumor marker is severely compromised by its apparent lack of restriction

Table 1

Central and Peripheral Nervous System Tumor-Associated Markers Detected by Monoclonal Antibodies[a]

Antigen detected[b]	Immunogen used[c]	Cell and tissue distribution[d]		Reference[e]
		Neoplastic	Normal	
Biochemically defined markers				
GFAP	Purified bovine GFAP	Glioma	Astrocytes, Bergmann glia	Eng et al., 1983
S-100	Purified bovine S-100	Glioma, melanoma, Schwannoma	Astrocytes, Bergmann glia, Schwann cells, melanocytes, Langerhans cells (epidermal), interdigitating reticular cells, chondrocytes	Golden and Gilespie, 1984
GD$_2$ ganglioside	Melanoma cell line M14	Glioma, melanoma, neuroblastoma	Fetal brain	Cahan et al., 1982 (OFA 1-2; human MA)
GD$_3$ ganglioside	Melanoma cell line SK-MEL-28	Glioma, melanoma	Fetal brain, lung muscle; adult brain	Pukel et al., 1982 (R24)
GD$_3$ ganglioside	Melanoma cell line SK-MEL-28	Glioma, melanoma, bladder carcinoma	Adult lung, kidney fibroblast	Nudelman et al., 1982 (4.2)
GQ ganglioside	Chick retina	Neuroblastoma, retinoblastoma, insulinoma	Adult brain, pancreatic islet cells	Eisenbarth et al., 1979 (A2B5)

Shared nervous system–lymphoid cell markers

HLA-DR (Ia-like antigens)	Cell line RPM1 8866	Glioma, osteosarcoma	Standard Ia distribution (Mitchell et al., 1980; Natali, et al., 1981)	Wikstrand et al., manuscript in preparation Lampson and Levy, 1980 (L-203, 227, 243)
HLA-DR	Daudi cell membranes	Glioma, melanoma, endometrial carcinoma	Standard Ia distribution (Mitchell et al., 1980; Natali, et al., 1981)	Carrel et al., 1982a (D1-12)
CALLA	Cell line NALM-1	Glioma, melanoma, lymphoblasts (C-ALL, CML)	Standard CALLA distribution (Metzgar et al., 1981)	Carrel et al., 1983 (A12)
CALLA	Pre B-ALL cell line NALM-6	Glioma	Standard CALLA distribution (Metzgar et al., 1981)	Wikstrand et al., manuscript in preparation (BA-3; Hybritech)
OKT-8	Human T lymphocytes	Glioma	T-suppressor cells oligodendroglia	Oger et al., 1982 Wikstrand et al., (manuscript in preparation)
Thy-1 $M_r = 25,000$	Human fetal 12-wk gestation brain	Glioma, neuroblastoma, rhabdomyosarcoma, leiomyosarcoma, teratoma	Brain, thymus, kidney, fibroblasts, myoblasts	Seeger et al., 1982a (390) Wikstrand et al., 1983 (390)
PNET (Peripheral neuroectodermal tumor)	PNET cell line SK-PN-DW	Melanoma, neuroblastoma, PNET, hepatoblastoma	Polymorphonuclear leucocytes	Helson et al., 1983 (DW-1)

(continued)

Table 1 (continued)

Antigen detected[b]	Immunogen used[c]	Cell and tissue distribution[a]		Reference[c]
		Neoplastic	Normal	
M22	Melanoma cell line SK-MEL-28	Glioma, melanoma, carcinoma	Adult brain, leucocytes	Dippold et al., 1980 (R-8)
P1153 $M_r = 30,000$	Neuroblastoma cell line 1MR-6	Glioma, neuroblastoma, retinoblastoma, null and B cell-ALL, B cell-CLL	Fetal brain, B lymphocyte lineage	Kennet et al., 1980; Seeger et al., 1982b
Shared neuroectodermal-oncofetal markers				
Neuroectodermal				
GE2 BF7 (48Kd)	Glioma cell line LN-18	Glioma, melanoma, meningioma, Schwannoma, carcinoma		Schnegg et al., 1981; De Tribolet, 1982
GMEM (230 Kd)	Glioma cell line U-251 MG	Glioma, melanoma, neuroblastoma, sarcoma, carcinoma	Adult spleen, liver, kidney	Bourdon et al., 1983 (81C6)
34.1 (250 Kd)	Melanoma cell line	Glioma, melanoma, neuroblastoma		Saxton et al., 1983
"Proteoglycan" (250 Kd)	Melanoma cell line M1733	Melanoma, carcinoma	Adult skin fibroblasts, nevi	Hellström et al., 1983 (48.7)
M19 (50-70 Kd)	Melanoma cell line SK-MEL-28	Glioma, melanoma, carcinoma	Adult kidney, fibroblasts	Dippold et al., 1980
Nu4B 19-19 (116,95,29,26 KD) complex	Melanoma cell line SW 691	Glioma, melanoma	Fibroblasts (Nu4B)	Herlyn et al., 1980

Antibody	Immunogen	Reactivity	Tissue distribution	Reference
Me 1-5 Me 1-14	Melanoma cell line Me-43	Glioma, melanoma, neuroblastoma	—	Carrel et al., 1982b
Oncofetal				
Q24 (150 Kd)	Melanoma cell line SK-MEL-28	Glioma, melanoma, carcinoma	Fetal brain, kidney and fibroblasts	Dipploid et al., 1980
K5 (95-97 Kd)	Melanoma call line SK-MEL-28	Glioma, melanoma, carcinoma, sarcoma	Fetal brain, lung, kidney, colon; adult gastrointestinal and urogenital organs, muscle	Saxton et al., 1983 (705 F6) Brown et al., 1981
7.51 7.60	Melanoma cell line CaCL 78-1	Glioma, melanoma, neuroblastoma, retinoblastoma	Fetal brain	Liao et al., 1981
376 175	Melanoma cell line M21	Glioma, melanoma, sarcoma (neuroblastoma; 376)	Fetal lung, kidney, intestine	Seeger et al., 1981
4C7 5B7	Glioma cell line D-54 MG	Glioma, melanoma (neuroblastoma; 4C7)	Fetal brain, thymus, spleen, skin fibroblast	Wikstrand et al., 1984
1H8 cl2	Human fetal 22-wk gestation brain	Glioma, neuroblastoma, medulloblatoma	Fetal brain, spleen, and fibroblasts	Wikstrand et al., 1982
1H8 cl3	Human fetal 22-wk gestation brain	Glioma, melanoma, neuroblastoma, medulloblastoma	Fetal brain, spleen, and liver; adult spleen	Wikstrand et al., 1982
4D2	Human fetal 22-wk gestation brain	Glioma, melanoma, neuroblastoma	Fetal brain, spleen, liver, and fibroblast; adult spleen	Wikstrand and Bigner, 1982

(continued)

Table 1 (*continued*)

Antigen detected[b]	Immunogen used[c]	Cell and tissue distribution[d]		Reference[e]
		Neoplastic	Normal	
7H10	Human fetal 22-wk gestation brain	Glioma, neuroblastoma, medulloblastoma, Hodgkins lymphomas	Fetal brain, thymus, spleen and liver; adult spleen	Wikstrand and Bigner, 1982
Putative tumor-restricted markers				
M4 M5 M8	Melanoma cell line	Melanoma	Newborn melanocytes	Houghton et al., 1982
2F3	Glioma cell line D-54 MG	Glioma	Fetal skin fibroblasts	Wikstrand et al., 1984
1D6 1A2 3B5	Autologous glioma cells (human hybrid)	Glioma	Incompletely characterized	Sikora et al., 1982
Markers of interest defined in animal model systems				
13GC 14BC	Chemically induced rat glioma cell line 79FR-G-41	Chemically induced rat glioma cell lines	Incompletely characterized	Stavrou et al., 1983

7G4 9F1 10E3 10E7	ASV-induced rat astrocytoma	Astrocytoma, neurinoma; virally and chemically induced neurogenic rat tumors	None	Lee et al., 1984
217C	Rat glioma cell line C6	Human and rat glioma cells; transformed rat astrocytes and oligodendrocytes, mouse and rat hepatomas	Rat hepatocytes, whole liver	Peng et al., 1982

[a]This table is not meant to be complete; it summarizes specificities of interest because of their pattern of occurrence as detected by monoclonal antibodies.

[b]If the antigen detected was not identified or named, an identifying characteristic or the designation of the monoclonal antibody detecting it has been listed.

[c]Original immunogen used to generate monoclonal antibody.

[d]Cell and tissue distribution are expressed as correctly concise as possible; some simplification resulted in the listing, primarily of normal tissue distribution. For complete description, see reference.

[e]The reference given is that which most comprehensively describes the antigen–MA system; it will refer to the original citation if it is a later publication.

to the nervous system (Golden and Gillespie, 1984); however, S-100 can be used to differentiate Schwannomas from other malignant spindle-cell tumors of neuronal origin. The absence of S-100 reactivity however, does not rule out a neuroectodermal origin for the tissue or tumor in question (Golden and Gillespie, 1984).

Cell surface markers which have been biochemically defined seem to be primarily gangliosides (glycolipids containing sialic acid) as reported by Eisenbarth et al., 1979; Cahan et al., 1982; Pukel et al., 1982; and Nudelman et al., 1982. Although Mab-detected galactocerebroside has been shown to be a developmental marker on the surfaces of oligodendrocytes and Schwann cells (Ranscht et al., 1982), the galactosphingolipids have not been heavily represented among Mab-detected neuroectodermal tumor markers. Eisenbarth et al. (1979) were the first to define the presence of GQ ganglioside as a marker for retina neuron cell bodies but not axons or dendrites, and for tumor cells of neuronal origin; interestingly, this marker is also characteristic of pancreatic islet cells. Using cultured melanoma cells as immunogen, other investigators have produced Mabs that react with a broader spectrum of HNTA. The OFA-1-2 cell surface antigen has been identified as the disialoganglioside GD2 (Cahan et al., 1982). Originally described by Irie et al. (1979) using monospecific human antibody produced in vitro by a lymphoblast cell line derived from a melanoma patient, OFA-1-2 is highly immunogenic in man, despite its presence in developing human fetal brain. The exquisite sensitivity inherent in these Mab-tumor cell surface antigen systems is illustrated well by the demonstration by Cahan et al. (1982) that anti-GD2 Mabs were totally nonreactive with gangliosides that differed by the addition of one galactose (GD1b), the loss of one sialic acid (GM2), or the loss of an N-acetylgalactosamine residue (GD3). This latter observation is especially notable in that GD3 has been demonstrated to be readily detected by Mabs produced against cultured melanoma cell line SK-MEL-28 by two separate groups (Pukel et al., 1982; and Nudelman et al., 1982). GD3, unlike GD2, is also expressed by carcinomas as well (Pukel et al., 1982; and Nudelman et al., 1982). Neither of these gangliosides is restricted to tumors, in that normal brain, retina, and kidney, for example, have high levels, yet absorb or directly label with anti-GD3 Mab AbR_{24} very weakly (Pukel et al., 1982). This discrepancy could be attributable to the predominantly intracellular location of GD3 in normal brain cells, or the relative nonavailability of the specificity on normal cell membranes for Mab binding (Pukel et al., 1982). Nudelman et al. (1982) have demonstrated that although the GD3 isolated from melanomas is distinct from normal brain-derived GD3 in that the ceramide of the former is characterized by longer chain fatty acids than the latter, the antigenic site detected by Mab 4.2 is on the identical terminal carbohydrate sequence [Neu Acα2$\rightarrow$8Neu Acα2$\rightarrow$3Galβ1$\rightarrow$4Glc$\rightarrow$].

2.2. Shared Nervous System–Lymphoid Cell Markers

Since the original report by Reif and Allen (1964) of a θ antigen (THY-1) on murine lymphocytes and brain cells, several investigators have reported the production of antisera in various species that react with a library of shared brain–lymphoid antigens of interspecies and restricted human specificity (for review, see Wikstrand and Bigner, 1980). These shared antigens are not necessarily confined to the T cell or thymic compartment of cells; early work with serum obtained from systemic lupus erythematosus patients showed that antigens common to normal human peripheral blood B and T cells and human brain were immunogenic in humans (Bluestein and Zvaifler, 1976). This pattern of reactivity has, not surprisingly, been repeated with Mabs.

2.2.1. Analysis of Neuroectodermal Tumors with Anti-Lymphoid Antigen Mabs.

Using standard HLA-A,B typing sera, Bigner et al. (1981) reported the readily detected presence of HLA-A,B, specificities on a panel of fifteen cultured glioma lines. In a more recent, rigorous study using Mabs against β-2 microglobulin and an invariant determinant on the HLA chain of all HLA-A,B, and C molecules, Lampson et al. (1983) have reported the relatively low expression of these molecules on four cultured neuroblastoma cells as compared to lymphoid cells or the oligodendroglioma-derived cell line CW1-TG1.

In contrast, the expression of HLA-DR (Ia-like) antigens by nonlymphoid tissues and tumor cell lines has been extensively investigated. Ia-like antigen expression in human tissues is not restricted to cells associated with immune functions, but has been shown to be expressed by "the epithelium of the gastrointestinal tract, urinary bladder, bronchial glands, thymic reticuloepithelial cells (entodermic origin); epithelium of mammary gland, acinar cells of the parotid, astrocytes (ectodermic origin); alveolar macrophages, Kupffer cells, glomerular and peritubular renal endothelium, endometrium, and Langerhans cells (mesodermic origin)" (Natali et al., 1981). It is not surprising, therefore, that Ia-like antigens have been demonstrated by Mabs on a wide variety of nonlymphoid human tumor cell lines including melanoma, carcinomas of the kidney, breast, stomach, prostate and vulva, hepatoma, sarcoma, and glioma (Pellegrino et al., 1981; Ng et al., 1981). Similarly, Howe et al. (1981) analyzed 27 tumor cell lines for Ia-like antigen expression, and could demonstrate reactivity with only 3/4 melanoma lines; significantly, 9/9 neuroblastomas, 3/3 gliomas, and 1 medulloblastoma did not express detectable Ia-like antigen. The absence of HLA-DR antigens on two additional neuroblastoma cell lines was also reported by Lampson et al. (1983) following their inability to detect binding of the anti-HLA-DR Mab 203 (Lampson and Levy, 1980).

Conversely, as with melanoma cell lines (Tai et al., 1983), Carrel et al. (1982a) readily demonstrated HLA-DR antigen expression by 3/8 glioma cell lines using the anti-IA-β chain Mab D1-12. This analysis was extended by Wikstrand et al. (manuscript in preparation) who, using the Lampson and Levy (1980) series of anti-HLA-DR Mabs 203, 227, and 243, demonstrated Ia-like antigen expression by subset populations of an additional 4/14 glioma lines. As demonstrated by Carrel et al. (1982a) and Mitchell et al. (1982), appropriate α and β chains of HLA-DR can be precipitated from glioma and melanoma cells, respectively; Mitchell et al. (1980) have some evidence that an additional, lighter 28 Kd molecule can be precipitated from solubilized melanoma cells by Mab 37-7.

Molecular weight heterogeneity of the Mab-defined antigen varying with tissue has also been reported for CALLA; estimated weight ranges from 95 to 110 Kd were obtained depending upon the antigen source (fibroblasts or granulocytes, respectively) (Braun et al., 1983). Using a rabbit anti-CALLA antiserum, Carrel et al. (1982a) demonstrated that the CALLA antigen precipitated from glioma cell lines LN-229 and LN-215 was of 100 Kd weight and apparently identical to that from NALM-1 cells. In a later study of 15 melanoma cell lines with the anti-CALLA Mab A12, this same group (Carrel et al., 1983) demonstrated that 6/15 lines were CALLA+, but that the level of 100 Kd precipitable antigen and the percentage of positive cells varied widely. Wikstrand et al. (manuscript in preparation) have similarly shown that 3/15 human glioma cell lines express CALLA; the percentage of positive cells per population was somewhat less variable, ranging from 80 to 100%.

Following the identification by Oger et al. (1982) of OKT-8 as a marker present on 50–86% of purified lamb oligodendrocytes as well as human T-suppressor cells, Wikstrand et al. (manuscript in preparation) demonstrated the presence of OKT-8 on small (8–12%) subpopulations of 3/8 glioma cell lines. The possibility that OKT-8 expression may be phase-specific in these cells is being investigated.

2.2.2. Analysis of Neuroectodermal Tumors with Anti-Nervous System Antigen Mabs Detecting Lymphoid Antigens

Perhaps the most extensively studied human "T"-related antigen is Thy-1. Seeger et al. (1982a) produced an anti-human Thy-1 Mab (390) using human 12-wk gestation age fetal brain for immunization; the antigen detected by Mab 390 was demonstrated to be Thy-1 by antigen distribution and absorption with purified human Thy-1. Using this Mab, Seeger et al. (1982a) demonstrated the expression of Thy-1 by glioma, neuroblastoma, rhabdomyosarcoma, leiomyosarcoma, and teratoma cell lines; in contrast, the expression of Thy-1 by medulloblastoma, melanoma, and carcinoma cell lines was insignificant. Wikstrand et al. (1984; manuscript in preparation) have demonstrated the presence of Thy-1 as detected by Mab 390 by 85–100% of the cells of all 14 glioma cell lines tested, as well as by the single medulloblastoma (TE-671) and osteosarcoma cell line tested. The ubiquitous presence of Thy-1 in these cultured lines raises the possibility, as suggested by Dales et al. (1983), that the detected sequence homology between murine Thy 1.2 and actin might be responsible for the observed extensive distribution of Thy-1. As anti-Thy 1.2 Mabs do react with human cells, this is indeed a possibility (Dales et al., 1983); the relative lack of binding of Mab 390 to melanoma and carcinoma cell lines could argue against this, or simply reflect the unavailability for antibody binding of this cross-reactive epitope on the actin molecule of these cells.

The first and now classical example of an anti-HNTA Mab was PI 153/3, described by Kennett and Gilbert in 1979; subsequent studies have shown that this glycoprotein with an $M_r = 30,000$ is present on neuroblastoma, glioma, and retinoblastoma cells, as well as null and B-cell ALL and B cell-CLL (Kennett et al., 1980). PI 153/3 is probably best summarized as a marker of fetal brain and B lymphocyte lineage (Seeger et al., 1982b) and has defined a general category which includes the anti-fetal brain Mabs described by Wikstrand and Bigner (1982) and Wikstrand et al. (1982), and the M22 antigen system described by Dippold et al. (1980).

Non-CNS tumors also share an antigen with lymphoid cells; the Mab DW-1 reported by Helson et al. (1983) was raised against the peripheral neuroectodermal tumor cell line SK-PN-DW. This Mab defines a specificity present only on peripheral neuroectodermal tumors, neuroblastoma cell lines, melanomas, and hepatoblastomas, as well as polymorphonuclear leucocytes. This apparent PNS-CNS antigenic segregation is quite interesting, in that the majority of Mab-detected HNTA described have not been so restrictive, as shown in the next section.

2.3. Shared Neuroectodermal–Oncofetal Markers

The antigens detected in this category can be loosely subdivided into two subgroups for ease of reference as shown in Table 1: (1) shared neuroectodermal tumor antigens, defined here as those antigens not detected on adult CNS or PNS or any fetal tissues, versus (2) oncofetal antigens, which are shared neuroectodermal tumor antigens also detected on human fetal tissues, including the fetal CNS and lymphoid systems. Rather than discussing each of the several studies reported in Table 1 that fall into this category, we intend to highlight various trends and exceptions.

As summarized by De Tribolet and Bigner (1982) following a workshop on Mab production to neuroectoderm-derived tumors, the general consensus is that shared, rather than restricted specificities appear to be most commonly detected within this system. This is strongly illustrated by the numerous recent publications having "shared" or "common" HNTA as the major theme (Cairncross et al., 1982; Carrel et al., 1982b; De Tribolet and Bigner, 1982; Herlyn et al., 1980; Kennet and Gilbert, 1979; Liao et al., 1981; Seeger et al., 1981; Wikstrand and Bigner, 1982; Wikstrand et al., 1982). In addition to the neuroectodermal vs oncofetal distinction outlined above, when the antigen–Mab systems are displayed as in Table 1, three other trends become apparent.

First, the tendency for described Mabs to react with carcinomas was largely confined to those within the "neuroectodermal" category, the primary immunogens being glioma or melanoma cell lines. The exceptions appear to be confined to immunization regimens involving the melanoma cell line SK-MEL-28 that has resulted in Mabs directed against antigens in all categories: GD_3 ganglioside (Nudelman et al., 1982); nervous-system lymphoid and shared neuroectodermal antigen series M22 and M19, respectively (Dippold et al., 1980); and oncofetal antigens Q24 (Dippold et al., 1980) and K5 (Saxton et al., 1983). Each of these Mabs react with carcinomas; the majority of Mabs within the shared brain–lymphoid and oncofetal categories do not. In contrast, anti-HNTA Mabs rarely react with sarcomas, the exceptions being anti-Thy-1 (Seeger et al., 1982a), 81C6 (Bourdon et al., 1983), and the anti-oncofetal Mabs K5 (Saxton et al., 1983) and 376 (Seeger et al., 1981). Of interest within this primarily neuroectodermal-reactive subset are Mabs GE2 and BF7 (Schnegg et al., 1981), the only anti-HNTA Mabs demonstrated to react with Schwannomas.

Second, and related to the first trend, is the observation that Mabs reacting with normal kidney are those that react with carcinomas and/or sarcomas; even reaction with fetal kidney (Seeger et al., 1981) occurs only under this condition. Although not surprising, this connection is significant in that localization to normal kidney is potentially hazardous when systemic administration to human patients is considered.

Third, the production of Mabs detecting cross-reactivity between HNTA and lymphoid tissues, fetal or adult, does not generally occur when melanoma cell line immunization is used, with the exception again of immunization with SK-MEL-28 (M22, Dippold et al., 1980). Immunization with any of a variety of immunogens (human fetal brain, PNET cells, neuroblastoma cells, or glioma cells; see Table 1) is capable of inducing lymphoid cell-reactive Mabs.

This category, shared neuroectodermal–oncofetal antigens, is the largest described here, due primarily to the large number of possible immunogens present in the complex antigen sources used. What is interesting is the relative consistency of observed response—the antigenic association primarily detected between gliomas, neuroblastomas, and melanomas; the relative lack of association between PNS and CNS tumors, most notably the relative paucity of reactivity for Schwannomas; and the impressive immunogenicity of shared brain–lymphoid markers. The specificity achievable by a panel of reagents reactive with specificities in this category is well illustrated by the panel of Mabs produced in this laboratory and presented in Table 2. The variation in reactivity profiles for tumor tissues of neoplastic origin reflects the antigenic complexity and heterogeneity inherent in these tumors, and underscores the necessity to continuously seek new markers in this system with additional Mabs.

2.4. Putative Tumor-Restricted Markers

In reality, this category consists of a family of both murine and human Mabs that have demonstrated highly restricted reactivity patterns, and that appear to be operationally specific for the designated tumor. As any hybridoma producer is aware, the range of specificity of any given Mab constantly changes as the panel of targets tested enlarges. However, the characteristic that each of the Mabs listed here has in common is a to-date-defined reactivity for only the tumor type of the immunogen used for its production, and could therefore be used as a specific probe for that tumor. It is anticipated that entry into and departure from this list shall be frequent in coming years; the advent of purified or partially purified antigen sources for immunization made possible by the Mabs listed here will hopefully increase the frequency of restricted specificity Mabs.

2.5. Markers of Interest Defined in Animal Model Systems

As introduced at the beginning of this section, initial work with the murine neuroblastoma C1300 tumor model system (Revoltella et al., 1982) was predictive of the antigenic specificities detected when human cells of neuroectodermal origin were used for immunization. Considering this, it is important to note a few recent studies in animal model systems that might have direct or indirect, predictive relevance to human studies. Although potential reactivity for normal tissues was not extensively tested, Stavrou et al. (1983) have reported the apparent detection of a specificity uniquely characteristic of nitrosourea induced-rat glioma cell lines. The specificity detected was not present on a small number of spontaneous canine or human gliomas, nor on rat brain or kidney cells or cultured human fibroblasts. These Mabs define a highly unique specificity potentially related to the inducing agent. Similar results were reported by Lee et al. (1984) who have isolated a small, soluble peptide (<1000 daltons) that is expressed on both virally and chemically induced neurogenic rat tumors. Extensive analysis with normal tissues and rodent, murine, and human tumor cell lines has established that this highly restricted specificity of ASV-transformed rat gliomas is characteristic of agent-transformed tumors, but potentially not of spontaneously transformed rat nonneurogenic

Table 2

Summary of the Reactivity Profiles of the Eight Monoclonal Reagents Generated in This Laboratory Against Cultured Glioma Cells Lines and Human Fetal Brain. Demonstration of Specificity.[a]

Target cell/or tissue	Anti-U-251 MG	Monoclonal antibody anti-D-54 MG			Anti-human fetal brain			
	81C6	2F3	4C7	5B7	1H8c12	1H8c13	4D2	7H10
Neoplastic tissue								
Glioblastoma	++	++	++	++	++	++	++	++
Medulloblastoma	–	–	–	–	++	++	–	++
Neuroblastoma	++	–	++	–	++	++	++	++
Melanoma	–	–	++	++	–	++	++	–
ALL, CML	++	–	–	–	–	–	–	–
Carcinoma[b]	++	–	–	–	–	–	–	–
Sarcoma[c]	++	–	–	–	–	–	–	–
Wilms' tumor	++	–	–	–	–	–	–	–
Normal tissue								
Adult brain (cortex, cerebellum)	–	–	–	–	–	–	–	–
Spleen	++	–	–	–	–	++	++	++

Lymph node
Thymus
Liver
Kidney
Skin fibroblast
Miscellaneous[c]

Fetal brain
Spleen
Thymus
Liver
Skin fibroblast

[a]The summary of specific reactivity of the monoclonal reagents listed here is compiled from Bourdon et al., 1983; Wikstrand et al., 1982; Wikstrand and Bigner, 1982; and Wikstrand et al., 1984, and presents data obtained by direct CS-RIA, absorption analysis, and immunohistochemistry (immunofluorescence and PAP). + indicates significant binding to a minimum of one sample of the tissue listed by the criteria for the assay used; − indicates lack of binding to the target tissue tested.

[b]Carcinomas tested include: colon, breast, prostatic, bladder, and adrenal cortex, ovarian, and cervical.

[c]Sarcomas tested include: osteogenic, soft tissue, rhabdomyo-, leiomyo-, and fibro-sarcoma.

[d]NT: not tested.

[e]Miscellaneous samples of adult human origin, none of which were reactive with any of the eight monoclonal reagents listed here include: normal adult muscle, lung, peripheral blood leucocytes, erythrocytes, gut.

[f]Negative on sample of 12-wk gestational age; positive on sample of 16-wk gestational age.

or human glial tumor cell lines. A transformation-associated specificity was also reported by Peng et al. (1982); a murine Mab raised against the C6 rat glioma cell line reacted with rat and human glioma cells, as well as rat and mouse hepatoma cells. Significantly, spontaneously transformed rat astrocytes or ENU-transformed rat oligodendrocytes were also reactive with Mab217. Although normal rat liver, specifically hepatocytes, reacts with this Mab, the marker defined may be associated with the early stage of transformation from normal to neoplastic. Given the previous correlation between animal tumor model studies and results with human tumor cells, there is strong basis to anticipate detection of similar specificities in human systems.

3. Current and Prospective Use of Marker–Mab Systems

The field of HNTA–Mab technology has moved very rapidly since the first report of an anti-HNTA Mab (Kennett and Gilbert, 1979). Within less than four years, investigators in the field have progressed from production and characterization of Mabs to biochemical isolation and purification, and ultimately, to the use in human patients of Mab for diagnostic, tumor localizing, and therapeutic regimens. As summarized by Bourdon et al. (1984a), the problems involved in the delivery of Mab to solid tumors are threefold: the vascularity of the tumor, the vascular permeability throughout the tumor, and the blood flow and extracellular fluid dynamics within the tumor. These factors provide a barrier problem for Mab localization; the second aspect of localization is the antigenic stability of the target that is complicated by the extensive antigenic heterogeneity of most human tumors investigated. Current research addressing these problems and their resolution are presented below.

3.1. The Problem of Antibody Localization and Delivery

Early studies of radiolabeled polyclonal antibody localization in brain tumor patients were performed by Marrack and McCardle (Marrack et al., 1967; McCardle et al., 1966) who demonstrated localization of ^{131}I-anti-fibrinogen antibody in 80% of primary and metastic brain tumors evaluated by radioscintigraphy. The major problems encountered, however, involved the non-specificity of the probe and the heterogeneous expression and distribution of fibrinogen within and between different brain tumors. The problem of specificity was addressed by Day and Mahaley (Day et al., 1964; Mahaley et al., 1965) with ^{131}I-rabbit anti-glioma antibodies; in 11/12 cases examined by presurgical radioscintigraphy and postsurgical tissue gamma counting and autoradiography, significant localization did occur; however, the inability to prepare sufficient amounts of specific, high affinity anti-glioma antibodies from heteroantisera made further experimentation impossible. The importance of these studies, however, is that they demonstrated that radiolabeled-antibody localization and imaging were possible and exploitable within the CNS.

The recent production and characterization of Mabs to glioma-associated antigens has renewed the feasibility of this approach. However, the current state of the art in CNS neoplasia is preclinical, primarily for two reasons: the paucity of antibodies of high specificity which are stable under labeling and in vivo administration conditions, and practical considerations of delivery, namely the blood–brain barrier (BBB). The aspects of antibody localization that must be addressed in logical order are: specificity of the Mab for the tumor target in the in vivo setting; accessability of the target to Mab by clinically achievable routes of administration; and in the case of CNS neoplasms, the potential of safe, well-tolerated blood–brain barrier disruption. A series of experiments have recently been undertaken to address these problems in a stepwise manner.

Bourdon et al. (1984b) have examined the localization of radiolabeled Mab 81C6 in human glioma cell line tumors growing subcutaneously and intracranially in athymic nude mice by paired label analysis, radioscintigraphy, and autoradiography. Mab 81C6 defines a glioma–mesenchymal extracellular matrix antigen (GMEM) present in the extracellular matrix of cultured human glioma cells, and in the basement membranes of hyperplastic and glomeruloid capillaries of human glioblastoma and glioma xenografts in nude mice (Bourdon et al., 1983). Paired-label experiments with ^{125}I-Mab 81C6 and ^{131}I-control Mab of the same IgG_{2b} type but nonreactive with any known antigen demonstrated high levels of specific localization of Mab 81C6 to GMEM-positive human gliomas in both subcutaneous and intracranial transplant sites in nude mice. Peak levels of localization were obtained within 24–48 h of intravenous administration, and persisted for 5–7 d before declining (Fig. 1); this allowed ready radioimaging throughout this period (Bourdon et al., 1984b). Specific localization was demonstrated, establishing this as a useful model with which to evaluate the pharmacokinetics of Mab localization. As reported by Groothuis et al. (1982) however, nude mouse-borne subcutaneous tumors derived from human glioma cell lines appear to be uniformly permeable to horseradish peroxidase, a measure of capillary permeability; and as Blasberg et al. (1984) demonstrated a variable distribution of Mab 81C6-detected antigen in intracranially transplanted tumors, it is necessary to control for accessability in studies of Mab localization.

The uneven distribution of abnormal blood vessels in gliomas correlates with *in situ* regional variability in vascular permeability in these tumors (Groothuis et al., 1982). Therefore, transport of a blood-borne Mab to brain or brain tumor tissue is directly determined by capillary surface area, permeability, and blood flow, and concentration of the Mab over time. The determination of blood-to-tissue transport and blood flow dy-

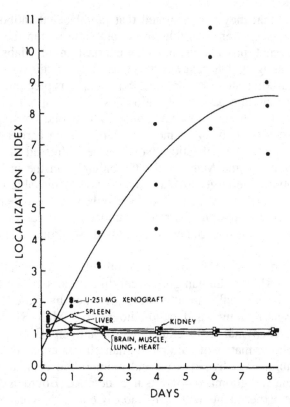

Fig. 1(a).   Paired-label analysis in U-251 MG glioma bearing mice with ^{131}I-Mab 81C6 and ^{125}I-Mab 45.6. Mab 81C6 localization index (LI) was calculated as the tissue specific to nonspecific cpm ratio in the tissue divided by the specific to nonspecific cpm ratio in the blood. The LI values are for 3 animals. The tumor L1 curve is a quadratic least squares regression fit ($p < 0.04$) of LI values.

namics in a series of experimentally induced gliomas in rats have been studied extensively by Blasberg et al. (1981) and Groothuis et al. (1982). Unidirectional blood-to-tissue transport was measured by the "trapping" of alpha-aminoisobutyric acid (AIB), a neutral amino acid with low lipid and high aqueous solubility, in brain or tumor cells following transport across the capillary; the rate of transport was expressed as a transfer constant (TC) dependent on capillary blood flow, permeability, and surface area (Table 3). The TC of AIB in normal brain was 0.001 mL/g/min; as shown in Table 3, the TCs of AIB in various experimentally induced tumors in rat brains ranged from 0.003 in the ENU-induced glioma model, a value only slightly higher than that for normal brain, to 0.075 for the D-54 human glioma cell xenograft model system. This intermodel variability was accompanied by marked intratumor variability in TC (Data reviewed in McComb and Bigner, 1984). As the observed differences in

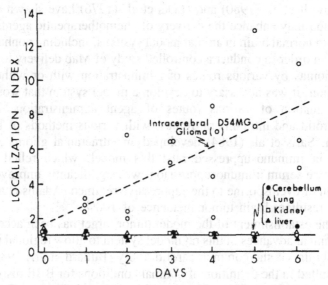

Fig. 1(b). Localization index time course in D-54 MG intracranial xenografts and normal tissues of tumor-bearing mice. Mice were injected with 7.5μCi/5μg ^{125}I-Mab 81C6 and 13μCi/5μg ^{131}I-Mab 45.6. Individual tumor localization index (0) and localization index linear regression curve ($p < 0.01$) (dashed line) are presented. (From Bourdon et al., 1984b).

blood flow between the various tumor model systems were relatively small, these results indicated that capillary permeability, and/or surface area, rather than blood flow, was the primary limiting factor in blood-to-tissue transfer for water-soluble agents such as Mabs.

Relative impermeability or intratumoral variation in permeability can potentially be overcome by reversible osmotic BBB disruption. Work

Table 3
Blood-to-Brain Transport and Blood Flow in Experimental Gliomas[a]

Tissue tumor model	Mean blood flow[b]	Transfer constant of AIB[b]
Normal white matter	0.40	0.001
ASV tumor	0.60	0.030
ENU tumor	0.45	0.003
MSV tumor	0.64	0.012
RG-2	0.84	0.037
RT-9	0.60	0.015
D-54 MG	0.45	0.075
WL-256	0.57	0.009

[a]Data from Groothuis, D., personal communication, 1984.
[b]Mean blood flow and transfer constant expressed as mL/g/min.

by Neuwelt et al. (1980) and Hicks et al. (1976) have shown that such disruption may enhance the delivery of chemotherapeutic agents or antibodies to normal brain in animal model systems, including nonhuman primates. In order to conduct a controlled study of Mab delivery to intracranial gliomas by various routes of administration with or without BBB disruption, it was necessary to develop a model system that would allow the evaluation of various routes of agent administration, including intracarotid and intratumoral routes, with various methods of BBB disruption. Saris et al. (1984) developed an intracranial glioma xenograft model in immunosuppressed rats; this model, which relied on antithymocyte serum immunosuppression, was significantly improved by the addition of cyclosporine to the suppressive regimen (Adams et al., 1984) with a resultant brain tumor incidence of 100%.

The establishment of the model tumor target has been accompanied by technical advances in this rat model system to allow regional perfusion of the brain via the common carotid artery (Bullard et al., 1984a). This has resulted in the definition of optimal conditions for BBB disruption by $1.4M$ mannitol or $1.6M$ arabinose within this model system (Bullard and Bigner, 1984), culminating in the recent demonstration that ^{125}I-Mab 81C6 could be delivered to the normal brain of rats by either intracarotid or intravenous routes of administration. The delivery of Mab to the brain was increased fivefold by previous hyperosmolar perfusion with mannitol or arabinose (Bullard et al., 1984b). The development of this model system has provided the basis for controlled studies of Mab localization in human gliomas in a xenograft model, and has demonstrated that many of the practical BBB-related problems: vascular permeability, Mab-conjugate half-life and transport, and BBB disruption, are ultimately resolvable in the rat, and translatably, in the human. The remaining problem to be addressed is that of target antigen heterogeneity.

3.2. The Problem of Antigenic Heterogeneity

The general phenotypic and genotypic heterogeneity of human neuroectodermal tumor cells, especially glioma cells, has been the subject of several recent reviews and papers (Bigner, 1982; Bigner et al., 1979; Bigner et al., 1981; Shapiro et al., 1981). It would be expected then, that a major reflection of this biological complexity would be antigenic heterogeneity. This is indeed the case, as demonstrated in the chemically induced rat glioma cell line-Mab system reported by Stavrou et al. (1983) and amply illustrated for human tumor antigens by the panel of Mabs described in Table 1. The variety of antigenic specificities expressed by the various target cells and tissues listed is large, and the variation in antigen expression between tumor cell lines or individual tumors is well documented (Bigner et al., 1981; Wikstrand and Bigner, 1982; Wikstrand et al., 1982; Liao et al., 1981; Dippold et al., 1980; Carrel et al., 1982b).

Of greater significance, however, is the repeated observation that heterogeneity in all its forms exists between individual cells in a single neoplasm. Genotypic heterogeneity has been demonstrated both within and among malignant human gliomas and cell lines derived from them (Bigner et al., 1983; Bigner and Mark, in press). Using karyotypes prepared directly or in short term culture these tumors can be divided into three groups: (1) those with only losses of one X or the Y chromosome, (2) near-tetraploid tumors, usually with losses of #22, and (3) near-diploid tumors with gains of #7 and often also losses of #10 (Bigner et al., 1984b, in press). The majority of individual tumors are heterogeneous containing one or more sidelines in addition to the stemline (Mark, 1971; Bigner et al., 1984b). These multiple populations are, however, closely related, usually differing from one another by one or two chromosomes or with one sideline representing an exactly doubled version of the stemline. When near-diploid gliomas are followed as they establish in culture the predominant population shifts continuously among the sidelines with the eventual dominance of a near-tetraploid clone that maintains the same marker types and general distribution seen originally (Bigner et al., 1984a). With further passage there is usually loss of individual chromosomes and often the appearance of new marker types. At this point there may not be a distinct stemline, but rather a cluster of karyotypically related cells, possibly being continually generated by nondisjunction. This type of karyotypic heterogeneity was also demonstrated in established human glioma derived cell line D-54MG and its single cell-derived clones (Wikstrand et al., 1984). The parent line and 2 of 3 karyotyped clones each contained a small number of cells with identical chromosomal composition including 18 distinctive markers. The majority of cells, however, differed from this common karyotype, but usually only by the gain or loss of a few normal or marker chromosomes. This demonstrated genotypic heterogeneity within a single tumor cell population has been shown to be reflected phenotypically—most pertinently, as antigenic heterogeneity. Using a panel of ten anti-HNTA Mabs, the complex antigenic heterogeneity of the glioma cell line D-54 MG and its eight single-cell derived clones was described by Wikstrand et al. (1984). With the exception of two clones, the antigenic profile of each clone was distinct, with the proportion of expressed antigens ranging from 2/10 to 10/10. The observation of relatively antigenically null cells in this study and of differential rates of antigenic loss (Yeh et al., 1981) is complicated also by the issue of cell-cycle or phase-dependent antigen expression (Sieverts et al., 1983), such that the antigenic profile of a single tumor could vary quantitatively and qualitatively from one time point to the next. This suggests, then, that for therapeutic or tumor-localizing studies, a panel of Mabs with demonstrated anti-HNTA activity would be most successful (Yeh et al., 1981); in addition it would be of value to determine if a correlation existed between cell surface markers and sensitivity to various therapeutic regimens (radiation, chemotherapy, targeted immunotherapy) in animal model systems (Wikstrand et al., 1983).

3.3. Current Use of Single Marker–Mab Systems

Despite the argument made above concerning the use of Mab panels, there are instances where the use of a single Mab of defined specificity can be of significant value. The most extensively described examples involve the use of Mabs directed against antigens defined by polyclonal antisera to be of use in neuropathological diagnosis: intermediate filament proteins (primarily NF and GFAP), S-100 protein, and neuron and nonneuronal specific enolases. The consensus of opinion of investigators in the area (Bonin and Rubenstein, 1984; Trojanowski and Lee, 1983a; and Hickey et al., 1983) is that Mabs to these specificities are not primarily of value in differential diagnosis of central and peripheral nervous system tumors, which can be performed primarily on morphological grounds, but rather as markers of the degree of differentiation or histogenesis of a given tumor.

Perhaps the most specific marker within this category is GFAP, which is currently used as a routine antigenic marker for normal, developing, and mature astroglial cells, and for pathologically altered astrocytes and ependymal cells in the central nervous system (CNS) (Bonin and Rubenstein, 1984). Until the recent production of GFAP-specific Mabs (Eng et al., 1983; Pegram et al., 1984), the most frequent complication of anti-GFAP polyclonal antibody use was the demonstration of true GFAP specificity, versus reactivity for cross-reactive specificities shared by the family of intermediate filament proteins (Gown and Vogel, 1982). Even given the existence of exquisitely specific anti-GFAP Mabs, however, as summarized by Bonin and Rubenstein (1984), several difficulties still remain regarding the use of anti-GFAP Mabs for the diagnosis of neurosurgical tumor biopsies, namely: the distinction between reactive and neoplastic astrocytes; false negatives resulting from delayed or improper fixation resulting in the disappearance or leaching of soluble GFAP; and the lack of total correlation between GFAP positivity and the demonstration of neuroglial fibrils.

Trojanowski and Lee (1983b) have reported the successful application of specific anti-NF Mabs to the division of tumors classically defined as of neuronal origin (pheochromocytomas, ganglioneuromas, ganglioneuroblastomas, and neuroblastomas) versus those of nonneuronal origin (astrocytic series, ependymomas, oligodendrogliomas, meningiomas, Schwannomas). The authors felt that the primary significance of the use of NF-specific Mabs was not as a histogenetic marker, but as an index of differentiation; this study demonstrated that a higher percentage of the more differentiated, benign samples (80% of the pheochromocytoma, ganglioneuroma, ganglioneuroblastoma group) contained NF-positive cells than did the less differentiated, malignant tumors (12.5% of the neuroblastoma, medulloblastoma group).

Despite the recent production of S-100 protein specific Mabs (Golden et al., 1984), S-100 protein is not considered a promising or reliable marker for diagnosis (Trojanowski and Lee, 1983a; Bonin and Rubenstein, 1984; Nakamura et al., 1982). Although polyclonal sera against S-100 have been used to differentiate Schwannomas from other extraaxial malignant spindle cell tumors, the wide distribution of this protein in cells not only of nervous system origin (Langerhans cells of the skin, interdigitating reticular cells of the lymph node, mesodermal chondrocytes) and the controversy surrounding its association with oligodendrocytes and sympathetic ganglia (Trojanowski and Lee, 1983a, Golden and Gillespie, 1984, Bonin and Rubenstein, 1984) compromise its utility.

As reviewed by Bonin and Rubenstein (1984), the initial hopes for the use of neuron-specific enolase (NSE), initially known as 14-3-2 protein, have not been maintained following the demonstration of the relatively widespread distribution of this enzyme (neuroblastomas, melanomas, APUD tumors, islet-cell tumors of the pancreas, medullary thyroid carcinomas, carcinoid tumors of diverse origins, lymphomas, and granular cell tumors). For these reasons, Bonin and Rubenstein (1984) felt that although anti-NSE Mab might identify normal neuronal and neuroendocrine cells and differentiate peripheral tumors of the APUD system, their usefulness in regard to central nervous system tumor diagnosis or localization is questionable.

There have been several demonstrations of the localization of single radiolabeled anti-HNTA Mabs to tumors of neuroectodermal origin, beginning with the localization of anti-melanoma (Ghose et al., 1982; Stuhlmiller et al., 1981) and anti-glioma Mabs (Bourdon et al., 1984b) in xenografts in nude mice. The ability to demonstrate significant, specific localization in tumor-bearing mice and the lack of toxicity of the radiolabeled Mabs in rabbits led Larson et al. (1983a and b) to attempt imaging in melanoma patients using ^{131}I-labeled Mab 8.2, specific for the melanoma-associated p97 antigen. Results were encouraging in that all patients had positive scans, with successful imaging of 88% of lesions larger than 1.5 cm. Although 3/6 patients did develop anti-mouse immunoglobulin antibodies, this did not have clinical sequelae, but resulted in more rapid clearance of injected labeled Mab, and a concomitant reduction in tumor uptake. Similar results were reported by Ferrone et al. (1983), using an Mab directed against a high molecular weight (>600,000) glycopeptide of melanomas. These investigators reported an apparent, but not established, superiority of Fab_2 fragments in these localization studies. Recently, successful imaging of Mabs to intracranial tumors in human patients has been reported. Farrands et al. (1982) successfully imaged a colorectal carcinoma metastasis to the brain with an ^{131}I-labeled Mab and image background subtraction. Phillips et al. (1983), using a putative anti-autologous glioma human Mab (Table 1, Sikora et al., 1982), were able to image a recurrent glioma. Specific localization was not demonstrated, nor was it shown that anything other than the "brain scanning" effect of normal immunoglobulin imaging was obtained. Nevertheless, no toxicity or complications occurred following administration of the radio-iodinated mouse or human immunoglobulin.

The logical progression is from imaging to targeted immunotherapy; initial animal model studies have been encouraging in that the human Mab OFA-1-2, when administered simultaneously with xenongeneic OFA-1-2+ melanoma cells, resulted in a significant prolongation of tumor-free interval (Katano et al., 1983). However, the only conditions under which the therapy was successful involved simultaneous administration of Mab and tumor. It appears that at the present time the most efficacious use of Mabs as cytotoxic or cytostatic agents might be in the context reported by Ritz et al. (1982), who used in vitro treatment with the anti-CALLA Mab J5 and complement to remove CALLA + cells from the bone marrow of leukemia patients prior to autologous marrow transplantation. This approach has been initiated for neuroblastoma patients; Byrd et al. (1982) have demonstrated the Mab-mediated detection of neuroblastoma cells in the bone marrow of neuroblastoma patients with radioscintigraphy, and Seeger et al. (1984) have reported in vitro toxicity of conjugates of Ricin A chain and Mab 390 for Thy-1 positive neuroblastoma cells.

3.4. The Use of Mab Panels

As introduced above, the problem of antigenic heterogeneity almost forces the use of multiple, differentially reactive Mabs in an attempt to completely "cover" all cells in a single neoplasm whether it be for descriptive, diagnostic, localizing, or therapeutic purposes. As mentioned above and discussed in detail by Osborn and Weber (1983), the use of panels of anti-intermediate filament Mabs for differential diagnosis, especially for neuroectodermal tumors and metastases to the CNS, is useful for determination of histogenesis (Ramaekers et al., 1982). Mabs of less defined specificity, however, are also useful in differential diagnosis panels; Kemshead et al. (1983) recently reported the use of a 12-member Mab panel to differentiate between the small-round-cell tumors of childhood. His group successfully used this panel to diagnose a CALLA + leukemia and a Thy-1 + neuroblastoma from bone marrow aspirates. Similarly, human cerebral tumors are difficult to differentiate between and from certain cerebral metastases. One Mab panel has been proposed for such differential diagnosis (Grahmann et al., 1983); one could as easily construct one from the Mabs listed in Table 1. Such a panel is presented in Table 4. Although the individual components might vary from panel to panel, the goal—to establish differential diagnosis—is essentially achievable with the Mab reagents produced to date.

Combinations of Mabs may also be used productively in cocktail form to achieve potential complete kill of heterogeneous tumor cell population. The successful use of this approach has been reported by LeBien et al. (1983) who showed that a cocktail of 3 Mabs + complement could be successfully used for the *ex vivo* elimination of residual leukemic cells in bone marrow to be used for autologous transplantation. Leukemic cells could be effectively lysed in the presence of a 100-fold excess of normal marrow cells in one-step, single assays that did not unduly stress bystander antigen negative cells, thus providing optimal conditions for marrow treatment. As clearance of neuroblastoma cells from a ninefold excess of normal marrow cells in a model system using anti-Thy-1 Mab 390 and anti-mouse immunoglobulin-coated polystyrene beads is already possible (Seeger et al., 1984), it is probable that a Mab cocktail approach would be equally as effective in this context.

4. Summary and Prospects

The advent of monoclonal antibody technology has, in the past 5 yr, revolutionized the approach to cancer biology. The fields of central and peripheral nervous system tumor immunology are, relatively speaking, still in their infancy as compared to leukemia research primarily because of the lack of established markers and in vitro methodology, and secondarily, to the much smaller number of laboratories devoted to this research. Given these factors, however, the progress over the past 5 yr has been impressive, and the directions and distance this research will take over the next 5 yr will be even more so.

The continual accrual of Mabs of murine and human origin is necessary to provide the ever more specific battery of reagents required for increased resolution in descriptive, localizing, and therapeutic regimens. The biochemical purification of relevant markers feeds back into this system by providing enriched substrates for immunization and assay standardization. As we have established that panels of Mabs are the most productive approach to all these applications, the constant isolation of new specificities is mandatory.

Localization and imaging studies with radiodlabeled anti-HNTA are well-underway, and significant localization in the absence of significant toxicity has been reported. The problems of antibody delivery, even for intracranial tumors, are being systematically studied (Bourdon et al., 1984b), so that the use of Mabs as carriers of radionuclides, drugs, or

Table 4
Proposed Monoclonal Antibody Panel for Differentiation of CNS Tumors[a]

Tissues reacting	Anti-intermediate filament Mabs			Anti-neuroectodermal Mabs				Anti-lymphoid cell Mabs	
	Anti-GFAP	Anti-NF	Anti-cytokeratin	GE2	PI 1153	1H8	2F3	Anti-Thy-1	Anti-common leucocyte antigen
Adult brain	+	+	-	-	+	-	-	+	-
Fetal brain	±	±	-	-	+	+	-	+	-
Glioma	±	-	-	+	+	+	+	+	-
Medulloblastoma	+	±	-	-	-	+	?	+	-
Ependymoma	-	-	-	-	-	?	-	?	-
Sympathetic-derived neuronal tumors	-	+	-	+	+	-	-	+	-
Choroid plexus papilloma	-	-	+	-	-	?	?	?	-
Meningioma	-	-	-	+	-	-	-	+	-
Metastic carcinoma	-	-	+	-	-	-	-	-	-
Cerebral lymphoma	-	-	-	-	±	-	-	-	+

[a]As in the panel used by Kemshead et al. (1983), multiple Mabs should be used for each category, as for example, not *all* gliomas may react with Mab 2F3, and so on. Reactions listed are not absolute; ? designates those Mab-tissue combinations where insufficient data is available to predict reactivity. Mabs listed are meant only as possible examples and are currently being used in a panel.

plant and bacterial toxins will soon be possible. This includes the potential use of a specifically localized [10]B-labeled Mab in situ followed by slow neutron activation of [10]B for extremely restricted local ionizing radiation (Bourdon et al., 1984a). In addition, recent results in animal model systems have shown that Mabs of the IgG_{2a} class have an increased cytolytic efficiency in antibody-dependent cell-mediated cytotoxic assays (Matthews et al., 1981; Langlois et al., 1981), thus suggesting possible approaches for specific, systemic passive immunotherapy.

References

Adams, C., D. Bullard, M. Clemons, S. H. Bigner, and D. D. Bigner (1984), (abstract) submitted.

Bigner, D. D. (1982), *Neurosurgery* **9**, 320.

Bigner, D. D., S. H. Bigner, J. Ponten, B. Westermark, M. S. Mahaley, E. Ruoslahti, H. Herschman, L. F. Eng, and C. J. Wikstrand (1981), *J. Neuropath. Exp. Neurol.* **40**, 201.

Bigner, D. D., D. Bullard, S. C. Schold, S. H. Preissig, and C. J. Wikstrand (1979), in *Multidisciplinary Aspects of Brain Tumor Therapy* (Paoletti P., M. D. Walker, G. Butti, and R. Knerich, eds.) Elsevier/North Holland Biomedical Press, pp. 329–333.

Bigner, S. H., and J. Mark (1984), *Brain Tumor Biology,* in press.

Bigner, S. H., J. Mark, and D. D. Bigner (1983), *Cancer Genet. Cytogenet.* **10**, 335.

Bigner, S. H., J. Mark, and D. D. Bigner (1984a), *Proc. A.A.C.R.*, in press.

Bigner, S. H., J. Mark, M. S. Mahaley, and D. D. Bigner (1984b), *Hereditas,* in press.

Blasberg, R. G., D. Groothuis, and P. Molnar (1981), *Sem. Neurol.* **1**, 203.

Blasberg, R. G., H. Nakagawa, M. A. Bourdon, D. Groothuis, C. S. Patlak, and D. D. Bigner (1984), submitted.

Bluestein, H. G., and N. J. Zvaifler (1976), *J. Clin. Invest.* **57**, 509.

Bonin, J. M., and L. J. Rubenstein (1984), *J. Neurosurg.*, in press.

Bourdon, M. A., R. E. Coleman, and D. D. Bigner (1984a), in *Progress in Experimental Brain Tumor Research,* Volume II (Rosenblum, M. and C. Wilson, eds.) Karger Basel.

Bourdon, M. A., R. E. Coleman, R. G. Blasberg, D. R. Groothuis, and D. D. Bigner (1984b), submitted.

Bourdon, M. A., C. J. Wikstrand, H. Furthmayr, T. J. Matthews, and D. D. Bigner (1983), *Cancer Res.* **43**, 2796.

Braun, M. P., P. J. Martin, J. A. Ledbetter, and J. A. Hansen (1983), *Blood* **62**, 718–725.

Brown, J., K. Nishiyama, I. Hellström, and K. E. Hellström (1981), *J. Immunol.* **127**, 539.

Bullard, D. E., and D. D. Bigner (1984), *J. Neurosurg.*, in press.

Bullard, D. E., M. A. Bourdon, and D. D. Bigner (1984a), submitted.

Bullard, D. E., S. C. Saris, and D. D. Bigner (1984b), *Neurosurg.*, in press.

Byrd, R. L., Z. L. Jonak, and R. H. Kennett (1982), *Prog. Cancer Res. Therapy* **21**, 219.

Cahan, L. D., R. F. Irie, R. Singh, A. Cassidenti, and J. C. Paulson (1982), *Proc. Natl. Acad. Sci. USA* **79**, 7629.

Cairncross, J. G., M. J. Mattes, H. R. Beresford, A. D. Albino, A. N. Houghton, K. O. Lloyd, and L. J. Old (1982), *Proc. Natl. Acad. Sci. USA* **79**, 5641.

Carrel, S., N. DeTribolet, and N. Gross (1982a), *Eur. J. Immunol.* **12**, 354.

Carrel S., N. DeTribolet, and J. P. Mach (1982b), *Acta Neuropathol.* **57**, 158.

Carrel, S., A. Schmidt-Kessen, J.-P. Mach, D. Heumann, and C. Girardet (1983), *J. Immunol.* **130**, 2456.

Dales, S., R. S. Fujinami, and M. B. A. Oldstone (1983), *J. Immunol.* **131**, 1332.

Day, E. D., M. S. Mahaley, B. Woodhall, and F. Pireher (1964), *J. Nucl. Med.* **5**, 357.

De Tribolet, N. (1982), *Bull. Schweiz. Akad. Med. Wiss.* **8**, 113.

De Tribolet, N., and D. D. Bigner (1982), *J. Neuroimmunol.* **3**, 237.

Dippold, W. G., K. O. Lloyd, L. T. C. Li, H. Ikeda, H. F. Oettgen, and L. J. Old (1980), *Proc. Natl. Acad. Sci. USA* **77**, 6114.

Eisenbarth, G. S., F. S. Walsh, and M. Nirenberg (1979), *Proc. Natl. Acad. Sci.* **76**, 4913.

Eng, L. F., C. N. Pegram, Y.-L. Lee, J. F. Glickman, and D. D. Bigner (1983), *Trans. Amer. Soc. Neurochem* **14**, 168.

Eng, L. F., J. J. Vanderhaeghen, A. Bignami, and B. Gerstl (1971), *Brain Res.* **28**, 351.

Farrands, P. A., M. V. Pimm, A. C. Perkins, J. D. Hardy, R. W. Baldwin, and J. D. Hardcartle (1982), *Lancet* **2**, 397.

Ferrone, S., P. Giacomini, P. G. Natali, G. Buraggi, L. Callegaro, and U. Rosa (1983), First Int. Symp. Neutron Capture Therapy, M.I.T., October, 1983.

Franko, M. C., C. L. Masters, C. I. Gibbs, and D. C. Gajdersek (1981), *J. Neuroimmunol.* **1**, 391.

Ghose, T., S. Ferrone, K. Imai, S. T. Norwell, S. J. Luner, R. H. Martin, and A. H. Blair (1982), *JNCI* **69**, 823.

Golden, P. S. and G. Y. Gillespie (1984), submitted.

Golden, P. S., G. Y. Gillespie, and J. M. Bynum (1984), submitted.

Gown, A. M., and A. M. Vogel (1982), *J. Cell Biol.* **95**, 414.

Grahmann, F. C., C. J. Wikstrand, and D. D. Bigner (1984), in *Neuroimmunology* (Behan, P., and Spreafico, F., eds.), Raven Press, New York, pp. 311–323.

Groothuis, D. R., J. M. Fischer, G. Lapin, D. D. Bigner, and N. A. Vick (1982), *J. Neuropath. Exp. Neurol.* **41**, 164.

Hawkes, R., E. Niday, and A. Matus (1982), *Proc. Natl. Acad. Sci.*, **79**, 2410.

Hellström, I., H. J. Garrigues, L. Cabasco, G. H. Mosely, J. P. Brown, and K. E. Hellström (1983), *J. Immunol.* **130**, 1467.

Helson, L., C. Helson, and C. Weinberger (1983), *Proc. Amer. Assn. Cancer Res.* **24**, 130.

Herlyn M., W. H. Clark, M. J. Mastrangelo, D. Guerry, D. E. Elder, D. LaRossa, R. Hamilton, E. Bondi, R. Tuthill, Z. Steplewski, and H. Koprowski (1980), *Cancer Res.* **40**, 3602.

Hickey, W. F., V. Lee, J. Q. Trojanowski, L. J. McMillan, T. J. McKearn, J. Gonatas, and M. K. Gonatas (1983), *J. Histochem. and Cytochem.* **34**, 1126.

Hicks, J. T., P. Albrecht, and S. I. Rapoport (1976), *J. Exp. Neurol.* **53**, 768.

Hirn, M., M. Pierres, H. Beagostini-Bazin, M. R. Hirsch, C. Goridis, M. S. Ghandour, O. K. Langley, and G. Gombos (1982), *Neuroscience* **7(1)**, 239.

Houghton, A. N., M. Eisinger, A. P. Albino, J. G. Cairncross, and L. J. Old (1982), *J. Exp. Med.* **156**, 1755.

Howe, A. J., R. C. Seeger, G. A. Molinaro, and S. Ferrone (1981), *J.N.C.I.* **66**, 827.

Irie, R. F., A. E. Giuliano, and D. L. Morton (1979), *J. Nat. Cancer Inst.* **63**, 367.

Katano, M., K. Irie, and R. F. Irie (1983), *Proc. Amer. Assn. Cancer Res.* **24**, 226.

Kemshead J. T., A. Goldman, J. Fritschy, J. S. Malpas, and J. Pritchard (1983), *Lancet* **1**, 12.

Kennett, R. H., and F. Gilbert (1979), *Science* **203**, 1120.

Kennett, R. H., Z. Jonak., and K. B. Bechtol (1980), in *Advances in Neuroblastoma Research.* (Evans, A. E., ed.), Raven Press, New York, pp. 209–217.

Lagenaur, C., I. Sommer, and M. Schachner (1980), *Der. Bio.* **79**, 367.

Lampson, L. A., C. A. Fisher, and J. P. Whelan (1983), *J. Immunol.* **130**, 2471.

Lampson, L. A., and R. Levy (1980), *J. Immunol.* **125**, 203.

Langlois, A. J., T. J. Matthews, G. G. Roloson, H. J. Thiel, J. J. Collins, and D. P. Bolognesi (1981), *J. Immunol.* **126**, 2337.

Larson, S. M., J. P. Brown., P. W. Wright, J. A. Carrasquillo, I. Hellström, and K. E. Hellström (1983a), *J. Amer. Med. Assn.* **249**, 811.

Larson, S. M., J. P. Brown, P. W. Wright, J. A. Carrasquillo, I. Hellström, and K. E. Hellström (1983b), *J. Nucl. Med.* **24**, 123.

LeBien, T. W., D. E. Stepan, and J. H. Kersey (1983), *Proc. Amer. Assn. Cancer Res.* **24**, 219.

Lee, V. M.-Y., C. D. Page, H.-L. Wu, and W. W. Schlaepfer (1984), *J. of Neurochemistry* **42**, 25.

Liao, S., B. J. Clarke, P. C., Kwong, A. Brickenden, B. L. Gallie, and P. B. Dent (1981), *Eur. J. Immunol.* **11**, 450.

Mahaley, M. S., J. L. Mahaley, and E. D. Day (1965), *Cancer Res.* **25**, 779.

Mark, J. (1971), *Hereditas* **68**, 61.

Marrack, D., M. Kubala, P. Corey, M. Leavens, J. Howze, W. Dewey, W. F. Bode, and I. L. Spar (1967), *Cancer* **20**, 751.

Matthews, T. J., J. J. Collins, G. G. Roloson, H. J. Thiel, and D. P. Bolognesi (1981), *J. Immunol.* **126**, 2332.

McCardle, R. J., P. V. Harper, I. L. Spar, W. F. Bale, G. Andros, and F. Jimenez (1966), *J. Nucl. Med.* **7**, 837.

McComb, R. D., and D. D. Bigner (1984), in *The Management of Central Nervous System Tumors.* (van der Schueren, E., ed.), Edward Arnold, in press.

McKay, R., M. C. Raff, and L. F. Reichardt (eds.) (1981), *Cold Spring Harbor Reports Neurosci.* **2**, 1.

Metzgar, R. S., M. J. Borowitz, N. H. Jones, and B. L. Dowell (1981), *J. Exp. Med.* **157**, 1249.

Mitchell, K. F., J. P. Fuhrer, Z. Steplewski, and H. Koprowski (1980), *Proc. Natl. Acad. Sci.* **77**, 7287.

Nakamura, Y., L. E. Becker, and A. Marks (1982), *Proc. Ninth Int. Cong. Neuropathol.*, p. 172 (abstract).

Natali, P., C. DeMartino, V. Quaranta, M. Nicotra, F. Freeza, M. Pellegrino, and S. Ferrone (1981), *Transplantation* **31(1)**, 75.

Neuwelt, E. A., E. P. Frenkel, and J. T. Hiehl (1980), *Trans. Am. Neurol. Assoc.* **104**, 1.

Ng, A.-K., M. Pellegrino, K. Imai, and S. Ferrone (1981), *J. Imm.* **127**, 443.

Nudelman, E., s. Hakomori, R. Kannagi, S. Levery, M.-Y. Yeh, K. E. Hellström, and I. Hellström (1982), *J. of Biol. Chem.* **257/21**, 12752.

Oger, J., S. Szuchet, J. Antel, and B. G. W. Arnason (1982), *Nature* **295**, 66.

Osborn, M., and K. Weber (1983), *Laboratory Investigation* **48**, 372.

Pegram, C. N., L. F. Eng, and D. D. Bigner (1984), submitted.

Pellegrino, M. A., J. F. Weaver, W. A. Nelson-Rees, and S. Ferrone (1981), *Transplant Proc.* **13**, 1935.

Peng, W. W., J. P. Bressler, E. Tiffany-Castiglioni, and J. De Vellis (1982), *Sci.* **215**, 1102.

Phillips, J., T. Alderson, K. Sikora, and J. Watson (1983), *J. Neurol. Neurosurg. Psych.* **46**, 388.

Pukel, C. S., K. O. Lloyd, L. R. Travassos, W. G. Dippold, H. F. Oettgen, and L. J. Old (1982), *J. Exp. Med.* **155**, 1133.

Ramaekers, F. C. S., J. J. G. Puts, A. Kant, O. Moesker, P. H. K. Jap, and G. P. Vooijs (1982), *Cell Biology International Reports* **6**, 652.

Ranscht, B., P. A. Clapshaw, J. Price, M. Noble, and W. Seifert (1982), *Proc. Natl. Acad. Sci.* **79**, 2709.

Reif, A. E., and J. M. Allen (1964), *J. Exp. Med.* **120**, 413.

Revoltella, R. P., R. Businaro, G. Lauro, and A. Tolsea (1982), *Cell. Immun.* **68**, 75.

Ritz, J., R. C. Bast, L. A. Clavell, T. Herrend, S. E. Sallan, J. M. Lipton, M. Fenney, D. G. Nathan, and S. F. Schosslman (1982), *Lancet* **II**, 60.

Saris, S. C., s. H. Bigner, and D. D. Bigner (1984), *J. Neurosurg.*, in press.

Saxton, R. E., B. Torbett, B. Nestor, M. Fairhurst, A. J. Cochran, F. R. Eilber, and M. W. Bunk (1983), *Proc. Amer. Assn. Cancer Res.* **24**, 894.

Schnegg, J. F., A. C. Diserens, S. Carrel, R. S. Accolla, and N. de Tribolet (1981), *Cancer Res.* **41**, 1209.

Seeger, R. C., Ugelstad, J., and G. P. Reynolds (1984), in *Advances in Neuroblastoma Research.* (Evans, A. E., Seeger, R. C., and G. D'Angio, eds.), Adam Liss, in press.

Seeger, R. C., Y. L. Danon, S. A. Bayner, and F. Hoover (1982a), *J. Immunol.* **128**, 983.

Seeger, R. C., H. M. Rosenblatt, K. Imai, and S. Ferrone (1981), *Cancer Res.* **41**, 2714.

Seeger, R. C., S. E. Siegel, and N. Sidell (1982b), *Ann. Int. Med.* **97**, 873.

Shapiro, J. R., W. A. Young, and W. R. Shapiro (1981), *Cancer Res*. **41,** 2349.
Sieverts, H., O. Alabaster, C. Janus, and R. G. Parsons (1983), *Proc. Amer. Assn. Cancer Res*. **24,** 207.
Sikora, K., T. Alderson, J. Phillips, and J. Watson (1982), *The Lancet,* vol. I, 1–14.
Stavrou, D., C. Süss, T. Bilzer, U. Kummer, and N. de Tribolet (1983), *Eur. J. Cancer Clin. Oncol*. **19,** 1439.
Stuhlmiller, G. M., D. C. Sullivan, C. E. Vervaert, B. P. Croker, C. C. Harris and H. F. Seigler (1981), *Ann. Surg*. **194,** 592.
Tai, T., M. Eisinger, S. Ogata, and K. O. Lloyd (1983), *Cancer Research* **43,** 2773.
Trojanowski, J. Q., and V. M.-Y. Lee (1983a), *Human Path*. **14,** 281.
Trojanowski, J. Q., and V. M.-Y. Lee (1983b), *Acta Neuropathol*. **59,** 155.
Wikstrand, C. J., and D. D. Bigner (1980), *Am. J. Pathol*. **98,** 515.
Wikstrand, C. J., and D. D. Bigner (1982), *Cancer Res*. **42,** 267.
Wikstrand, C. J., S. H. Bigner, and D. D. Bigner (1983), *Cancer Res*. **43,** 3327.
Wikstrand, C. J., S. H. Bigner, and D. D. Bigner (1984), *J. Neuroimmunol*. (in press).
Wikstrand, C. J., M. A. Bourdon, C. N. Pegram, and D. D. Bigner (1982), *J. Neuroimmunol*. **3,** 43.
Yeh, M.-Y., I. Hellström, and K. E. Hellström (1981), *J. Immunol*. **126,** 1312.

Chapter 17

Human Monoclonal Antibodies

Humoral Immune Response in Patients with Cancer

ALAN N. HOUGHTON AND RICHARD J. COTE

Memorial Sloan-Kettering Cancer Center, New York, New York

1. Introduction

The monoclonal antibody technology has had a major impact on the serological and biochemical analysis of human tumor antigens. Monoclonal antibodies have rapidly led to the identification and characterization of a large number of antigenic determinants on cancer cells. To date, most of these monoclonal antibodies have been of mouse or rat origin. Antigens recognized by these reagents have therefore been defined generally by their immunogenicity in the mouse or rat, and they do not necessarily correspond to antigens that are immunogenic in humans.

There has been a need to extend this technology to the production of human monoclonal antibody. Questions about the humoral immune response and B cell repertoire in diseases such as cancer or autoimmune states can be directly addressed by studies with human monoclonal antibody. Human monoclonal antibodies have two potential applications in the study of human cancer beyond that offered by mouse or rat monoclonal antibody: (1) to define the humoral immune response of patients with cancer, (2) to provide diagnostic and therapeutic agents for adminstration to patients with cancer, under the presumption that human monoclonal antibodies are less immunogenic in humans than heterologous antibody.

399

1.1. Serological Evidence of Tumor Immunity in Humans

An underlying assumption of tumor immunology has been that cancer cells can be distinguished from normal cells by the presence of distinctive antigens on their cell surface, and that these antigens can serve as targets for recognition and rejection by the immune system (Old, 1981). To address this question, serological techniques have been primarily used as a way to study the host's ability to recognize antigens on the surface of cancer cells. Serological methods are most advanced in terms of sensitivity and precision, and have yielded most of our present knowledge about human cancer antigens. It must be kept in mind, however, that certain antigens may not elicit a humoral immune response but rather recognition may be in the realm of cellular immunity. Given this caveat, techniques to produce human monoclonal antibodies can be applied to extend studies of the humoral immune response of cancer patients.

The evidence supporting the view that hosts can immunologically respond to their tumor comes from transplantation experiments in mice and rats with tumors induced by chemical carcinogens or viruses. In these experiments, immunization with a given chemically induced tumor or tumor induced by an oncogenic virus such as polyoma was able to elicit transplantation resistance resulting in rejections of tumor (Foley, 1953; Prehn and Main, 1957; Sjogren et al., 1961; Habel, 1961). A feature of chemically induced tumors was the expression of individually distinct antigens that elicited transplantation resistance to that tumor, but not to other tumors. In these experimental systems, progress has been made towards the serological characterization of these antigens (DeLeo et al., 1977, 1979). Despite the experimental evidence for immunogenic tumor-specific antigens, there remains a dearth of critical evidence for tumor-specific antigens in human cancers. Most of our present information of cell surface antigens of human cells is derived from analyses using heterologous antibodies or allogeneic sera and lymphoid cells. To date, most restricted tumor cell surface antigens have turned out, on futher analysis, to belong to the category of differentiation antigens—antigens characteristically expressed on normal cells at some phase of differentiation (Boyse and Old, 1969; Houghton et al., 1982). Interpretation of studies using sera or lymphocytes from one individual and tumor cells from another have been complicated by the frequent participation of alloantigens (e.g., blood group or major histocompatibility complex antigens) in the observed reactions.

The most direct approach to the question of whether patients with cancer recognize tumor-specific antigens has been the serological approach referred to as autologous typing. This serological method involves testing sera from cancer patients against cultured tumor cells and normal cells from the same individual. Absorption analysis is then used as a sensitive method to determine the absence or presence of antigen on a panel of cells from a variety of sources, including autologous normal cells, as well as allogeneic and xenogeneic normal and malignant cells. This study has led to the definition of three classes of surface antigens recognized by antibodies in cancer patient: Class 1, unique antigens restricted to autologous tumor cells; Class 2, shared antigens present on autologous and some allogeneic tumor cells; and Class 3, widely distributed normal cell surface antigens or components acquired from the heterologous serum used in cell culture. Using autologous typing, antibodies to Class 1 and/or Class 2 antigens have been found in patients with malignant melanoma (Carey et al., 1976; Shiku et al., 1976; Albino et al., 1981; Real et al., 1983), astrocytoma (Pfreundschuh et al., 1978), renal cancer (Ueda et al., 1979) and acute leukemia (Garrett et al., 1977). These serological studies suggest that some tumor cell surface molecules can be immunologically recognized by humans, and Class 1 antigens remain the best candidates for tumor-specific antigens. However, further studies of the biochemical nature of these molecules and the genetic loci coding for these antigens have been difficult, hindered in part by the necessity of using low titer human sera that contain many unrelated antibodies.

1.2. Clinical Evidence of Tumor Immunity in Humans

Several clinical observations suggest that immunological factors affect the course of human cancer, including well-documented cases of spontaneous complete regression (Everson and Cole, 1966) and the frequent waxing and waning of tumor lesions without treatment. Too much emphasis cannot be placed on these observations since clearly non-immunological factors can influence the growth and spread of tumors. A second line of evidence comes from the excessive incidence of several types of cancer in patients who are immunosuppressed, including lymphoid neoplasms (Penn, 1970) and malignant melanoma (Fraumeni and Hoover, 1975).

The observation that primary tumors are often infiltrated or surrounded by lymphocytes has raised analogies to the historical appearance of rejection of transplanted allogeneic tissues. This lymphocyte response could provide a clue to the host-immune response, but lymphocytes found in the region of tumors have generally been inaccessible for study. The first positive correlation between lymphocytic infiltration and prognosis was made by Moore and Foote in 1949 in their study on the favorable prognosis of medullary carcinoma of the breast. Even prior to this study, Russel (1908), Murphy (1931), and Ewing (1940) had indicated that the lymphocytic infiltrates seen in association with some tumors may represent an immune response by the host directed against the tumor.

Since Moore and Foote's original paper, there have been many studies concerned with the significance of lymphocytic infiltration in tumors. Most of these have concentrated on the relationship of tumor filtrates to prognosis and on prognostic significance of lymphocytic responses in lymph nodes in the region of the tumor. The results of these studies have been inconsistent and for most tumor types it is unclear whether or not changes in lymphocytic or histiocytic populations can be related to prognosis. Malignant melanoma exemplifies this confusion, with several contradictory studies concerning the relationship of lymphocytic infiltration to prognosis (Thompson, 1973; McLean et al., 1979; Larson and Grude, 1978). Recently, however, there is evidence that for certain stages of the disease, lymphocytic infiltration does indeed correlate with an improved prognosis (Day et al., 1981). There are a few other tumor types for which this correlation also exists, among them medullary carcinoma of the breast.

1.3. In Vivo Applications of Human Monoclonal Antibodies

Results of initial clinical trials with mouse monoclonal antibodies have suggested that toxicity resulting from hypersensitivity to heterologous protein is not an overwhelming problem (Ritz et al., 1981; Miller et al., 1983; Sears et al., 1982). A more insidious side-effect of passive administration of mouse antibody may be the elicitation of antibodies to mouse immunoglobulins (Miller et al., 1983; Sears et al., 1982). It is clear that many, if not the majority, of patients receiving systemically administered mouse antibody develop antibodies to mouse immunoglobulins. An anti-mouse Ig response could produce rapid clearance of monoclonal antibody from the circulation and could inhibit antibody–antigen interactions or effector functions of the antibody molecules (e.g., complement fixation or mediation of antibody-dependent cellular cytotoxicity). Since an anti-mouse Ig response may prevent effective binding of the monoclonal antibody to target tumor cells, this feature could ultimately limit therapeutic applications of heterologous monoclonal antibodies. This limitation of mouse monoclonal antibodies is a strong incentive to develop human monoclonal antibodies for eventual in vivo therapeutic or diagnostic applications. Despite the prediction that human monoclonal antibodies would be less immunogenic in humans, it is likely that some human antibodies would elicit a response to allotypic determinants or to the antibody idiotype [i.e., antigenic determinant on the antibody variable region (Kunkel et al., 1963)]. An anti-idiotype response has been reported in patients receiving mouse monoclonal antibodies for treatment of T-cell lymphoma (Miller et al., 1983). The outcome of an anti-idiotype response is uncertain. Anti-idiotype antibodies may bind to antibody combining sites, interfering directly with antibody–antigen interaction. As proposed by Jerne (1974), idiotype–anti-idiotype reactions could also regulate specific immune responses. In experimental systems anti-idiotype antibodies have been shown to induce a specific immune response in mice exposed to trypanosomes (Sacks et al., 1982) or hepatitis

B surface antigen (Kennedy and Breesman, 1984). Depending on dose and schedule of injection, anti-idiotype antibodies can either suppress or augment an immune response to the antigenic determinant recognized by the idiotype (Rajewsky and Takemori, 1983). Thus, the consequence of an anti-idiotype response to human monoclonal antibody could be positive or negative: anti-idiotypes could inhibit antibody binding to antigen, or alternatively, anti-idiotype responses could play a role in initiating and establishing an active immune response (Koprowski et al., 1984), although such an effect is still speculative.

2. Approaches to the Generation of Human Monoclonal Antibodies

The production of human monoclonal antibodies has relied on two basic approaches: the immortalization of B lymphocytes by infection with Epstein-Barr virus (EBV) and the fusion of B lymphocytes to established myeloma or lymphoblastoid cell lines using the hybridoma technology. Advances in the field of B cell growth and differentiation may eventually offer a third approach, but so far it has been difficult to manipulate B cell proliferation and differentiation in vitro to the degree necessary to produce sufficient quantity of human antibodies. No single technique has clearly established itself as the optimal method to generate human monoclonal antibodies. Each method has advantages and disadvantages. For this reason, a combination of approaches is being explored, with the hope that the strengths of one method will overcome the weakness of another method. In addition to the discussion below, the reader is referred to more detailed reviews of results using the different methods to produce human monoclonal antibodies (Cote et al., 1984; Kozbor and Roder, 1983).

2.1. Immortalization of B Lymphocytes by Epstein-Barr Virus

One of the earliest approaches to the production of human monoclonal antibodies was the establishment of continuous lymphoblastoid cell lines by transformation with the lymphotrophic herpes virus, Epstein-Barr virus. In this technique, lymphocytes are infected with EBV particles, usually derived from the B-95-8 marmoset lymphocyte line (Miller and Lipman, 1973). The B-95-8 cell line was developed by transforming marmoset lymphocytes with EBV produced by a lymphoblastoid cell line derived from a patient with infectious mononucleosis (Shope et al., 1973). Typically after exposure to EBV there is polyclonal proliferation of B cells with concomitant secretion of polyclonal immunoglobulins. EBV is selective for the cell types that it can infect; receptors for EBV so far have been found on only a proportion of B cells and on epithelial cells derived from the nasopharynx. Thus, in mixed populations of lymphocytes, only a proportion of B cells are infected and transformed. Which population of cells is eventually immortalized by EBV is not completely clear, and therefore efforts to select B cells secreting antibodies of defined specificity may not necessarily enrich for populations of B cells that are transformed by EBV.

The strategies most generally used either alone or in combination for establishing B cell lines transformed by EBV are (1) enrichment for specific antibody-producing cells, and (2) selection and cloning to establish stable, clonally-derived cell lines. Enrichment for B cells of defined specificities has usually taken the approach of selecting lymphocytes that bind to a specific antigen, by rosetting, and subsequent separation of lymphocytes using erythrocytes coupled to antigen, by panning techniques, or by fluorescence-activated cell sorting with antigen labeled with fluorescein. An interesting alternative approach has been depletion of B cells that do not bind antigen by capping antigen-specific surface immunoglobulin of B cells binding antigen, followed by removal of cells retaining surface Ig (Kozbor and Roder, 1981). In an initial report of the EBV technique for production of human monoclonal antibodies by Steinitz et al. (1977), a B cell line secreting IgM antibodies to the hapten NNP was established. In subsequent studies, the EBV method has been used to obtain antibodies to the hapten TNP (Kozbor et al., 1979), antibody against the D determinant of Rh blood group antigen (Koskimies, 1979; Boylston et al., 1980; Crawford et al., 1983a), antitetanus toxoid (Zurawski, 1978; Kozbor and Roder, 1981), antidiphtheria toxin (Tsuchiya, 1980), antiphosphorylcholine (Yoshie and Ono, 1980), rheumatoid factor (Steinitz and Tamir, 1982), antiacetylcholine receptor (Kamo et al., 1982), anti-influenza virus nucleoprotein (Crawford et al., 1983b), and antiglycoprotein D of herpes simplex virus (Seigneurin et al., 1983).

Although EBV transformation of B cells was the first method to be used widely to produce human monoclonal antibodies, there are several drawbacks to the methodology. Despite the occasional establishment of stable, long term B cell lines secreting high levels (5 μg/mL) of IgG or IgM antibodies of known reactivities, most EBV-derived cell lines produce low quantities of antibody (<1 μg/mL), and antibody secretion of EBV cell strains is relatively unstable. After the initial polyclonal expansion, usually only a few transformed B cells can be grown under conditions used for single cell cloning. For instance, Crawford et al. (1983a) were able to capture one stable, cloned B cell line secreting anti-Rh antibody after infecting 10^5 preselected lymphocytes, and Winger et al. (1983) produced 1 antibody-secreting clone/10^4 preselected lymphocytes transformed, although stability of antibody production was not followed.

Since the yield of lymphocytes after preselection procedures rarely exceeds 0.1% of the initial lymphocyte population, the frequency of antibody-secreting cell lines probably ranges from 1 clone/10^7 to 1 clone/10^8 starting lymphocytes. These results suggest an alternate strategy for the EBV methodology: initial polyclonal expansion of preselected B cell populations that can then be used as partners to produce hybridomas, by somatic cell hybridization techniques. Kozbor and Roder (1983) have followed this approach in an effort to increase the efficiency of capturing rare antigen-specific B cells (see below).

2.2. Strategies Using the Hybridoma Technology

Despite the rapid advances in the development of hybridomas secreting mouse immunoglobulins, the methodology to produce hybridomas secreting human immunoglobulin has lagged behind. The early report in 1973 by Schwaber and Cohen had demonstrated that somatic cell hybrids could secrete both mouse and human immunoglobulins. However, the potential of the hybridoma technique was not recognized until two years later deriving from the seminal work of Kohler and Milstein (1975). This study established a standard approach to developing antibody-secreting hybridomas. A critical component of the system is a drug-marked fusion partner, a cell line rendered deficient in hypoxanthine-guanine phosphoribosyl transferase (HGPRTase). The fusion partner has three characteristics: (1) the ability to grow in tissue culture; (2) the inability to remain viable in selective conditions, such as medium containing HAT (hypoxanthine–aminopterin–thymidine); and (3) the potential to fuse with other cells to produce synkaryons. Recently there has been considerable success in generating hybridomas secreting human antibodies. Human B cells have been hybridized to HAT-sensitive mouse myeloma cell lines (mouse × human hybrids) or human myeloma or lymphoblastoid cell lines (human × human hybrids).

2.2.1. Fusions with Mouse Myeloma Cell Lines

From the beginning of the development of the hybridoma methodology, mouse myeloma cell lines have been used for fusion partners. Because of availability of these mouse cell lines, it seems natural that human B cells would be fused with mouse fusion partners, especially in view of the scarcity of appropriate drug-marked human fusion partners. Fusions of human lymphocytes with mouse myeloma cell lines have had some success. Mouse × human hybridomas can be generated at a relatively high frequency using lymphocytes from peripheral blood, spleen, tonsil, lymph nodes, and tumor infiltrates (40–60 clones/10^7 lymphocytes fused), grow rapidly, and usually can be readily subcloned (Cote et al., 1983). In particular, mouse × human hybrids have favorable growth characteristics when compared to EBV-transformed lymphocytes or human × human hybrids (see below). There is a general impression, however, that immunoglobulin secretion of mouse × human hybrids is very unstable due to a predilection to segregate human chromosomes in heterohybrids. In spite of this problem, mouse × human hybrids that stably secrete human immunoglobulin can be generated, possibly because human chromosome 14 (site of immunoglobulin heavy chain genes) and chromosome 22 (site of lambda light chain genes) are preferentially retained in these interspecies hybrids (Croce et al., 1980; Erikson et al., 1981). Instability of human immunoglobulin secretion need not be due only to loss of genetic loci coding for immunoglobulin chains. Problems in immunoglobulin gene regulation or posttranscriptional events may also lead to loss of secretion in hybrid cells. This may be a problem that is not restricted to mouse × human hybrids, but may also be prevalent in human × human hybrids. Recently, Raison et al. (1982) have shown that immunoglobulin genes can be retained in Ig⁻ hybrids and that nonsecreting hybrids can be rescued to secrete Ig by stimulation with mitogens such as lipopolysaccharide. The problem of instability in mouse × human hybrids means that aggressive subcloning is often required to establish stable secreting cell lines. The use of mitogens to rescue Ig secretion in heterohybrids has not yet been tested on a large scale.

Ultimately, the success of a method will depend on its ability to generate cell lines secreting antibodies of defined specificities. The first human monoclonal antibody reported to be produced by the hybridoma technique was derived from a fusion between human splenocytes immunized in vitro with influenza virus and the mouse myeloma cell line NS1 (Nowinski et al., 1980). Surprisingly, an antibody was found that was directed against the glycolipid Forssman antigen. These workers and others (Sikora and Phillips, 1981; Sikora and Wright, 1981) have noted that many clones studied were unstable secretors of antibodies and required extensive subcloning to establish stable secreting cell lines. Other reports have suggested that instability of Ig secretion is not an overwhelming problem (Volkman et al., 1982; Cote et al., 1983; Houghton et al., 1983); 25–50% of mouse × human hybrids have been reported to continue to produce Ig 3–6 mo after fusion with aggressive subcloning (Cote et al., 1983; Houghton et al., 1983). Human monoclonal antibodies of predetermined specificity have been generated by fusing peripheral blood lymphocytes from immunized donors, including antibodies to keyhole limpet hemocyanin (Lane et al., 1982), tetanus toxoid (Butler et al., 1983; Kozbor et al., 1982a; Gigliotti and Insel, 1982) and diptheria toxoid (Gigliotti and Insel, 1982a). Peripheral blood lymphocytes obtained 5–7 d after immunization seemed to yield the highest frequency of antibody-positive clones (Butler et al., 1983; Gigliotti and Insel, 1982). In one study, preincubation of lymphocytes with a low-dose of the soluble antigen tetanus toxoid increased the number of antigen-positive clones by a factor of two (Butler et al., 1983).

2.2.2. Fusion with Human Cell Lines of B Cell Origin

The assumption that human × human hybridoma systems offer advantages over mouse × human hybrids arises from the observed stability of human intraspecies hybrids. In order to retain the desired phenotypic characteristic of immunoglobulin-secretion in hybrids, the human fusion partner should be derived from the B cell lineage. In mouse hybridoma systems, the best fusion partners are myeloma tumor cell lines corresponding to the ultimate stage of B cell differentiation, the plasma cell. Mouse plasmacytomas can be readily induced after injection of mineral oil and are frequently adapted to growth in tissue culture after explantation. Mouse myeloma cell lines that work well in hybridoma systems grow rapidly (doubling times 24 h) and can be cloned readily.

Human myeloma cells have been difficult to establish as continuous cell lines. Myeloma cells can be characterized as usually aneuploid, EBNA⁻, and containing extensive Golgi complex and rough endoplasmic reticulum, few free polyribosomes and many mitochondria (Kozbor and Roder, 1983). Only a handful of *bona fide* myeloma cell lines have been grown in long term tissue culture, and only one myeloma cell line, SKO-007 (IgE, lambda light chain), a derivative of the U266 cell line (Nilsson et al., 1970), has been drug-marked (rendered HGPRTase⁻) and shown to produce hybridomas after fusion (Olsson and Kaplan, 1980; Cote et al., 1983; Houghton et al., 1983). The original SKO-007 cell line was subsequently shown to be contaminated with mycoplasma, and most attempts to reproduce the initial results were not successful. Mycoplasma-free variants of SKO-007 have been made, and these cell lines have been shown to fuse and produce hybrids, albeit at a low frequency (1 clone/10⁷ lymphocyte fused) (Cote et al., 1983; Houghton et al., 1983; Abrams et al., 1983). Although other myeloma cell lines have been established (Moore and Kitamura,1968; Karpas et al., 1982; Togawa et al., 1982; Houghton et al., unpublished results), these either have not been drug-marked or have not yet been clearly shown to produce hybrids after fusion (Abrams et al., 1983). One problem that has occurred is contamination or mixup between human cell lines and cells of nonhuman origin. In particular, certain sublines of the RPMI 8226 human myeloma cell line have been shown to be of rodent (Pickering and Gelder, 1982) or nonhuman primate origin (Zeijlemaker et al., 1982).

The dearth of human myeloma cell lines has led to the use of other available human cell lines of the B cell lineage. Most of these immature B cell lymphoblastoid lines are infected with EBV that can be detected by expression of EBV nuclear antigen (EBNA). Given the larger number of drug-marked lymphoblastoid cell lines that are available, it is not surprising that most published human × human hybridomas are derived from a EBNA⁺ lymphoblastoid fusion partner. The contribution of EBV to the fusion frequency must be considered in the case of fusions with lymphoblastoid cell lines. The first human lymphoblastoid cell line to be used as a fusion partner was GM1500 6TG-2 (IgG_2, kappa) (Croce et al., 1980). Subsequently, derivatives of this cell line have been used, including GM4672 (Schoenfeld et al., 1982). Another lymphoblastoid cell line that has been successfully fused to produce human × human hybrids is the LICR-Lon-HMy2 cell line (IgG, kappa), a derivative of the ARH 77 cell line (Edwards et al., 1982; Cote et al., 1983; Houghton, et al., 1983). A third group of cell lines have been generated from the parent lymphoblastoid cell line, WIL-2 (IgM, kappa), including clone H35.1 (Chiorazzi et al., 1982) and the cell lines UC729-6 (Glassy et al., 1983) and HF2 (a clone of UC729-6) (Abrams et al., 1983). Other lymphoblastoid cell lines that are in use include HFB-1 (secretes no detectable Ig, demonstrates no surface Ig) (Hunter et al., 1982), GK-5 (Satoh et al., 1983), Mc/Car (Ritts et al., 1983), and LTR 228 (IgM, Kappa) (Larrick et al., 1983). Recently, a human B cell lymphoma cell line designated RH-L4 (IgG, kappa) has been used as a fusion partner (Olsson et al., 1983; Olsson et al., 1984); the EBV status of this cell line has not been reported.

An issue that is debated in monoclonal antibody circles is the choice of fusion fusion partner for producing human × human hybridomas. Performance of a fusion partner can be measured in several ways: (1) outgrowth of clones after fusion, usually reported as number of clones/10^6 or 10^7 lymphocytes fused; (2) levels and class of immunoglobulin produced by clones; (3) stability of immunoglobulin secretion over time; (4) efficiency of subcloning; and (5) detection of antibodies reactive to antigens of interest. No fusion partner has clearly established itself as superior in human hybridoma systems. Reports of the performance of a single fusion partner from individual laboratories are hard to interpret. Fusion methods, identification of clonal outgrowth after fusion, assays for immunoglobulin secretion and antibody reactivity, and methods for subcloning differ from laboratory to laboratory. We have reported comparative studies of 235 fusions using lymphocytes from lymph nodes, spleen, peripheral blood, and tumor infiltrates (Cote et al., 1983; Houghton et al., 1983). In these studies, four fusion partners were compared: NS1 (mouse myeloma cell line), SKO-007 (human myeloma cell line), GM 4672 (human lymphoblastoid cell line), aud LICR-Lon-HMy 2 (human lymphoblastoid cell line). A number of factors in the fusion procedure were found to influence results, although there can be great variability from fusion to fusion. For any hybridoma procedure, the condition of the fusion partner is critical. Fusion partners maintained in logarithmic growth phase and at maximum cell viability gave optimal results. Lymphocyte to fusion partner ratios from 1:1 to 2:1 generated 2–8 times greater clonal outgrowth than ratios of 5:1 or 10:1. When the addition of selective HAT medium was delayed to 24 h after fusion, clones grew out more vigorously. Finally, different lots of fetal calf serum in the growth medium produced substantial differences in the frequency of clonal outgrowth.

The amount of Ig produced by clones generated in these studies ranged from 500 ng/mL to greater than 10 µg/mL. Although the mechanisms regulating the levels of Ig production are unknown, it does not appear to be a feature that is conferred on the hybrid clone by the myeloma or lymphoblastoid fusion partner. A comparison of the source of lymphocytes also did not reveal any consistent difference in the amount of Ig produced after fusion. However, as might be expected, the proportion of clones secreting different Ig classes varied with the source of lymphocytes used for fusion. A greater percentage of IgA-secreting clones was obtained with lymphocytes from lymph nodes and IgM-secreting clones with lymphocytes, from peripheral blood lymphocytes.

The hybrid character of clones derived from fusions of NS1 with human lymphocytes has been clearly established; the presence of human and mouse chromosomes and the secretion of human Ig are unequivocal signs of a hybrid cell. The situation with clones derived from LICR-Lon-HMy2, GM4672, and SKO-007 fusions is less clear, because EBV transformation as well as hybrid formation can give rise to growing cell populations secreting human Ig. This is particularly pertinent in the case of LICR-Lon-HMy2 and GM4672, which are EBNA$^+$ lymphoblastoid lines and therefore a potential source of transforming EBV. Although EBV transformants are less likely to emerge in fusions with SKO-007 (which does not harbor the EBV genome), they may still arise from pre-existing B cells infected by EBV in the host. In theory, the distinction between EBV transformants and hybrid cells should be straightforward. EBV-transformed cell lines clone poorly, are usually diploid (Nilsson and Ponten, 1975), and secrete only one species of light and heavy Ig chains. On the other hand, hybrid cells should clone easily, have a tetraploid DNA content, and produce (with fusion partners that secrete Ig) more than one type of light and heavy chain. Experience has taught that these distinctions are not absolute. For instance, some EBV-transformed cell lines are tetraploid, and we have found that the majority of mouse × mouse hybridomas have a subtetraploid DNA content. In addition, human × human hybrid cells tend to be difficult to subclone and generally have a subtetraploid DNA content. Because of problems in interpreting clonal ploidy, the most useful evidence for a human × human hybrid cell is production of distinct Ig chains. We have shown this for a series of human × human hybrids by intracytoplasmic immunofluorescence and by polyacrylamide gel electrophoretic analysis of secreted products (Cote et al., 1984).

In a comparison of fusion frequencies, clonal outgrowth appeared most frequently after fusion with the NS1 mouse myeloma line (25–60 clones/10^7 lymphocytes fused) and the frequency of clonal outgrowth was similar with lymphocytes from lymph node and peripheral blood. In addition, mouse × human clones appeared sooner and generally subcloned with higher efficiency than human × human clones. From 3 to > 25 times lower frequency of growing clones was obtained after fusion with four human cell lines, UC729-6 (Cote, unpublished results), LICR-Lon-HMy2, GM4672, and SKO-007. In the case of lymphocytes from lymph node, fusions with LICR-Lon-HMy2 and UC729-6 resulted in a higher frequency of clonal outgrowth (5–10 clones/10^7 lymphocytes fused) than fusions with SKO-007 or GM4672 (1 clone/10^7 lymphocytes fused). Uniformly poor results have been obtained in human × human fusions with peripheral blood as a source of lymphocytes (≤ 1 clone/10^7 lymphocytes fused). Since peripheral blood is usually the most readily available source of lymphocytes, this low yield is a limiting factor in the application of human fusion partners. There are several explanations for this observation, including (a) the low percentage of B cells in peripheral blood; (b) the possibility that the differentiation stage of B cells in the peripheral blood is not optimal for hybrid formation or hybrid stability in human × human systems; and (c) destruction of hybrid cells by cytotoxic effector cells elicited by histocompatibility alloantigens contributed by the human fusion partner. If the last possibility is involved in low frequency of clonal outgrowth, removal of T cells before fusion should increase the frequency of Ig-positive clones. Initial experiments indicate that this may be the case (Houghton et al., 1983). Depletion of cells from peripheral blood lymphocytes before fusion has resulted in 10 to greater than 20 times higher frequency of growing clones, suggesting that T cells from peripheral blood are cytotoxic for hybrid cells. In fusions performed with peripheral blood lymphocytes, mouse × human systems seem to be preferable to most human × human systems studied to date. Mouse × human fusions generally generate greater than 20-fold more hybridomas than human × human fusions (Cote et al., 1983; Houghton et al., 1983).

2.2.3. Analysis of B Cell Specificity Using Human Monoclonal Antibodies

With techniques available which consistently permit the construction of Ig-secreting hybrids, this methodology is being used to analyze the immune response and immune repertoire of humans and to study autoimmune disorders and infectious diseases. Both the fields of tumor immunology and autoimmune disease require the identification of antibodies to cellular antigens. In a screen for human antibodies to cellular antigens, we have found that antibodies reacting with cell surface antigens are rare (<1% of clones secrete antibodies to cell surface components) whereas antibodies to intracellular structures occur at a significantly higher frequency (3–9% of clones) (Cote et al., 1983;

Houghton et al., 1983). This finding could have several explanations, including (a) greater polymorphism of cell surface antigens vs intracellular antigens, requiring a larger variety of cell lines and cell types in a screening panel to identify antibodies reacting with cell surface antigens; (b) greater range of antigenic determinants within the cell than on the cell surface; (c) loss or low expression of certain cell surface antigens on cells in vitro vs cells in vivo; and (d) immunological tolerance that restricts autoantibodies to cell surface antigens to a greater degree than to intracellular antigens. Human × human fusions with lymphocytes of patients with autoimmune disorders have yielded clones secreting IgM antibodies to islet cells (Eisenbarth et al., 1982) and to multiple other endocrine tissues including anterior pituitary and thyroid (Satoh et al., 1983). Several of these antibodies react with cytoskeletal elements, most likely intermediate filaments, although none of these antigens were biochemically identified (Satoh et al., 1983). Since human monoclonal antibodies to cytoskeletal antigens can be derived from lymphocytes of normal individuals (Cote et al., 1983), the relationship of such autoantibodies to the pathogenesis of autoimmune disease remains to be established. Human monoclonal antibodies to DNA and platelets have been generated using lymphocytes from patients with systemic lupus erythematosus (Schoenfeld et al., 1982; Schoenfeld et al., 1983). In keeping with previous studies in the mouse (Lafer et al., 1981), human monoclonal autoantibodies to DNA were found to react with determinants present on both nucleic acids and the phospholipid cardiolipin. The presence of this antigenic determinant on different molecules suggests that multiple serological reactions may detect the same anti-DNA antibodies and that DNA is not necessarily the primary immunogen in these patients. An antibody that seems to react with the idiotype of a mouse monoclonal antibody to the acetylcholine receptor was developed from a fusion with lymphocytes of a patient with myasthenia gravis (Dwyer et al., 1983).

Another series of human monoclonal antibodies have been generated by human × human fusions to cell components or products of infectious agents. These include antibodies to measles virus nucleocapsid (Croce et al., 1980), tetanus toxoid (Chiorazzi et al., 1982; Larrick et al., 1983) and type B capsular polysacchride of influenza virus (Hunter et al., 1982).

3. Further Experimental Strategies

Application of human monoclonal antibodies to the study of the human immune response and human diseases is now possible. However, a more successful approach is needed to capture individual clones of B cells. Even in the hyperimmunized host, the frequency of B cells reactive to a specific antigen is usually <1 clone/10^5 lymphocytes. The best fusion frequencies in human hybridoma systems are on the order of 1 hybridoma generated/10^5 lymphocytes fused. If one assumes that fusion and outgrowth of hybridoma clones are random events, then the chances of obtaining a specific antigen-reactive hybridoma is $<1/10^8$ lymphocytes fused. The outlook may not be quite so grim; it is likely that proliferating B cells or antigen-primed B cells fuse and form stable hybrids preferentially. In any case, these figures imply that a great deal of work might be necessary to capture a desired B cell clone. The EBV technique is able to capture many more B cells than the hybridoma method, but these cell lines characteristically produce low quantities of antibody and growth is unstable. A number of approaches are being considered to improve the construction of cell lines secreting specific antibody: (1) a combination of EBV transformation to expand antibody-secreting B cell populations followed by somatic cell fusion; (2) expansion of populations of B cells in tissue culture using B cell growth factors; (3) in vitro systems to expand specific B cell populations by antigen stimulation; (4) establishment or construction of new cell lines for fusion partners; (5) new methods for somatic cell fusion; and (6) application of the recombinant DNA technology including gene transfer and engineering of immunoglobulin genes.

3.1. The EBV-Hybridoma Approach

Kozbor et al. (1981, 1982a, 1982b) have sequentially applied the EBV technique and the hybridoma technology to construct cell lines secreting human antibody. An EBV-transformed cell line, designated B6, producing antibody to tetanus toxoid, was fused to the mouse myeloma cell line P3X63Ag.8v.653 (Kozbor et al., 1982b). Hybrid cells were selected in HAT to kill nonfused mouse myeloma cells, whereas ouabain was used to kill nonfused EBV-transformed human cells (ouabain-resistance is a dominant trait and mouse cells are resistant to 10^3–10^4 higher concentrations of ouabain than human cells). Hybrid clones were produced that secreted 2 μg/mL of antibody, whereas the original EBV-transformed B6 cell line produced 0.85 μg/mL for only a 10 mo period. These heterohybrids continued to secrete anti-tetanus toxoid antibody for 6 mo, but subsequently ceased to produce antibody.

To overcome the instability of interspecies hybrids, the B6 EBV clone was fused to a human fusion partner (Kozbor, 1982a). In order to construct an appropriate fusion partner, the HAT-sensitive human lymphoblastoid cell line GM1500 6TG-2 was modified to select a ouabain-resistant variant designated KR-4. When KR-4 cells were fused to B6 EBV-transformed cells in the presence of HAT and ouabain, only hybrid cells survive. HAT selected against KR-4 cells and ouabain against B6 cells, whereas hybrid cells were resistant to both ouabain and

HAT. Human × human hybrids produced 3–6 μg/mL of antitetanus toxoid antibody and, as hoped, remained stable for over 1 yr.

The disadvantages of the techniques of EBV-transformation or somatic cell fusion may be overcome by using these systems in combination. In many cases it may be easier to expand specific B cell populations by EBV-stimulation and transformation. EBV-transformed B cells have been reported to be more susceptible to hybridization than resting lymphocytes (Kozbor and Roder, 1983) and fusion experiments can be planned and repeated when EBV-transformed cultures are used.

3.2. Growth of Nontransformed B Cells in Culture

Advances in understanding the growth and differentiation of lymphocytes hopefully will lead to strategies for continuous growth of nontransformed B cells in culture. In contrast to T cells that can be maintained in culture in the presence of the T cell growth factor, interleukin 2, B cells have been more difficult to adapt to long-term culture, despite the recent definition of several B cell growth factors (Howard and Paul, 1983). One strategy has been to use a combination of factors: first to expand the B cell population by stimulation with mitogens such as pokeweed mitogen, protein A, or phytohemagglutinin, and then to propagate B cell colonies by stimulation with conditioned media from human peripheral blood mononuclear cells (Sredni et al., 1981). Systems to expand B cell populations have not yet been routinely used, however, despite their potential to augment the number of B cells from a given source for subsequent in vitro stimulation by antigen, EBV-transformation, or somatic cell fusion.

3.3. Preselection of B Cells In Vitro: Systems for In Vitro Stimulation by Antigen

There is a general impression that systems to expand minor populations of antigen-primed B cells in vitro would greatly enhance the application of the human monoclonal antibody technology. The success of the mouse hybridoma methodology depended to a great deal on hyperimmunization of animals with a chosen antigen, followed at a carefully timed interval by somatic cell hybridization of immune splenic B cells. In humans, adequate primary or secondary immunization is not always possible and optimal timing for fusion has been reported only in a few selected experimental systems (Butler et al., 1983). Preincubation of human B cells with antigen, either prior to EBV-transformation (Crawford et al., 1983b) or fusion with mouse myeloma cells (Butler et al., 1983), has been found in some circumstances to increase the frequency of human monoclonal antibodies to predetermined antigens. However, reproducible in vitro systems for immune stimulation of B cells have proved to be complex, involving multiple steps to elicit primary or secondary immune responses (Hoffman, 1980; Misiti and Waldman, 1981; Cavagnaro and Osband,

1983). Many parameters need to be considered for in vitro sensitization of B cells: concentration of antigen, use of accessory cell populations, length of time for sensitization, and density of B cells. Finally, the majority of studies have been performed using soluble antigens, such as tetanus toxoid, although systems for sensitization to cellular antigens are more pertinent to the development of human monoclonal antibodies to antigens on cancer cells.

3.4. Fusion Partners and Fusion Conditions

Because no fusion partner has clearly emerged as superior for human hybridoma systems, the search continues for new fusion partners. An optimal fusion partner should be a human cell line of the B cell lineage that grows rapidly and subclones at high efficiency. Fusion partners that do not secrete their own immunoglobulins, but that support high levels of immunoglobulin secretion in hybrids, are desirable. Although many B lymphoblastoid cell lines are available, only a handful of human myeloma cell lines have been established. Using a variety of growth conditions, we have attempted to culture over 70 bone marrow specimens from patients with plasma cell neoplasms. Only two long-term myeloma cultures have been established, both from patients with plasma cell leukemia. One cell line, designated SK-My-1, has been mutagenized and adapted to growth in $1 \times 10^{-5}M$ 6-thioguanine. This cell line was established from a patient with kappa light chain myeloma, and the cell line secretes only kappa light chain. This experience points out that, although myeloma cells are extremely difficult to adapt to long term cell culture, neoplastic plasma cell lines may be more readily establish patients with plasma cell leukemia. This variant of multiple myeloma is highly malignant, and the malignant phenotype of plasma cells in this condition may be more suitable for adaptation to tissue culture and maintenance of growth vigor.

An alternative strategy is the engineering of new cell lines using the technique of somatic cell fusion and/or the recombinant DNA technology. Teng et al. (1983) have constructed mouse × human heteromyeloma fusion partners. A HAT-sensitive mutant subline of the U266 human myeloma cell line was transfected with a recombinant plasmid vector pSV2-neo[R] that carries a dominant trait conferring resistance to the antibiotic neomycin. A neomycin-resistant clone of U266 was then fused to a nonproducer, antibiotic-sensitive mouse myeloma cell line, X63-Ag8.653, and hybrid clones were selected in ouabain and antibiotic. Heteromyeloma fusion partners retained only a small number of human chromosomes, did not secrete mouse or human immunoglobulin chains, and generated hybridomas in a variety of fusion systems.

Methods for cell fusion presently rely on conditions which disrupt cell membranes, leading to the formation of heterokaryons and subsequently synkaryons. The process of fusion requires the chance opposition of two or more cells, and the frequency of generating viable hybrid cells is usually < 1 hybridoma/5×10^4 cells fused. Although most fusion techniques rely on selectable genetic markers (e.g., HGPRTase⁻ cells as fusion partners), fusion methods have been described where growth of the fusion partner is prevented by exposure to irreversible biochemical inhibitors such as iodoacetamide or diethylpyrocarbonate (Wright, 1978). In this method fused cells receive a complement of undamaged cell products and are able to survive. A novel fusion technique has been reported that uses an alternating, nonuniform electric field of low strength to oppose neighboring cells, followed by short electrical pulses of high intensity to produce cell fusion (Zimmerman and Vienken, 1982). This method has been reported to give a high yield of fused cells (up to 50–80% of lymphocytes fused), although the actual yield of growing hybrids have yet to be determined. Given high rates of viable hybrid cells, selection methods such as HAT sensitivity might not be required. In addition, very high fusion frequencies would have definite advantages in systems that preselect B cells for fusion; small numbers of antigen-reactive B cells could be selected and captured as hybridomas.

3.5. Immunoglobulin Genes

The recombinant DNA technology has provided detailed insight into the process of immunoglobulin gene organization and expression. The diversity of immunoglobulin molecules arise from several mechanisms including the presence of 100–1000 variable segment germ-line genes, DNA rearrangements, and somatic mutations. The techniques for splicing and cloning genes and for transfecting genes into eukaryotic cells provide new strategies for manipulation and expression of specific immunoglobulin genes. Cloned genes are available for major classes and subclasses of human immunoglobulin (Honjo, 1983). Cloned light and heavy chain mouse immunoglobulin genes have been transfected and expressed in various plasmacytoma and hybridoma cell lines (Oi et al., 1983; Ochi et al., 1983a; Ochi et al., 1983b). However, at least one study has suggested that cells of the B cell lineage are more likely to express transfected immunoglobulin genes (Stafford and Queen, 1983). Genetic engineering technique can be applied in several areas of human monoclonal antibody research:

(1) Antibody properties can be changed by manipulating genes that code for constant and variable regions of the antibody molecule. For instance, antibody classes or subclasses that determine antibody effector functions (e.g., complement fixation) can be switched by gene splicing techniques, or genes coding for antibody fragments can be cloned and expressed.

(2) Immunoglobulin genes can be linked to genetic markers that can be amplified and selected. These constructions can be introduced into eukaryotic cells by transfection or protoplast fusion or used for transformation of bacteria.

(3) B cell clones could be immortalized by genes known to transform human cells. This strategy is an extension of the technique of EBV transformation. It remains to be seen whether genes such as oncogenes can efficiently and stably transform cells of the B cell lineage and whether this approach would offer advantages over EBV transformation or hybridoma techniques.

4. Human Monoclonal Antibodies Derived from Lymphocytes of Patients with Cancer

Now that methods are available to generate human monoclonal antibodies, a fine analysis of the humoral immune response to cancer in humans has begun. Initial studies have started to explore the specificity of lymphocytes from cancer patients using the hybridoma technique and EBV-transformation. Immunoglobulins produced by lymphocytes from peripheral blood, lymph nodes, and tumor infiltrates have been screened for reactivity to cell surface and intracellular antigens, in the hope of identifying antibodies to cellular products. In over 500 fusions using lymphocytes from patients with breast cancer, kidney cancer, lung cancer, and malignant melanoma, <1% of clones secreted antibodies reacting with cell surface antigens, whereas 3–9% of clones produced antibodies to intracellular antigens (Cote et al., 1983; Houghton et al., 1983; Cote and Houghton, unpublished observations). A tentative conclusion that can be drawn is that human monoclonal antibodies reacting to intracellular structures occur at a significantly higher frequency than antibodies to cell surface components (Cote et al., 1983; Houghton et al., 1983). In these studies, a panel of tissue culture cell lines was used as targets. It will be important to extend this screen to a larger panel of tissue culture target cells and to noncultured cells, since a particular cell population may be lacking from the panel and since antigen loss may occur during tissue culture.

The cell surface reactivities in this initial screening did not conform to any known antigenic systems. For example, an IgG antibody, designated Ri37, derived from a fusion of lymphocytes from an axillary lymph node of a patient with breast cancer and the mouse myeloma NS1, detected a cell surface antigen expressed on nontransformed B cells and certain cancer cell lines. Likewise, specificity testing of an IgM antibody Ma4, derived from a fusion between lymph node lymphocytes of a patient with malignant melanoma and the human lymphoblastoid cell line LICR-

Lon-HMy2, did not show any recognizable reactivity pattern. The Ma4 antibody reacted with a glycolipid antigen on 6 of 61 tumor cell lines tested, with no predilection for any particular cell type, but Ma4 antibody did not react with cultures derived from normal cells.

In contrast, Irie et al. (1982) have analyzed a human antibody secreted by EBV-transformed peripheral blood lymphocytes of a patient with melanoma that reacted with an antigen expressed by cells of neuroectoderm origin. This antibody, designated OFA-I-2, detects a cell surface glycolipid, GD2 ganglioside, expressed on melanoma cells (Cahan et al., 1982). The reactivity of OFA-I-2 antibody corresponds to antibody reactivities found in the sera of a small proportion of patients with malignant melanoma and astrocytoma by autologous typing (Shiku et al., 1976; Watanabe et al., 1982; Pfreundschuh et al., 1978) and in occasional normal individuals (Houghton et al., 1980). The antigen detected by the human monoclonal antibody OFA-I-2 seems to be identical to the Class 2 AH and AJ antigens (Shiku et al., 1976; Watanabe et al., 1982) and OFA-1 antigen (Irie et al., 1976) detected by human sera. A second human monoclonal antibody, designated OFA-I-1, also produced by EBV-transformed peripheral blood lymphocytes of a patient with melanoma, has been shown to react with the ganglioside GM2. OFA-I-1 antigen is found on a wide variety of human cancer cells and on fetal brain. Olssen et al. (1984) analyzed an antibody, designated aml-18, derived from a fusion between lymphocytes of a patient with acute myeloid leukemia and the human lymphoma partner RH-L4. The aml-18 antibody reacted with a proportion of acute myeloid and acute lymphoblastic leukemia samples and showed weak binding to normal human bone marrow cells. This antigen possibly represents a differentiation antigen present on precursor cells in the bone marrow.

The serological dissection of intracellular structures by human monoclonal antibodies permits a new level of precision in the study of autoimmune recognition of normal and malignant cells. A range of intracellular structures have been identified by human monoclonal antibodies, including nuclei, nucleoli, Golgi complex, cytoskeletal elements and other cytoplasmic components (Cote et al., 1983; Houghton et al., 1983). Intracellular antigens have been identified by antibodies derived from lymphocytes of normal individuals and patients with cancer, suggesting that these autoantibodies need not be related to overt disease (Cote et al., 1983). A number of these human monoclonal antibodies detect intermediate filament components in cultured cells including vimentin, glial fibrillary acidic protein, and several species of cytokeratins (Thomson, Cote, and Houghton, unpublished observations).

A series of other studies have generated human monoclonal antibodies from lymphocytes of patients with cancer. An IgM antibody, derived from a fusion between lymphocytes from regional lymph nodes of a breast cancer patient and the mouse myeloma NS1, was analyzed by Schlom et al. (1980). This antibody was found to react with primary and metastatic breast cancers, a proportion of benign breast lesions, and a variety of nonbreast malignancies (Schlom et al., 1980; Wunderlich et al., 1981; Teramoto et al., 1982). Sikora's group has generated human monoclonal antibodies from tumor infiltrates of malignant gliomas (Sikora and Phillips, 1981; Sikora et al., 1982) and draining lymph nodes from patients with lung cancer (Sikora and Wright, 1981). Although antibodies produced by mouse × human hybrids were not analyzed in these studies because of the instability of immunoglobulin secretion, reactivity to human glioma cells was found after human × human fusions. These reactivities were not extensively analyzed, however. Tumor infiltrating B cells of metastatic melanoma lesions have been EBV-transformed, and antibodies have been detected in preliminary screens that reacted to melanoma cells (Watson et al., 1983). Fusions between lymphocytes of regional lymph nodes from cancer patients and the UC729-6 human lymphoblastoid cell line generated human monoclonal antibodies that bound to carcinoma cell lines, but not normal fibroblast cultures (Glassy, 1983).

5. Conclusions

Human monoclonal antibodies will have a range of applications in the study of cancer. The monoclonal antibody technology permits the fine analysis of the humoral immune response of a patient with cancer, including the specificity of previously inaccessible B cells located in lymph nodes in the region of the tumor and in tumor infiltrates. Human monoclonal antibodies may have distinct advantages over mouse antibodies for clinical applications. Although the immune response to mouse antibodies may limit their usefulness for in vivo application in humans, human antibodies should be less immunogenic. Thus far, only a small number of well-characterized human monoclonal antibodies have been reported that react with cell surface antigens. Extensive specificity testing and biochemical analysis will be required to fully characterize any antigen system, in particular to identify potentially immunogenic tumor antigens and candidates for tumor-specific antigens.

Acknowledgments

We are grateful to Yvette Johnson for help in preparation of this chapter and to Dr. Lloyd Old for his support and comments. The research was supported in part by grants IM-333 from the American Cancer Society and NCI CA-34079 from the National Cancer Institute, National Institutes of Health.

References

Abrams, P. G., J. A. Knost, G. Clarke, S. Wilburn, R. K. Oldham, and R. A. Foon (1983), *J. Immunol.* **131,** 1201.

Albino, A. P., K. O. Lloyd, A. N. Houghton, H. F. Oettgen, and L. J. Old (1981), *J. Exp. Med.* **154,** 1764.

Boyse, E. A. and L. J. Old (1969), *Ann. Rev. Genet.* **3,** 269.

Butler, J. L., C. Lane, and A. S. Fauci (1983), *J. Immunol.* **130,** 165.

Boylston, A., B. Gardner, R. L. Anderson, and N. C. Hughes-Jones (1980), *Scand. J. Immunol.* **12,** 355.

Butler, J. L., H. C. Lane, and A. S. Fauci (1983), *J. Immunol.* **130,** 165.

Cahan, L., R. F. Irie, R. Singh, A. Cassidenti, and J. C. Paulson (1982), *Proc. Nat. Acad. Sci. USA* **79,** 7629.

Carey, T. E., T. Takahashi, L. A. Resnick, H. F. Oettgen, and L. J. Old (1976), *Proc. Nat. Acad. Sci. USA* **73,** 3278.

Cavagnaro, J., and M. Osband (1983), *Biotech* **1,** 31.

Chiorazzi, N., R. L. Wasserman, and H. F. Kunkel (1982), *J. Exp. Med.* **156,** 930.

Cote, R. C., A. N. Houghton, H. F. Oettgen, and L. J. Old (1984), in *Human Hybridomas and Monoclonal Antibodies.* Plenum Publ. Corp., New York.

Cote, R. C., D. Morrissey, A. N. Houghton, E. J. Beattie, H. F. Oettgen, and L. J. Old (1983), *Proc. Nat. Acad. Sci. USA* **80,** 2026.

Crawford, D., M. Barlow, J. Harrison, L. Winger, and E. Huens (1983a), *Lancet* **i,** 386.

Crawford, D., R. Callard, M. Muggeridge, D. Mitchell, E. Zanders, and P. C. Beverley (1983b), *J. Gen. Virol.* **64,** 697.

Croce, C. M., A. Linnenbach, W. Hall, Z. Steplewski, and H. Koprowski (1980), *Nature* **288,** 488.

Croce, C., M. Shander, J. Martinis, L. Cicurel, G. G. D'Ancona, and H. Koprowski (1980), *Eur. J. Immuno.* **10,** 486.

Day, C. L., A. J. Sober, R. A. Lew, M. C. Mihm, T. B. Fitzpatrick, A. W. Kopf, M. N. Harris, S. L. Gumport, J. W. Raker, R. A. Malt, F. M. Golomb, W. C. Wood, P. Casson, S. Lopransi, F. Gorstein, and A. Postel (1981), *Cancer* **47,** 955.

DeLeo, A., G. Jay, G. Appella, G. C. DuBois, L. W. Law, and L. J. Old (1979), *Proc. Nat. Acad. Sci. USA* **76,** 2420.

DeLeo, A., H. Shiku, T. Takahashi, M. John, and L. J. Old (1977), *J. Exp. Med.* **146,** 720.

Dwyer, D. S., R. J. Bradley, C. K. Urguhart, and J. F. Kearney (1983), *Nature* **301,** 611.

Edwards, P. A., C. M. Smith, A. M. Neville, and M. J. O'Hare (1982), *Eur. J. Immunol.* **12,** 641.

Eisenbarth, G. S., A. Linnenbach, R. Jackson, R. Searce, and C. Croce (1982), *Nature* **300,** 264.

Erikson, J., J. Martinis, and C. M. Croce (1981), *Nature* **294,** 173.

Everson, T. and W. Cole (1966), *Spontaneous Regression of Cancer,* Saunders, Philadelphia, PA.

Ewing, J. (1940), *Neoplastic Diseases,* Saunders, Philadelphia, PA.

Foley, E. J. (1953), *Cancer Res.* **13,** 835.

Fraumeni, J. F. and R. Hoover (1975), *Immunosurveillance and Cancer,* Natl. Cancer Inst. Monogr., Washington, D.C.

Garrett, T. J., T. Takahashi, B. D. Clarkson, and L. J. Old (1977), *Proc. Nat. Acad. Sci. USA* **74,** 4578.

Gigliotti, F. and R. A. Insel (1982), *J. Clin. Inv.* **70,** 1306.

Glassy, M. C., H. H. Handley, H. Hagiwara, and I. Royston (1983), *Proc. Nat. Acad. Sci. USA* **80,** 6327.

Habel, K. (1961), *Proc. Soc. Exp. Biol. Med.* **106,** 722.

Hoffman, M. (1980), *Proc. Nat. Acad. Sci. USA* **77,** 1139.

Honjo, T. (1983), *Ann. Rev. Immunol.* **1,** 499.

Houghton, A. N., H. Brooks, R. J. Cote, M. C. Taormina, J. F. Oettgen, and L. J. Old (1983), *J. Exp. Med.* **158,** 53.

Houghton, A. N,, M. Eisinger, A. Albino, J. G. Cairncross, and L. J. Old (1982), *J. Exp. Med.* **156,** 1755.

Houghton, A. N., M. C. Taormina, H. Ikeda, T. Watanabe, H. F. Oettgen, and L. J. Old (1980), *Proc. Nat. Sci. Amer. USA* **77,** 4260.

Howard, M. and W. Paul (1983), *Ann. Rev. Immunol.* **1,** 307.

Hunter, Jr., K. W., G. W. Fischer, V. G. Hemming, S. R. Wilson, R. J. Hartzman, and J. N. Woody (1982), *Lancet* **ii,** 798.

Irie, R. F., K. Irie, and D. L. Morton (1976), *Cancer Res.* **36,** 3510.

Irie, R., L. L. Sze, and R. E. Saxton (1982), *Proc. Nat. Acad. Sci. USA* **79,** 5666.

Jerne, N. K. (1974). *Ann. Immunol. (Paris) 125C,* 373.

Kamo, I., S. Furukawa, A. Tada, Y. Mano, Y. Iwasaki, and T. Furuse (1982), *Science* **215,** 995.

Karpas, A., P. Fischer, and D. Swirsky (1982), *Science* **216,** 997.

Kennedy, R. C. and G. R. Breesman (1984), *J. Exp. Med.* **159,** 655.

Kohler, G. and C. Milstein (1975), *Nature* **256,** 495.

Koprowski, H., D. Herlyn, M. Lubeck, E. DeFreitas, and H. F. Sears (1984), *Proc. Nat. Acad. Sci. USA* **81,** 216.

Koskimies, S. (1979), *Scan. J. Immunol.* **10,** 37.

Kozbor, D., A. Lagarde, and J. C. Roder (1982a), *Proc. Nat. Acad. Sci. USA* **79,** 6657.

Kozbor, D. and J. C. Roder (1981), *J. Immunol.* **127,** 1275.

Kozbor, D., J. C. Roder, (1983), *Immunol. Today* **4,** 72.

Kozbor, D., J. C. Roder, T. H. Chang, Z. Steplewski, and H. Koprowski (1982b), *Hybridoma* **1,** 323.

Kozbor, D., M. Steinitz, G. Klein, S. Koskimies, and O. Makela (1979), *Scand. J. Immunol.* **10,** 187.

Kunkel, H. G., M. Mannik, and R. C. Williams (1963), *Science* **140,** 1218.

Lafer, E. M., J. Rauch, C. Andrejewski, Jr., D. Mudd, B. Furie, R. S. Schwartz, and B. D. Strollar (1981), *J. Exp. Med.* **153,** 897.

Lane, H. C., J. H. Shelhamer, H. S. Mostowski, and A. S. Fauci (1982), *J. Exp. Med.* **155,** 333.

Larrick, J. W., K. E. Truitt, A. A. Raubitschek, G. S. Senyk, and J. C. N. Wang (1983), *Proc. Nat. Acad. Sci. USA* **80,** 6376.

Larsen, T. E. and T. H. Grude (1978), *Acta Pathol. Microbiol. Scand.* **86,** 523.

McLean, D. I., R. A. Lew, A. J. Sober, M. S. Mihm, and T. B. Fitzpatrick (1979), *Cancer* **43,** 157.

Miller and Lipman (1973), *Proc. Nat. Acad. Sci. USA* **70**, 190.

Miller, R. A., A. R. Oseroff, P. T. Stratte, and R. Levy (1983), *Blood* **62**, 998.

Misiti, J. and T. Waldman (1981), *J. Exp. Med.* **154**, 1069.

Moore, G. E. and H. Kitamura (1968), *N.Y. State J. Med.* **68**, 2054.

Moore, O. S. and F. W. Foote (1949), *Cancer* **2**, 634.

Murphy, J. B. (1921), *J. Exp. Med.* **33**, 423.

Nilsson, K., H. Bennich, S. G. O. Johansson, and J. Ponten (1970), *Clin. Exp. Immunol.* **7**, 477.

Nilsson, K. and J. Ponten, (1975), *Int. J. Cancer* **15**, 321.

Nowinski, R., C. Berglund, J. Lane, M. Lostrom, I. Bernstein, W. Young, and S. Hakomori (1980), *Science* **210**, 537.

Ochi, A., R. G. Hawley, T. Hawley, M. J. Shulman, A. Traunecker, G. Kohler, and N. Hozumi (1983a), *Proc. Nat. Acad. Sci. USA* **80**, 6357.

Ochi, A., R. G. Hawley, M. J. Shulman, and N. Hoyuni (1983b), *Nature* **302**, 340.

Oi, V. T., S. L. Morrison, L. A. Herzenberg, and P. A. Berg (1983), *Proc. Nat. Acad. Sci. USA* **80**, 825.

Old, L. J. (1981), *Cancer Res.* **41**, 361.

Old, L. J. and E. A. Boyse (1964), *Ann. Rev. Med.* **15**, 167.

Olsson, L., R. B. Anderson, A. Ost, B. Christensen, and P. Biberfeld (1984), *J. Exp. Med.* **159**, 537.

Olsson, L. and H. Kaplan (1980), *Proc. Nat. Acad. Sci. USA* **77**, 5429.

Olsson, L., H. Kronstrom, A. Cambon-De Mouzon, C. Honsik, T. Brodin, and B. Jakobsen (1983), *J. Immuno. Methods* **61**, 17.

Penn, I. (1970), *Malignant Tumors in Organ Transplant Recipients*, Springer-Verlag, New York.

Pfreundschuh, M., H. Shiku, T. Takahashi, R. Ueda, J. Ransohoff, H. F. Oettgen, and L. J. Old (1978), *Proc. Nat. Acad. Sci. USA* **75**, 5122.

Pickering, J. W. and F. B. Gelder (1982), *J. Immunol.* **129**, 406.

Prehn, R. T. and J. M. Main (1957), *J. Natl. Cancer Inst.* **18**, 769.

Raison, R. L., K. Z. Walker, C. R. E. Halnan, D. Briscoe, and A. Bastan (1982), *J. Exp. Med.* **156**, 1380.

Rajewsky, K. and T. Takemori (1983), *Ann. Rev. Immunol.* **1**, 569.

Real, F. X., J. M. Mattes, A. N. Houghton, P. L. Livingston, K. O. Lloyd, H. F. Oettgen, and L. J. Old (1983), *Proc. Am. Assoc. Cancer Res.* **24**, 686.

Ritts, R. E., A. Ruiz Arguello, K. G. Weyl, A. L. Bradley, B. Weihmeir, D. J. Jacobssen, and B. L. Strehlo (1983), *Int. J. Cancer* **31**, 133.

Ritz, J., J. M. Pesando, S. E. Sallon, L. A. Clavell, J. Notis-McConaty, P. Rosenthal, and S. Schlossman (1981), *Blood* **58**, 141.

Russel, B. R. (1908), *Third Scientific Report, Imp. Cancer Res. Fund* **3**, 341.

Sacks, D. L., K. M. Esser, and A. Sher (1982), *J. Exp. Med.* **155**, 1108.

Satoh, J., B. S. Prabhakar, M. V. Haspel, F. Ginsburg-Fellner, and A. L. Notkins (1983), *N. Engl. J. Med.* **309**, 217.

Schlom, J., D. Wunderlich, and Y. A. Teramoto (1980), *Proc. Nat. Acad. Sci. USA* **77**, 6841.

Schoenfeld, Y., S. C. Hsu-Lin, J. E. Gabriels, L. E. Silberstein, B. C. Furie, B. Furie, B. D. Stollar, and R. S. Schwartz (1982), *J. Clin. Inv.* **70**, 205.

Schoenfeld, Y., J. Rauch, H. Massicote, S. K. Datta, J. Andre-Schwartz, B. D. Stoller, and R. S. Schwartz (1983), *N. Eng. J. Med.* **308**, 414.

Schwaber, J. and E. P. Cohen (1973), *Nature* **244**, 444.

Sears, H. F., B. Atkinson, J. Matis, C. Ernst, D. Herlyn, Z. Steplewski, P. Hayry, and H. Koprowski (1982), *Lancet* **1**, 762.

Seigneurin, J. M., C. Desgranges, D. Seigneurin, J. Paire, J. C. Renversez, B. Jacquemont, and C. Micouin (1983), *Science* **221**, 173.

Shiku, H., T. Takahashi, H. F. Oettgen, and L. J. Old (1976), *J. Exp. Med.* **144**, 873.

Shope, T., D. Dechairo, and G. Miller (1973), *Proc. Nat. Acad. Sci. USA* **70**, 2487.

Sikora, K., T. Alderton, J. Phillips, and J. Watson (1982), *Lancet* **i**, 11.

Sikora, K. and J. Phillips (1981), *Br. J. Cancer* **43**, 105.

Sikora, K. and R. Wright (1981), *Br. J. Cancer* **43**, 696.

Sjogren, H. O., I. Hellstrom, and G. Klein (1961), *Exp. Cell Res.* **23**, 204.

Sredni, B., D. G. Sieckmann, S. Kumagai, S. House, I. Green, and W. E. Paul (1981), *J. Exp. Med.* **154**, 1500.

Stafford, J. and C. C. Queen (1983), *Nature* **306**, 77.

Steinitz, M., G. Klein, S. Kosimies, and O. Makela (1977), *Nature* **269**, 420.

Steinitz, M. and S. Tamir (1982), *Eur. J. Immunol.* **12**, 126.

Teng, N., K. S. Lam, F. C. Riera, and H. S. Kaplan (1983), *Proc. Nat. Acad. Sci. USA* **80**, 7308.

Teramoto, Y. A., R. Mariani, D. Wunderlich, and J. Schlom (1982), *Cancer* **50**, 241.

Thompson, P. G. (1973), *Pigm. Cell* **1**, 285.

Togawa, A., N. Inoue, K. Miyamoto, H. Hyodo, and M. Namba (1982), *Int. J. Cancer* **29**, 495.

Tsuchiya, S., S. Yokoyama, O. Yoshie, and Y. Ono (1980), *J. Immunol.* **124**, 1970.

Ueda, R., H. Shiku, M. Pfreundschuh, T. Takahashi, L. T. C. Li, W. F. Whitmore, H. F. Oettgen, and L. J. Old (1979), *J. Exp. Med.* **150**, 564.

Volkman, D. J., S. P. Allyn, and A. S. Fauci (1982), *J. Immunol.* **129**, 107.

Wantanabe, T., C. S. Pukel, H. Takeyama, K. O. Lloyd, H. Shiku, L. T. C. Li, L. R. Travassos, H. F. Oettgen, and L. J. Old (1982), *J. Exp. Med.* **156**, 1884.

Watson, D. B., G. F. Burns, and I. R. Mackay (1983), *J. Immunol.* **130**, 2442.

Wright, W. E. (1978), *Exp. Cell Res.* **112**, 395.

Wunderlich, D., Y. A. Teramoto, C. Alford, and J. Schlom (1981), *Eur. J. Cancer Clin. Oncol.* **17**, 719.

Yoshie, O. and Y. Ono (1980), *Cell Immunol.* **56**, 305.

Zeijlemaker, W. P., G. C. Asaldi, M. C. Janssen, E. A. Striker, and R. F. Tiebout (1982), *Immunobiology* **163**, 368.

Zimmerman, U. and J. Vienken (1982), *J. Membrane Biol.* **67**, 165.

Zurawski, V. R., E. Haber, and H. P. Black (1978), *Science* **199**, 1439.

INDEX

423